Praise for
BEAT AUTOIMMUNE

"Now is the time to take back your health! Autoimmune conditions are reversible, but you need to address root causes head-on. Palmer Kippola used to have MS, and now she's on a mission to help anyone who is eager to reverse or prevent any autoimmune condition. *Beat Autoimmune* is an empowering and actionable guidebook that simplifies the steps back to health. Highly recommended!"

—**Izabella Wentz**, PharmD, FASCP, and #1 *New York Times* bestselling author of *Hashimoto's Protocol*

"Palmer Kippola not only raises our awareness of the important mechanisms underlying the dramatic increase in autoimmune diseases worldwide but, in addition, *Beat Autoimmune* is wonderfully prescriptive, providing the reader with a powerful action plan to reverse and even prevent these issues."

—**David Perlmutter**, MD, FACN, and author of *New York Times* #1 bestseller *Grain Brain and Brain Maker*

"It's time for a root cause revolution! *Beat Autoimmune* is a fantastic field guide for anyone seeking real solutions to this modern-day epidemic. Palmer Kippola simplifies the steps to health so you can beat autoimmune and thrive."

—**Frank Lipman**, MD, *New York Times* bestselling author of *How to Be Well*

"An excellent resource for those who want to use an integrative and Functional Medicine approach to support their healing journey!"

—**Terry Wahls**, MD, clinical professor of medicine, and author of *The Wahls Protocol: How I Beat Progressive MS Using Paleo Principles and Functional Medicine*

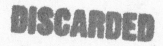

"*Beat Autoimmune* serves up proven ways to address the root causes of autoimmune disorders. If you're ready to reclaim your health, I highly recommend reading this book and following the steps that Palmer has laid out. It could transform your life."

—**Dr. Josh Axe**, DNM, DC, CNS, author of *Eat Dirt: Why Leaky Gut May Be the Root Cause of Your Health Problems and 5 Surprising Steps to Cure It*

"Palmer offers easy, digestible nuggets blending her lived experience and insights with the science of Functional Medicine—a super accessible read and an important tool in the toolbox for patients facing autoimmune disease."

—**Donna Jackson-Nakazawa**, award-winning science journalist and author of *Childhood Disrupted: How Your Biography Becomes Your Biology and How You Can Heal* and *The Autoimmune Epidemic: Bodies Gone Haywire in a World out of Balance—and the Cutting-Edge Science that Promises Hope*

"This book may be your first introduction to health information that flies in the face of conventional wisdom and Western medical advice—that autoimmune conditions are "incurable." The frenzied pace of modern scientific discovery has left many mainstream medical professionals in the past. As a scientist who has studied chemistry, biochemistry, nutrition, and metabolism, I can attest to the staggering amount of research that gets published every month. It's no wonder that new discoveries take too long to filter into practice. But there's good news about autoimmunity, and Palmer is here to share it. She's not just writing about a topic from a knowledge perspective; she's lived with an autoimmune diagnosis and personally experienced the debilitating effects of the disease—until she did something about it. Now you can, too."

—**Steven Wm. Fowkes**, organic chemist, biohacker, health educator, and author

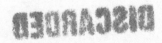

"With the emerging field of research into the gut microbiome and re-pairing intestinal permeability, new avenues of treatment for autoimmunity will no doubt develop in the near future. In the mean-time, Palmer Kippola's common-sense suggestions to improve your autoimmune condition through lifestyle changes in diet, restorative sleep, and other areas provides a welcome approach for many with these conditions."

> —**Alessio Fasano**, MD, director of the Center for
> Celiac Research and Treatment, Massachusetts
> General Hospital

"Palmer has done a fantastic job bringing to light the importance of food and a leaky gut in the rise of autoimmunity and in giving us practical tools to reverse the equation!"

> —**Jill C. Carnahan**, MD, ABFM, ABIHM, IFMCP

"This book provides just the right measure of hope and targeted heal-ing protocols to overcome or ward off any autoimmune condition. Since autoimmune disease is currently an increasingly insidious epi-demic, Palmer Kippola's book is loaded with exactly the right information we all need to support our immunity each and every day. The environmental and inherited challenges we all face don't stand a chance with Palmer's advice to guide us."

> —**Ann Louise Gittleman**, PhD, CNS, award-winning,
> *New York Times* bestselling author of over thirty
> books on health and nutrition, including *Radical
> Metabolism*, *The New Fat Flush Plan*, and *Guess
> What Came to Dinner*

"Palmer takes a deep dive into the root causes of disease and disorder to provide us with an evidence-based, integrative approach to re-building our health and as a result restoring our resilience. A must-read!"

> —**Heidi Hanna**, PhD, executive director, American
> Institute of Stress, and *New York Times* bestselling
> author of *The SHARP Solution* and *Stressaholic*

"Autoimmune and chronic inflammatory conditions are on the rise and something needs to be done about it! In this book, Palmer Kippola lays out why we have an inflammation epidemic and what we can do. This book is comprehensive and covers key lab tests to get to root causes, diet and lifestyle strategies, and supplements to heal the gut and balance the immune system. I would highly recommend this book for anyone looking to improve their health and for practitioners who desire to get better healing results with their patients and clients."

—**David Jockers**, DNM, DC, MS

"*Beat Autoimmune* is an essential book for anyone with an autoimmune condition who wants not only to feel better but understand—and heal—their root causes. Palmer so elegantly combines cutting-edge research with personal experience to create an approachable guide that'll change your life."

—**Deborah Anderson**, ND, Functional Medicine
doctor and autoimmune disease expert

"Doctors have failed patients by focusing on symptoms of chronic disease and not root causes. Thankfully, we now know how to treat and prevent autoimmune conditions at the source. *Beat Autoimmune* provides a clear path for people suffering with autoimmune conditions and a friendly approach that's equal parts comprehensive and comprehensible. Palmer's zeal and zest for life will inspire readers to change their long-held habits and finally achieve true well-being!"

—**Dr. Sarah Myhill**, MB, BS, and autoimmune expert

"Autoimmune illness really is optional! In this superb guide, Palmer Kippola gathers everything you need to know to make these diseases go away. Offering both her personal experience of recovering and the guidance of numerous world-class experts, she puts it all together in an easy-to-read book. Autoimmune disease used to be rare. Now it's an epidemic. With this book it can become rare again. And optional!"

—**Jacob Teitelbaum**, MD, author of *The Fatigue and Fibromyalgia Solution* and *Diabetes Is Optional*

"Millions of people deal with symptoms related to inflammation and autoimmunity, and just sifting through all the information on the subject is nothing short of daunting. I know because I personally struggled with my own autoimmune disorder for years before I was able to heal with the help of detox and the Modern Paleo Diet. That's why I'm thrilled to have discovered *Beat Autoimmune*. Palmer Kippola has created a resource with everything you need to know about healing your gut, reducing your stress levels, addressing hormone imbalances, and truly reclaiming your health—using action steps you can start today!"

—**Wendy Myers**, FDN-P, NC, CHHC, and founder of Myers Detox™

"Before working with Palmer, I had trouble just getting through the day. I had tummy pain and IBS-symptoms so bad I could barely leave the house. I was so tired I would frequently fall asleep at work, and I didn't have the energy to exercise. My hormones were so out of whack I had debilitating monthly cycles and extra weight that wouldn't budge. By following Palmer's anti-inflammatory food plan, taking targeted supplements, and detoxing slowly, I was able to heal my gut and reverse all symptoms of celiac disease and Hashimoto's thyroiditis. Now I'm running 5Ks with my daughter and enjoying life instead of dreading it. If I can beat autoimmune, you can too!"

—**Wendy McCarter**, accountant/office manager, mom, and horse lover

"Palmer Kippola's attack on autoimmunity in this comprehensive volume makes for a solid cover-to-cover read for those who seek the big picture while being a useful reference to return to in the future when a specific detail is needed."

—**Ken Sharlin**, MD, MPH, IFMCP, neurologist, and author of *The Healthy Brain Toolbox: Neurologist-Proven Strategies to Avoid Memory Loss and Protect Your Aging Brain*

"The power of lowering inflammation and healing autoimmunity is now in your hands! This book puts all together in an easy, concise, and evidence-based approach to healing disease from the inside out."

—**Madiha Saeed, MD**, "HolisticMom, MD," and author of *The Holistic Rx: Your Guide to Healing Chronic Inflammation and Disease*

"Palmer's commitment to not let others suffer like she did is truly inspiring and certainly succeeds with this book. I would highly recommend this book to my patients."

—**Anna M. Cabeca**, DO, FACOG, ABAARM, ABoIM and author of *The Hormone Fix*

"Palmer Kippola shares a moving and beautiful chronicle of how she learned to reverse her 26-year history of serious multiple sclerosis, a disease that is widely believed to be irreversible in traditional medicine. The nutritional and Functional Medicine approach that Palmer applied will be helpful not only for people suffering from MS but for anyone grappling with chronic illness of any kind."

—**Kat Toups**, MD, DFAPA, IFMCP, Alzheimer's researcher and author of the forthcoming book *Dementia Demystified*

"Working with Palmer changed my life. I was diagnosed with MS on Nov 1, 2016, and had the good fortune to begin working with her that same week. By following Palmer's advice, I started to heal by removing inflammatory foods, gluten, dairy, corn, sugar, and soy, and by following a Paleo template diet. Within weeks, my MS symptoms subsided, and I felt ready to address stress and childhood traumas that had been plaguing me for decades. Today my family and friends view me as a role model for health and well-being. The approaches in this book changed my and my family's lives, and I have every reason to believe they will change yours too."

—**April Saenz**, executive assistant, wife, mother of two, former MS sufferer

BEAT
Autoimmune

*The 6 Keys to Reverse Your
Condition and Reclaim
Your Health*

PALMER KIPPOLA

Foreword by
Mark Hyman, MD

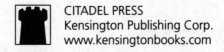
CITADEL PRESS
Kensington Publishing Corp.
www.kensingtonbooks.com

CITADEL PRESS BOOKS are published by

Kensington Publishing Corp.
119 West 40th Street
New York, NY 10018

PUBLISHER'S NOTE
The reader is advised that this book is not intended to be a substitute for an assessment by, and/or advice from, an appropriate medical professional(s). This book contains general information regarding health and should be viewed as purely educational in nature.

The author has made diligent efforts to include Internet addresses that are accurate at the time of publication, however neither the author nor the publisher is responsible for inaccurate or incomplete addresses, or for changes occurring after this book was printed and published. Moreover, the publisher and the author have no control over any such third-party Internet sites or the content contained thereon, and are not responsible for any such content.

All Kensington titles, imprints, and distributed lines are available at special quantity discounts for bulk purchases for sales promotions, premiums, fund-raising, educational, or institutional use. Special book excerpts or customized printings can also be created to fit specific needs. For details, write or phone the office of the Kensington sales manager: Kensington Publishing Corp., 119 West 40th Street, New York, NY 10018, attn: Sales Department; phone 1-800-221-2647.

CITADEL PRESS and the Citadel logo are Reg. U.S. Pat. & TM Off.

ISBN-13: 978-0-8065-3894-5
ISBN-10: 0-8065-3894-5

First trade paperback printing: May 2019

10 9 8 7 6 5 4 3 2 1

Printed in the United States of America

Library of Congress CIP data is available.

Electronic edition: May 2019

ISBN-13: 978-0-8065-3895-2 (e-book)
ISBN-10: 0-8065-3895-3 (e-book)

For my parents, Ed and Beverly Beyer Rabey,
who loved and believed in me more than anything.

For Tom, my soul mate,
strategic adviser, and biggest supporter.

For anyone who has been diagnosed with
an "incurable" autoimmune disease
and told there is nothing to do
except "take medication."
This book is for you.

CONTENTS

FOREWORD:
YOU HAVE THE KEYS TO YOUR HEALTH

by Mark Hyman, MD

One in five Americans, or about ten percent of the world's population, suffers from one of the more than a hundred autoimmune diseases. To put the problem in perspective, the prevalence and cost of autoimmune disease is greater than cancer, heart disease, and diabetes *combined*, and it's one of the top ten causes of death in women under age sixty-four.

The list of autoimmune diseases is long and growing, and includes Hashimoto's thyroiditis (hypothyroid), Graves' disease (hyperthyroid), type 1 diabetes, inflammatory bowel disease (IBD), Crohn's disease, multiple sclerosis (MS), celiac disease, rheumatoid arthritis (RA), scleroderma, Sjögren's syndrome, lupus, eczema, psoriasis, and vitiligo. Even chronic Lyme disease and some types of heart disease have recently been classified as autoimmune. Symptoms range from frustrating to debilitating and may show up years before a diagnosis is made. Profound fatigue, insomnia, brain fog, body aches and pain, numbness and tingling, hair loss, swelling, and stubborn extra weight are among the most common complaints.

Thanks to a dramatic increase of toxicants in our environment, diets filled with sugar and simple carbohydrates, an over-emphasis on antibiotics and an underemphasis on basic stress-relief practices, it's no surprise we are facing an autoimmune epidemic. These days it's not uncommon to see ten-year-olds in my clinic with hypothyroid issues and even rheumatoid arthritis.

While Western medicine excels at *acute* care for conditions such as heart attacks, trauma, and broken bones, unfortunately, it's not well-matched to address *chronic* health conditions like autoimmune diseases. While steroids, immunosuppressive drugs, and strong pain killers may provide temporary symptom relief, they are devastating to the body long-term, and can even lead to autoimmune disease and cancer!

If you're dealing with mysterious symptoms or one or more diagnosed autoimmune diseases and have not had much luck with Western medicine, or been told there's nothing you can do to heal, you may be eager to embrace natural approaches that work.

Fortunately, there's another way. For the past two decades I've been at the forefront of a relatively new type of medicine that is perfectly suited to address autoimmune disorders. It's called Functional Medicine (FM)—a whole-person-based scientific approach that addresses and resolves health challenges at the *root-cause* level.

We have the science, the information, and methods for reversing and preventing autoimmune disorders right now. Contrary to once-popular belief, autoimmune disease is not a one-way street. Thanks to groundbreaking research in the last decade, we now have an autoimmune equation to reverse and prevent them: detect and remove your inflammatory root causes and heal your gut.

While autoimmune diseases appear to be numerous, they are really just one disorder with countless variations based on your genetic weak link. Every autoimmune condition is an immune system challenge driven by chronic inflammation. My biggest source of inflammation was mercury toxicity; that's what set the stage for my debilitating chronic fatigue syndrome. I recovered by finding and removing the mercury and healing my gut. Following these time-tested principles, hundreds of patients in my own clinic have healed, and numerous physicians and health practitioners have personally recovered and now guide their clients back to health.

When Palmer was diagnosed with MS at age nineteen, thankfully she wasn't satisfied with the answer, "There's nothing you can do." By doggedly pursuing the answer to why she developed MS in the first place, she found and then addressed her root causes head-on.

This is what Functional Medicine teaches us. By working at the root-cause level and seeking the source(s) of our inflammation, we find the keys to our recovery. My biggest root cause was mercury; Palmer's were gluten and chronic stress. Yours might be different, but chances are they fall in one of six categories that Palmer calls "F.I.G.H.T.S.," for food, infections, gut health, hormone balance, toxins, and stress.

Palmer is the ideal guide as you embark on your healing journey, because she was once in your shoes, searching for answers and desperate to feel better, wishing she had the book you're reading right now. After reversing her MS, researching autoimmune root causes and solutions, and becoming certified as a Functional Medicine Health Coach, she's made it her life's work to help those who continue to suffer. And she wants to make the path to wellness as painless as possible. In *Beat Autoimmune*, Palmer simplifies the science and provides a framework for healing that I've seen work again and again.

By reducing inflammatory lifestyle factors and adding in nourishing ones, you tip the balance of health in your favor. Healing at the root requires proactive choices, and Palmer breaks it down into actionable and manageable steps everyone can follow. For example, to take the bad stuff out: reduce your toxic load of processed foods; remove chemicals in home and personal care products; and address toxic stress. And to add the good stuff in: eat real, whole, foods; prioritize sleep; and adopt easy daily relaxation practices. In other words, give your body what it needs and it will repair, restore, and even thrive, whether you're dealing with an autoimmune condition or are just looking to stay well.

You have in your hand the keys to reversing your condition and reclaiming your health. It's up to you to use these keys so that you can unlock your health and thrive.

BEAT AUTOIMMUNE

My Story

*Not everything that is faced can be changed; but nothing can
be changed that is not faced.*
      —JAMES BALDWIN, American writer and social activist

In July 1984, I was a fun-loving and hard-working 19-year-old college student, back home in Los Angeles for the summer working as a hostess for a local restaurant. I didn't have much planned beyond graduation, still a few years away, but my future seemed promising whatever it held. Or so I thought.

One morning on my way to work, I felt a tingling sensation in the soles of my feet. You know that "pins and needles" feeling you have after you've sat on a limb too long and the blood flows back all tingly? Only that morning, the blood didn't flow back. No matter how hard I shook my feet, the prickling persisted.

Within a few hours the tingling crept up my legs. When it reached my knees, I called my parents. By the time we sat in the neurologist's office that afternoon, the feeling had wrapped around my abdomen. The neurologist checked my reflexes, had me walk across the room heel-to-toe tightrope-style, and watched while I touched the tip of my nose with my eyes closed. Within minutes, she diagnosed me. "I am 99 percent certain that you have multiple sclerosis," she said.

Multiple what?!

We were stunned and confused. The doctor continued, "We'll schedule an NMR (a nuclear magnetic resonance image was the scary precursor name for the MRI) to confirm, but if I'm right, there's nothing you can do." We left with little information and a bleak outlook.

That evening my feet started going numb. In bed, the scary lack of sensation ascended and enveloped me like a fog. By the time I fell asleep, the numbness had enshrouded my body. I would remain completely numb from the neck down for a full month and a half.

It was a terrifying time, but my parents didn't let on that they were scared. Instead, my dad encouraged my can-do attitude by often repeating the refrain, "We're going to beat this thing." I mostly believed him, but sometimes I got weepy when I worried about the future. Thankfully my mom was quick to empathize and nurture. She helped me research and plan for a very different future than we ever could have imagined. Together, we envisioned how I might be able to attend a local university in a wheelchair.

I was so grateful for good friends who weren't scared off by this mysterious disease and who visited or called daily. Some hung out and watched movies with me and some brought books. Another friend brought me a gift that didn't seem like a gift at the time. It came in the form of a question. She asked me, "Why do you think you got the MS?"

Pow! Packed into that short question were so many implications. Was there a lesson to be learned? Did I do something to *cause* the MS? How dare she insinuate that I was responsible! But was I? If I unknowingly brought it on, perhaps there was something I could do to usher it out. Little did she or I know that question would become my North Star for the next thirty years.

One Question, Four Experiments

A week later, I lay on the couch, chewing the question over in my mind when an answer appeared in a flash. I had been adopted as a baby by loving parents, but my dad had been a fighter pilot whose way was invariably the "right way," and we butted heads often. He was judgmental and opinionated, and he yelled a lot. My mom was a softer personality who perpetually struggled with her weight. My dad must have thought if he yelled louder, she might slim down.

It's telling that one of my earliest memories is my dad shouting at my mom, who was crying behind her bedroom door. I stood in the hallway, age three or four, with my small fists clenched, threatening my dad. The words are blurry, but the message I shouted remains clear: "If you don't shut up, I'm going to make you!"

Always ready to protect my mom, I was a hyperdefensive child. Lying on the couch, reflecting on the reasons for the MS, I realized that my immune system must have become hyperdefensive, too. The way I saw it, my immune system's soldiers were primed to defend and protect at the smallest trigger. And if they didn't have a real battle to fight, they would create a fake one, even if that resulted in friendly fire, with my own body as the victim. As it turns out, a revved up and runaway immune response can result in an autoimmune condition like MS, where the body's own immune system ends up attacking our bodies' own tissues. In the case of MS, the immune system attacks and damages the myelin sheath, the protective coating that insulates nerve fibers.

That first hypothesis I had on the couch in 1984 was that chronic stress was at the root of my MS. That still rings true for me today, even though I now know there's more to the story.

The type of MS I had was "relapsing-remitting," meaning that symptoms came and went, which can be the case with many autoimmune disorders (although many can grow progressively worse over time). So, six weeks after that dreadful first day, my body began to wake up. The numbness started its retreat, neck to feet, and slowly, over more than two years, the numbness *finally* lifted. In the meantime, I returned to college for my sophomore year with relief and cautious optimism that life would return to normal. I was right, as it turned out, although it would take much longer than I anticipated to get there.

Over the course of twenty-six years, I saw six neurologists, each of whom told me, "There's nothing you can do." Except, of course, take medication. But as my dad reminded me, I could beat the MS; I just needed to figure out how. As time passed, I began to conduct informal experiments, more than a dozen in total, and I want to share the four biggies.

Experiment #1: Stress Reduction

After my epiphany on the couch in the wake of my MS diagnosis, the first experiment was obvious: stress reduction. Back at school, I noticed right away that when stress was high, symptoms escalated. When the pressure of exams or my heavy workload weighed me down, within a week I would develop a flare-up. Sometimes these symptoms were sensory, like numbness or tingling; sometimes I felt tightness like a hundred rubber bands wrapped around my torso; and sometimes the only sign was profound fatigue. I also developed a disturbing symptom called *Lhermitte's sign*: whenever I bent my neck forward, a bolt of electricity coursed down my spine.

Later, while working in a stressful job at AT&T Network Systems in New Jersey, I took a very relaxing Caribbean vacation. The moment I walked back into the corporate building with its glaring fluorescent lights, I was struck blind in my left eye. Searing pain persisted for two weeks and it took two visits to the emergency room, plus a visit to an MS expert at Johns Hopkins Hospital in Baltimore, to be diagnosed with optic neuritis, a hallmark symptom of MS.

After years of living with on-again-off-again MS symptoms, it became painfully clear that stress led to more symptoms, so I actively searched for practical ways to relax. I tried numerous techniques and most helped to the degree I stuck with them. I attended my first yoga class in 1987 and was soothed by the instructor's calming voice encouraging me to "let it gooooo." Later, a friend introduced me to meditation; I found that meditating was easier with other people, so I joined a weekly meditation group. I saw a psychologist to help me deal with anger issues and underlying sadness. He taught me to pay attention to my thoughts, catch and challenge distorted ones that were leading to negative emotions, and replace them with more accurate and, inevitably, less stressful ones.

But even when yoga, meditation, and mindfulness practices became habits, the MS symptoms never went away entirely.

Experiment #2: Low-Fat, Vegetarian Diets

Growing up, I ate big bowls of cereal with nonfat milk every morning, peanut butter and jelly sandwiches on whole wheat bread for lunch, and some variation of meat and potatoes for dinner. We followed the food pyramid, with loads of grains at the foundation and minimal fats on top.

I thought it was normal to feel minor discomfort after eating, so I ignored messages from my tummy and continued to follow what we believed was a pretty healthy American diet.

Early on, I intuited that diet might play an important role in helping me to beat the MS, so I searched the library for guidebooks. I found Phyllis

Balch's *Prescription for Nutritional Healing* and the *Multiple Sclerosis Diet Book* by Roy Laver Swank. Both authors were adamant that low-fat, vegetarian diets were the way to go, so I decided to give it a try. I replaced animal protein with tofu, tempeh, and rice and beans. I tried the macrobiotic diet, adding sea veggies to platefuls of brown rice or quinoa. I read *The China Study*, which linked consuming animal proteins with cancer, so I went vegan for a time.

Not only did I notice no reduction in my symptoms, I had worsening tummy discomfort: more grumbling after meals and ongoing constipation. I was told, "constipation is a symptom of the MS" and I should "learn to live with it by taking laxatives as needed." It would take years of GI discomfort before I figured out what was truly to blame.

Experiment #3: Medication

For years I saw neurologists, and each of them insisted that medication would be the best insurance policy to protect me from a potentially dreadful future with MS. Averse to taking medication and to needles, I resisted as long as I could, until an especially persistent neurologist at Stanford said I needed to pick one of the top three MS medications, known colloquially as the "A, B, C drugs." I chose one purported to have the fewest side effects, and for four years, I injected myself with this medication every night.

I didn't notice any symptom reduction, likely because by this point I was managing the MS pretty well with relaxation practices. I did, however, *gain* three additional symptoms that I call the "three strikes."

The first strike was lipoatrophy—literally a disappearing of fat. Everywhere I injected myself in the fatty places of my body, the fat didn't bounce back. The injections produced deep divots in my thighs, hips, and tummy—unappealing, but perhaps not worth forgoing a supposed life-extending medication. However, the second strike was far more concerning. Fifteen minutes after I injected myself one evening, my heart started racing uncontrollably. I felt constriction and pain in my chest; I went cold and clammy and thought I was having a heart attack. The medication nurse had forewarned me that heart attack symptoms are, in fact, a common side effect of this particular medication, but I took little comfort in her words during the terrifying experience. The third and final strike was an infection in an injection site on my hip. It took six months and as many visits to a wound care clinic—and several more months of attending to the wound—to finally heal. I still have a scar as an unpleasant reminder of that experience.

Given how well I was managing the MS with stress reduction and given the additional symptoms that came with the injections, I decided to quit the medication. I knew right then I would have to find a solution outside the limitations of modern medicine to beat this thing. Fortunately, the best experiment was right around the corner.

Experiment #4: Gut Healing

The fourth and final experiment is what I call "gut healing." While I didn't know at the time that addressing my tummy troubles would lead to MS healing, that's, in fact, what happened. In the fall of 2010, my MS symptoms were very present, despite my relaxation efforts. Each morning when I woke, my legs felt as heavy as lead. Just walking from my bed to the bathroom felt like plodding through waist-deep water. And most days, I had that tight sensation of rubber bands constricting my torso.

By then, I had learned enough about nutrition through my own research to know that food, even supposed health foods, might be causing my tummy trouble, so I decided to see a Functional Medicine nutritionist. A series of tests showed that I was sensitive to gluten, a protein found in wheat, many grains, and even soy sauce. My nutritionist educated me about the perils of gluten and how gut inflammation led to its leakiness and, finally, to autoimmunity. She guided me through a thirty-day elimination diet and gut healing protocol. I went cold turkey on gluten that day and within a week my tummy troubles vanished for good.

Within a month of removing gluten, I stopped having any and all MS symptoms. The feeling of heavy legs on waking lifted completely and the tightness around my torso just stopped. I call this my "eureka experiment."

I was cautiously optimistic at first. How could it be that something as simple as making a dietary change and healing my gut could arrest an "incurable" disease, when a half-dozen neurologists had insisted there was nothing I could do? I puzzled and pondered and returned to the question that had started this journey nearly three decades earlier: *Why do I think I got the MS?*

The more I've learned, the more complex, but clear, the answer to this question has become. It wasn't *just* a result of childhood stress, as I first thought all those years ago. Nor was gluten solely to blame. I now believe my MS was brought on by a collection of root causes which, together, inflamed my gut, disrupted the balance of my microbiome, breached my gut lining, and triggered an autoimmune reaction that didn't stop until I removed the inflammatory triggers.

Have you heard of "the total body burden"? It's the cumulative load of toxins that we have in our bodies. Imagine that each of us carries within us a bucket that fills with toxins that accumulate faster than we can eliminate them. Inflammatory factors like processed foods, infections, metals, plastics, and chronic stress fill the bucket, until one too many stressors causes our bucket to overflow. At this point, our detoxification system becomes overwhelmed, our immune system gets impaired, and we develop hyperpermeable intestines, commonly called a *leaky gut*. When large protein and other molecules breach the gut barrier, our immune system reacts, attacking food particles and other invaders, and our own tissues get caught in the attack. That's a simplified summary of the autoimmune cascade. My genes gave me a tendency for MS, so that's what got expressed when my bucket overflowed.

What was in my toxin bucket? Beyond chronic stress and gluten, my biggest culprits included a mouthful of mercury and a gut filled with *Candida* thanks to my massive sweet tooth, extra vaccines for international travel, and significantly imbalanced hormones, including high cortisol, low vitamin D, and insulin resistance.

How did I heal? By emptying my toxin bucket and healing my gut. I identified my inflammatory triggers and removed them the best I could, thereby modifying the expression of my genes and stopping the autoimmune attack.

Before and After

Over twenty-six years, between 1984 and 2010, I had a half dozen MRIs that revealed numerous white lesions on my brain, including lesions that formed the MS telltale pattern of plaques called *Dawson's finger*; I experienced myriad symptoms, including full-body numbness, Lhermitte's sign, optic neuritis, and sensory challenges in my torso and limbs; and my symptoms came and went, flaring up most noticeably following stressful events. While symptoms ebbed and flowed, I always felt like I was plugged into an electrical socket, with errant energy running haywire throughout my body.

Since 2010, I've been symptom-free and no longer feel that electrical hum. More modern testing revealed my sensitivity to gluten and a leaky gut. Nowadays, antibody tests can show whether or not your immune system is mounting an autoimmune attack on your own tissues, like myelin sheath, the protective nerve covering that is the target of attack in MS. A blood test in 2014 confirmed that my antibodies to myelin sheath were all in the "normal" range—which meant my immune system was no longer attacking my myelin sheath. And an MRI of my brain in 2017 showed not only no new lesions, but also a reduction and disappearance of old ones. Today, all signs point to vibrant health. My neurologist said, "It couldn't be a better story."

So how does my story end? It turns out reversing MS was just the beginning. I quit my job in 2012 to study how it's possible that I beat an incurable disease, and I have since discovered both scientific studies and numerous healing stories that prove reversing autoimmune conditions is possible. I started www.BeatAutoimmune.com as an online resource to share the heart, science, and stories of people transcending autoimmune conditions naturally. I've become certified as a Functional Medicine Health Coach (FMCHC) and now collaborate with the same Functional Medicine practitioner who helped me heal in 2010. Together we serve clients who actively seek to heal from autoimmune conditions.

This book is the accumulation of everything I've learned during my own journey and put into practice with my clients. In other words, it's everything I wish I had known at nineteen. Now I hope that by condensing and sharing what I've learned, I can help you, too, to fully heal, and in a fraction of the time it took me.

Overview

Illness doesn't just happen; illness has causes, so to resolve illness, find and resolve the causes.
—W. Lee Cowden, integrative MD,
cardiologist, and health educator

Once free of symptoms and disease markers on lab tests, I dove into the research, trying to learn as much as I could about why people develop MS and other autoimmune conditions. I spent my days immersed in PubMed.gov—an endless online resource of biomedical studies—and I dug into dense scientific journals like the *Journal of Autoimmunity*. I read Donna Jackson Nakazawa's important *Autoimmune Epidemic*, which makes a compelling case that increasing environmental toxins may be the primary reason for the massive rise in these disorders; I devoured Dr. David Perlmutter's *Grain Brain: The Surprising Truth about Wheat, Carbs, and Sugar—Your Brain's Silent Killers*, which taught me about how grains inflame and damage our brains and bodies; and I learned from Dr. Bruce Lipton's groundbreaking book *The Biology of Belief* about the first of three exciting scientific findings, epigenetics.

Good News #1: Epigenetics Supersedes Genetics

For two decades, University of Wisconsin School of Medicine professor and cell biologist Bruce Lipton, Ph.D., taught his students what he calls "the Central Dogma"—that our genes are our destiny. In other words, the belief that whatever your parents had will likely befall you, too. But, while on sabbatical at a medical school in the Caribbean in 1985, Dr. Lipton had a profound insight: while he was reviewing research on cells, it dawned on him that a cell's life is controlled by its physical and energetic environment and not by its genes.

While this perspective would be seen as heretical by those unwilling to consider the new biology, Dr. Lipton's research at Stanford University a few years later would confirm his hypothesis. Dr. Lipton placed identical stem cells into three separate petri dishes, each containing a different culture medium—the only variable in his experiment. Those who embraced the old biology theory of predetermined genetic destiny would have expected to find a growing number of identical cells across the three petri dishes. The results told a different story: each petri dish held a *different* cell type. In one dish, bone cells were growing, in another, fat cells, and in the third, muscle cells. It turns out it wasn't the nucleus (the "brain" of the cell where the genetic matter is housed) that predetermined the destiny of those cells. It was the medium—that is, the *environment*—that made the difference.

The emerging science that explains this phenomenon of the environment directing our genes is called *epigenetics*. The word *epigenetics* literally means "above the genes." Imagine your genome (all your genes) as computer hardware; the epigenome is the software program that directs how the computer works.

In 2014, I was introduced to the Institute for Functional Medicine (IFM) by the Functional Medicine nutritionist who helped me heal. We attended the annual IFM conference where biologist Randy Jirtle, Ph.D., was given the Linus Pauling Award for his extraordinary role as the "father of environmental epigenomics."

In one of the most compelling demonstrations of epigenetics in action, the Agouti Mouse Study, Dr. Jirtle and his post-doc student, Dr. Robert Waterland, were able to show that nutrition fed to genetically identical pregnant mice could change the physical appearance and disease susceptibility of their newborn mice. *Agouti* is the name of a gene that, when expressed, makes mice fat, yellow, and prone to chronic disease. In their experiment, Jirtle and Waterland fed pregnant mice vitamins including B12, choline, and SAMe. The control pregnant mice that didn't get the vitamins gave birth to yellow mice pups who were obese, diabetic, and prone to other diseases thanks to that Agouti gene, while the mice pups born to the vitamin-enriched mama mice were lean, brown, and less prone to obesity and disease. It turns out the nutrients turned off the harmful Agouti gene in the offspring—and it stayed silenced for *life*!

That's the power of epigenetics. It means *we* get to influence which genes get turned on or off by our lifestyle choices, including and especially the multiple daily decisions we make about what to eat and drink—but we'll get to that in the next chapter.

Finding Functional Medicine

Once I tasted Functional Medicine, I was hungry for more. I signed up (and must have slid in under the radar) for one of IFM's meaty multiday courses on immune dysfunction. When the emcee asked for a show of hands from the audience of several hundred how many were medical doctors, and then how many were naturopaths, osteopaths, nurses, chiropractors, nutritionists, and down the line, I sat still as a church mouse in the back. Just about every hand shot up but mine. The doctor to my left whispered to me, "Who are you?" To which I replied, "Someone who reversed her MS and wants to learn how that's possible." She smiled and introduced me to a number of people who shared resources and encouragement. I may not have had a bunch of credentials (e.g., MD or Ph.D.) after my name, but I was welcomed into the tribe.

It was at this IFM course that I learned the second of three exciting scientific findings.

Good News #2: Our Environments Matter Way More Than Our Genome

To kick things off, Mark Hyman, MD, taught us that Functional Medicine is the science of creating health so that disease goes away as a side effect of those healthy habits. He described health as a state of whole-system balance, which could be as simple as removing the causes of imbalance and adding what creates balance. He then put up a slide that stated that *90 percent of chronic disease is driven,* not by the genome, but *by "the exposome,"* or the cumulative number of disease-causing factors we are exposed to in our environments.[1] Ha! I silently cheered, more evidence that we are far more in control of our health outcomes than we ever imagined.

In the five years since attending the IFM immune dysfunction course, I've seen more evidence of the 90/10 environment vs. genes assertion, including a review of cancer research called "Cancer Is a Preventable Disease That Requires Major Lifestyle Changes," which attributes only 5 percent to 10 percent of cancer risk to defective genes and 90 percent to 95 percent to environmental and lifestyle factors.[2] Even the CDC has acknowledged the supremacy of environmental factors: "Unfortunately, genetics has been found to account for only about 10 percent of diseases, and the remaining causes appear to be from environmental causes. So, to understand the causes and eventually the prevention of disease, environmental causes need to be studied."[3]

So, what are these environmental causes leading an increasing number of people to develop autoimmune disorders? That question would drive me to dig deeper once I learned about the third piece of good news: the autoimmune equation.

Good News #3: An Autoimmune Equation Gives Us the Answer for Reversing Autoimmune Conditions

Before the 2000s, the two ingredients of autoimmune disease were thought to be genes and environmental factors. The question that no one could explain was: how do these two worlds collide to unleash autoimmunity? In 2008, Alessio Fasano, MD, renowned pediatric gastroenterologist and research scientist at Massachusetts General Hospital for Children, published a study that revealed a necessary third element in the autoimmune disease equation: increased intestinal permeability, commonly known as a *leaky gut*.

The study abstract supplies the myth-shattering good news: "This new paradigm subverts traditional theories underlying the development of autoimmunity . . . and suggests that *the autoimmune process can be arrested if the interplay between genes and environmental triggers is prevented by reestablishing intestinal barrier competency*."[4]

Dr. Fasano's findings offer both hope and guidance to anyone seeking to heal from autoimmune conditions with a simple equation:

Genes + environmental triggers + leaky gut = autoimmune condition(s)

**Detect and remove the environmental triggers + heal your gut =
free of autoimmune expression!**

Buoyed by the exciting science, I spent my days researching the offending environmental triggers. I thought that if people had a simple way to understand what might be harming their guts and creating the pathway to autoimmunity, maybe they would have an easier time recovering their health. I compiled a chart of the harmful environmental elements and their counterparts, the nourishing solutions. Ready with my autoimmune root-cause reversal checklist, I sought feedback from numerous autoimmune experts, including Functional Medicine doctors, practitioners, and scientists, who were generous with their time and supportive of my mission.

To simplify the myriad environmental triggers, I came up with a mnemonic, a device that would help people remember the six major areas that need to be addressed for full healing: **F**ood, **I**nfections, **G**ut health, **H**ormone balance, **T**oxins, and **S**tress. F.I.G.H.T.S.™ I wish it spelled PEACE, but alas, the universe supplied a word that resonated with the can-do attitude that my dad fostered in me when he reminded me that I could "beat the MS."

I then interviewed and compiled healing stories from more than a dozen autoimmune experts—doctors, authors, and Functional Medicine practitioners—who themselves suffered from what were thought to be irreversible autoimmune diseases and mysterious inflammatory conditions:

celiac disease, Crohn's disease, Graves' disease, Hashimoto's thyroiditis, lupus, chronic Lyme, chronic fatigue, fibromyalgia, and progressive MS.

Each person had been told some version of misinformed medical opinion, including:

"There's nothing you can do."
"It's all in your *head*."
"You'll need to be on medication for life."
"You're just depressed."
"*Diet* has nothing to do with this."
or "I'd like you to see a psychiatrist."

Thankfully, each person pushed past the myopia of modern medicine, sought and found complete healing in some combination of natural solutions. Although everyone's circumstances differed, each person healed by addressing their root causes head-on, removing inflammatory triggers, and adding nourishing elements.

Everyone also healed their guts. Why? Because the integrity of the gut lining is ground zero for the battlefront of health and disease—a vulnerable membrane between your body and the outside world. Turns out inflammatory triggers like toxic foods, chemicals, medications, and even stress harm the gut, causing it to become leaky, and that's the fast track to autoimmunity. Over time, inflammation moves from being a local response to a body-wide problem, and that overburdens the immune system—the very system that is supposed to promote healing.

And what's the biggest inflammatory factor that harms the gut? Our steady, daily and multiple daily doses of processed and chemical-laden foods. When I asked each expert what their number one recommendation is for those dealing with an autoimmune issue, they all said, *start with food*. More specifically, they emphasized, *eliminate sugar, gluten, and dairy*. So that's where we'll begin, but before we do, a few notes of orientation.

Getting the Most out of This Book

- You may notice that chapters 1–6 are not in the order that F.I.G.H.T.S. is spelled. That's because the chapter titled "Heal Your Gut" must naturally follow the one titled "Start with Food." The only other deliberately placed chapter is "Balance Your Hormones," which is last because hormones are downstream from the other subjects. While each chapter can be read and worked as a stand-alone subject, I recommend reading them in order.

- This book is meant to be used as an action-oriented resource. Grab a pen and make margin notes, bookmark pages, highlight the sentences and concepts that speak to you, use a journal—write down anything that resonates in the stories, the science, or the toolkits. And, note your efforts and results as they happen.

- You may choose to read all the way through and return to work the toolkits one by one; or, if you're moved to action right away, go for it!

- I offer lots of tools in the toolkits. Please know this is meant to provide you with a variety of options for your consideration. If you resonate with a few of the suggestions, try those. The name of the game is experimentation. You are searching for *your* unique triggers and causes.

- While there is so much you can do on your own, you will hear me suggest again and again the importance of working with a functional/integrative/naturopathic expert. You'll naturally want to find doctors that fit into your health insurance plan, but unfortunately, the experts skilled in guiding their patients back to health don't neatly fit into our modern medical paradigm of the six- to fifteen-minute doctor visit. Instead, these holistic experts usually offer sixty- to ninety-minute initial visits, and while many may bill your insurance company, they expect cash payment for their services. Do what you can on your own and do what you can to work with an expert, too.

- You'll notice some overlap in recommendations throughout, like certain supplements, the push to eat more fiber, and the encouragement to relax more. That's intentional but shouldn't be seen as additive. For example, in the Food chapter, I recommend taking up to 4,000 mg of omega-3 fatty acids per day as part of an overall autoimmune supplement regime. Omega-3s are also discussed in the Gut and Hormone chapters. View the additional recommendations as new information on a familiar idea and not as a suggestion to add another 8,000 mg of omega-3s.

- You may be wondering how long it's going to take to heal. The best expectation I can offer is that if you follow the recommendations in the Food and Gut chapters, you may feel somewhat better, much better, or eureka better within the first three months. Some people feel much better and even *lighter* within a few weeks of removing sugar. As you probably know, autoimmune conditions don't happen overnight. It can take five or ten years, and sometimes decades, of environmental triggers to build up before autoimmunity is expressed. In fact, autoimmune conditions develop along a spectrum: from silent autoimmunity, where antibody levels are increasing but no symptoms are felt, to autoimmune expression where symptoms start to be felt, and finally to autoimmune disease, where symptoms may worsen and tissue damage may occur. How long it takes you to heal depends on several variables, including where you are on the autoimmune spectrum; how much, if any, tissue damage has already occurred; your mind-set; and devotion to your health and well-being above all. My biochemistry mentor, Steve Fowkes, has a rule of thumb that autoimmune conditions can usually be reversed in about a tenth of the time it took to cause them. For example, if something's been brewing for ten years, it should take about a year to heal.

- If after working the Food and Gut toolkits, you are still feeling bad, I'll encourage you to get tested for infections and heavy metals. Reducing those burdens will take time. Detoxification experts say that it may take a few years to get the lead and mercury out. And, if you've worked through all of F.I.G.H.T.S. and you're *still* not getting better, check out the Advanced Considerations in the Appendix.

If you've been struggling with your health for some time, it's normal to feel skeptical or even discouraged. But before we begin, I ask you to let the possibility of hope back into your life. If you believe that healing is possible, you'll open the door not only to wellness but to a different, and often better, life. It may sound hokey, but when I asked each practitioner I interviewed about the silver lining of their illness, nearly everyone said, "Waking up." Each person viewed their journey back to health as an invitation to embrace wholeness and discover their authentic selves. That's the gift.

Stress can have a positive effect if you believe it makes you stronger. Your attitude may be your most important healing influence. If you believe you can, chances are far better that you will!

Now, more than ever before, we have the opportunity to reverse and prevent these previously deemed "incurable" autoimmune conditions. I've strategically used the term *conditions* instead of *diseases* to show that these disorders are conditional and largely depend on how we live—our personal *environments*. We have the science, the inspiration, the lab tests, and a growing number of functional/integrative/naturopathic medicine practitioners and health coaches to support our journeys back to health. It's possible to recover our health faster than ever and certainly in a more cost-effective way than the many people profiled in this book who at times spent more than a decade and/or over half a million dollars attempting to heal.

Great! But how?

Let's begin with your next meal.

CHAPTER 1

Start with Food

Food is how we get terribly sick; or it's how we can restore our health.

—TERRY WAHLS, MD

The importance of food in autoimmune diseases cannot be overstated and yet is often hard for people to understand. How could something so ordinary, so ubiquitous, so simple and so basic be a *cause* or *remedy* for such drastic and debilitating conditions? If this seems counterintuitive to you, you are not alone. I had no idea that my "pretty healthy" diet, low in fat and high in whole grains, could have been a major contributing factor in my developing MS. But our daily bread, so to speak, can be the cause of our debilitating autoimmune conditions—*and, conversely, the very remedy our bodies need to heal.* It was fortunate that I found out I had non-celiac gluten sensitivity, and crazy to me that by removing that one culprit I was able to turn the tide on a twenty-six-year course of relapsing-remitting multiple sclerosis, largely by changing what I ate.

Can it be so simple? That complex, chronic, and often debilitating autoimmune conditions can be reversed or significantly healed by removing a few foods? The short answer is yes, for many people. What I've learned from dozens of practitioners and by observing my own clients is that people with autoimmune issues often heal 60 percent to 100 percent just by changing what they eat. For some, like me, it can be 100 percent.

17

You may be thinking that giving up your favorite foods sounds too daunting to even attempt. But taken one step at a time, any journey, no matter how steep, is surmountable. That's where the Healing Foods Toolkit comes in handy. My step-by-step guide will help you to approach the process one manageable bite at a time—with me by your side. Need more convincing? Let's examine food's essential role in our health.

What's Wrong with What We Eat?

Answering this seemingly simple question requires a quick review of human evolution and the advent of chronic disease. For the vast majority of our time on planet Earth, we humans were hunter-gatherers, eating fresh, whole foods harvested or hunted in the wild. There were few grains, no pesticides, no herbicides, few processed foods, and no genetically modified foods. The topsoil teemed with beneficial organisms, plants grew at a natural pace, and trace minerals were recycled back into the soils for next year's season; plants and animals provided nourishing, nutrient-dense food; and chronic disease was virtually nonexistent.

While our ancestors may not have lived long lives (due to infectious illness and trauma), they were mostly free of inflammatory and degenerative diseases. This phenomenon has been chronicled by anthropologists like Weston A. Price, a Canadian dentist who sought to understand how traditional cultures avoided both tooth decay and chronic disease. Turns out that people of traditional cultures who ate local food were naturally healthy and fit. Had they not succumbed to tuberculosis or the elements, they might have lived to seventy or beyond.

Modern Foods and Human Biology: An Evolutionary Mismatch

Fast forward to the Industrial Revolution, which eventually ushered in mass agriculture and machinery for large-scale production to feed a growing American population after World War II. Vast quantities of processed cereal grains like wheat, corn, rice, and soy provided a cheap and easy source of calories. Procuring fast, frozen and packaged foods, after all, is way more efficient than foraging for sustenance.

But convenience has come at a cost.

As we've become great mass-producers of grains, oils, and animals, we've also gotten really sick. Today, chronic illnesses afflict nearly half of all adults, cause the most deaths and disability in the United States, and are a leading driver of health care costs.[1] Most tragically, these diseases, once rare or associated with old age, now affect children and especially women in their prime. Food sensitivities, mysterious and frequently debilitating symptoms, insulin resistance, obesity, and chronic illnesses are becoming the norm.

It turns out that our modern lifestyle is at the root of autoimmune conditions; and modern foods are one of the biggest culprits. As people have shifted from eating a diverse diet of foraged foods to eating only a few staple crops, the population has experienced an overall decline in health and longevity. We have also shifted from intermittent food availability to constant food availability (packaged, processed foods), and from seasonal eating to year-round obtainability (imported or greenhouse-grown) foods. The shortcuts provided by fast and cheap packaged foods are not a good match for human biology. Our bodies are rebelling against these unnatural foods, and we're developing modern, chronic diseases that were extremely rare or absent prior to the agricultural era. Some call these modern, chronic illnesses "mismatch disorders" for that reason. In other words, the standard American diet (SAD)—a.k.a. Western diet—loaded with sugars and chemically produced products, is a fast track to insulin resistance, obesity, cancer and autoimmunity.

The Return to Health

The great news is that a return to health and vitality usually follows a return to more traditional ways of eating. Often in a short time, too.

We know that people from traditional cultures who adopt Western diets suffer the same health consequences as people who grow up eating a Western diet. Even a temporary SAD diet can lead to diabetes, obesity, and heart disease—each risk factors for autoimmune conditions. Nutrition researcher Kerin O'Dea studied Australian aboriginals who had left their native home in the bush for the more Westernized town of Derby, Australia. With access to refined carbohydrates and a more sedentary lifestyle, it wasn't long before they became obese and diabetic. O'Dea conducted a seven-week study to see what would happen if the aboriginals returned to their bush habitat and their customary diet of fish, shellfish, birds, kangaroo, tubers, and bush honey. Sure enough, as the aboriginals returned to eating their native foods, they lost weight and experienced remarkable health improvements. Markers of inflammation and diabetes all improved or resolved, *in just seven weeks!*

Does this mean you're going to have to sharpen your spear and roam the wild to find your own food? Metaphorically speaking, that's the right direction. Practically speaking, you'll just need to become a savvy, modern-day huntress-gatherer to find the most evolutionarily appropriate foods for you. As you align your food choices to those better suited to your biology, remarkable things happen: signs and symptoms of chronic disease begin to fade, replaced by shoots and blooms of vibrant health and well-being. The more you heal, the easier it becomes to make the right food choices, until one day it's simply second nature.

Food and the Three Invisible but Powerful Forces Inside You

To understand the significance of your food choices, it helps to have an appreciation for what's happening in your body. Your moment-to-moment daily decisions—what you eat, drink, think, and do—directly affect whether you are moving toward health or toward disease. Three of the biggest impacts on health or disease exist at a microscopic level inside each of us and exert their influence multiple times a day. These three invisible yet powerful forces are *epigenetics*, the *microbiome*, and *mitochondria*. Each of these forces responds in real time to the foods you eat daily. Awareness of their significance is a huge first step. Let's consider each separately before we look at the bigger picture.

You know the cliché "You are what you eat." The latest science proves that this old refrain is absolutely true. The foods we eat not only become the building blocks of new cells, they also write our personal health stories, bite by bite. To understand the *epigenetics* of food, imagine it's lunchtime and you're eating a burger with one hand. Envision your other hand on a light switch. If your burger is made with typical GMO-produced, corn-fed, antibiotic-laden meat cooked at high heat in industrial oils and comes with a bun, flip the switch up. You've just turned on your disease-promoting genes. What if you decide instead to have a 100 percent grass-fed burger cooked in ghee (clarified butter) on medium heat and wrapped in organic lettuce? Your hand on that light switch just flipped the switch down. Congratulations! You've just turned off disease-promoting genes—and turned *on* health-promoting genes.

What you choose to eat directly determines the composition and function of your *microbiome*. Sugar and processed foods feed non-beneficial fungi that produce mycotoxins and yeast infections (*Candida*), whereas probiotic-rich foods like fermented vegetables feed health-promoting bacteria, which help maintain beneficial microbial balance. With each food decision, you choose what instructions get directly delivered to your genes—harm or heal—and you choose the balance of microbes you feed—disease-promoting or health-promoting.

You've heard that food is fuel, well, here's how: *Mitochondria* are the tiny but mighty factories in each of your cells that turn the food you eat into energy. They produce 90 percent of your cellular energy, so they are definitely mighty! The number and efficiency of your mitochondria reflect a microcosm of your health and well-being. When your mitochondria function well, you'll feel better and have more energy. The opposite is also true: when your mitochondria experience harm inflicted by stress, infections, toxins, and SAD foods, your energy producers are given reasons to go on strike.

KEY CONCEPT: *With each meal, you control whether harmful or healing genes get expressed.*

Mitochondrial expert and neurologist Bruce H. Cohen, MD, says that one of the biggest reasons our mitochondria deteriorate is that we eat too many poor-quality foods and not enough healthy ones. He warns that unless we eat plenty of phytonutrients, antioxidants, healthy fats, proteins, and fiber, our bodies don't get the basic tools they need to heal and generate life.

Now that you understand the significant invisible forces within you, you may have a greater appreciation for how consequential your food choices are. You're literally eating for trillions—*microbes*, that is. For some, the prospect of exerting such direct control over their health outcomes will come as a huge relief, while for others, the impact of everyday choices might feel more like unwanted pressure. If you fall into the latter category, remember that you don't have to start from scratch or go it alone. The foods described in the Healing Foods Toolkit will be your map and I'll be your guide on the path to wellness, one step at a time. Right now, what's most important is your willingness to examine and, eventually, optimize your food choices.

The Recipe for Healing with Food

So, where do you start? How do you determine what foods to avoid and what to eat to optimize your health? Fortunately for me, a Functional Medicine nutritionist helped guide me on my journey back to health. She educated me about toxic foods, assisted me in uncovering my personal food sensitivities, and led me through a gut-healing protocol. Within thirty days, I had identified and removed my personal food triggers, I had added in nourishing foods that would help heal my gut, and I was free of digestive and autoimmune symptoms.

The same straightforward process I used to go from decades of autoimmune symptoms to vibrant health is the one I use with my coaching clients and the one I'll guide you through now. First, I'll help you understand the connection between food and autoimmune conditions. We'll look at specific examples of how food can trigger and perpetuate autoimmunity for years or even decades, and also how food can serve as the greatest healer, even if it's not your primary trigger. (We'll address other common triggers in the following chapters.) Many people have succeeded in healing with food. If I can do it, so can you.

Before we jump to solutions, let's first look at how food can trigger autoimmune conditions. After you see the connection, you'll likely feel even more motivated to remove the culprits that may be causing you harm.

The Harmful Side of Food

As previously mentioned, the standard American diet (SAD), or Western diet, is a massive factor in creating the autoimmune epidemic today. Processed foods, refined sugars, gluten, grains, conventionally grown and factory-farmed animal products, and unhealthy fats like hydrogenated (chemically altered) oils and most vegetable oils are the primary inflammatory culprits in launching and perpetuating autoimmune disorders. Here's how:

About 75 percent of your immune system resides in your gut—specifically inside the lining of your small intestines—and autoimmunity is an immune system problem. We'll look at inflammation more closely in the Gut chapter, but for now, what's most important to know is that anything that inflames or harms your gut harms your immune system. Inflammatory SAD foods create imbalances in gut bacteria (microbiome dysbiosis or gut imbalance), nutritional deficiencies, and intestinal hyperpermeability (a.k.a. "leaky gut"), which is the gateway to autoimmunity.

Leaky Gut and Food Sensitivities

A leaky gut—literally large openings in the lining of your intestines (think rips in a fishing net)—allows large, undigested food particles to cross into the bloodstream. Once in the bloodstream, large protein molecules like gluten, casein (a dairy protein), or egg whites may be tagged and targeted as dangerous invaders by the immune system, which creates antibodies (missiles) to attack these "dangerous" food particles. Once food particles have been tagged for attack, every time you eat those foods, as long as your gut is permeable, your immune system will continue to attack the foods, resulting in multiple food sensitivities and worse. Eventually, in susceptible people, the immune system will turn its attack on tissues in your body that resemble the food protein molecules the immune system is attempting to destroy.

Research shows that many things can lead to a leaky gut: foods including gluten, dairy, and sugar; infections like *Candida* and Lyme disease and coinfections; toxins including pesticides and medications like antibiotics; and ongoing or traumatic stress. But consider the case of gluten. At a cellular level, the gluten molecule happens to look like a thyroid molecule. Continue eating gluten, and if you're predisposed, you may wind up with Hashimoto's thyroiditis. That's the autoimmune cascade: environmental factor(s) including food, infections, toxins, and stress lead to a leaky gut, which leads to immune system reactions like food sensitivities, autoimmune expression, and finally, full-blown autoimmune disease.

You may currently experience delayed allergic reactions to many of the foods you eat and not even know it. If you assume, like many do and like I did, that these symptoms are just a normal part of life, you won't make the connection between the foods you eat and the discomfort you experience. When you can't tell cause and effect between the foods you eat and body aches or brain fog, it may take years, if ever, for you to make the connection. If you keep eating foods that cause your gut to be inflamed and your immune system to overreact, the symptoms you experience will likely worsen in an attempt to grab your attention.

Autoimmune conditions don't develop overnight. It's a gradual and typically stealthy process that builds over five, ten, or more years, often simmering below conscious awareness until minor symptoms express as unmistakable signs of autoimmune disease.

What You Don't Know *Can* Harm You

I know lots about silent but harmful food toxins and resulting autoimmunity. Throughout my childhood, daily breakfasts of cereal with milk and school lunches of peanut butter and jelly sandwiches on whole wheat bread were, unbeknownst to me, steadily inflaming my gut, disrupting the balance of my microbiome, harming my mitochondrial function, and damaging my metabolism.

Looking back, it's hardly surprising that an undiagnosed gluten sensitivity led to immune system imbalances, a leaky gut, and, ultimately, a diagnosis of MS at age nineteen. Because I continued to eat gluten-containing grains until I was forty-five, I unknowingly perpetuated the autoimmune response and the MS persisted.

What we consume can be an autoimmune trigger, but it's an equally powerful healer. In fact, according to multiple experts, *food offers the highest healing potential of any solution yet identified*. Many who have addressed this root cause head-on—by removing the most harmful foodstuffs like sugar, processed foods, gluten, and dairy, and replacing them with nourishing foods like organic leafy greens, healthy fats, and moderate amounts of protein—have found that numerous autoimmune symptoms fade and never return.

When I discovered that I had non-celiac gluten sensitivity (NCGS) in 2010, I went cold turkey on gluten and healed my leaky gut; all my digestive issues and MS symptoms ended for good. A blood test later confirmed that I no longer had elevated antibodies to myelin sheath—the tissues previously under autoimmune attack—and a recent MRI showed a history of MS but no evidence of active MS in my body. The MRI confirmed not only the absence of new lesions, but also the disappearance of old ones.

Whatever the Cause, *Start with Food:*
Two Short Stories

Food doesn't have to be your primary root cause to be your primary solution. Whether your primary root cause is stress, an infection, or exposure to toxins—all of which we'll explore in other chapters—you may experience remarkable healing by starting with food. Here are two examples of people who achieved remarkable healing with food even though their primary triggers were stress and toxins, respectively:

Michelle Corey, Functional Medicine practitioner, suffered for years from the effects of ongoing physical and emotional trauma in childhood. The long-term abuse she endured activated a deep sense of unworthiness and resulted in unhealthy coping strategies. By her thirties, Michelle developed two full-blown autoimmune disorders: Hashimoto's thyroiditis and lupus. A host of symptoms plagued her, including hair loss, rashes "everywhere," a puffy face, aching joints, and melasma—a skin pigmentation disorder often present in women with Hashimoto's. While Michelle addressed the childhood trauma with deep emotional healing work, she didn't fully recover until she identified and eliminated her food triggers: gluten, grains, and nightshades (tomatoes, peppers, eggplants, potatoes, goji berries, chili peppers, and dried spices made from peppers, including cayenne, chili powder, and paprika). Once she removed those foods for good, all of her autoimmune symptoms vanished. As a bonus, she finally lost those "last ten pounds."

Terry Wahls, MD, who was diagnosed with a devastatingly progressive form of MS, believes her primary triggers were long-term exposure to toxic pesticides and herbicides while growing up on a farm—that, plus the cumulative stress she endured while attending medical school, including erratic sleep, lack of sunlight, and ongoing exposure to the embalming fluid formaldehyde. Terry feels the key to her recovery was changing her food from a grain-heavy, vegetarian diet to a nutrient-dense Paleo diet, rich with seaweed and colorful vegetables and targeted supplements. Within five years, she went from wheelchair-bound to bicycling and has become an icon for victorious healing with food. (You'll read more about Dr. Wahls's and Michelle's healing journeys in the Toxins and Stress chapters.)

You may not have made the connection between mysterious symptoms or outright autoimmune challenges and food, but a lot of people have, including me. Many of us have taken our health into our own hands and healed from disorders and conditions that we had been told and believed were incurable, untreatable, or hopeless. Fear not! No matter how long or intensely you have been suffering, there is almost always a new level of healing when you simply remove inflammatory foods and add in nourishing ones. You can do it, too; and in the next pages we'll dig into the details of how to heal with food.

Healing Foods Toolkit

It's natural to be intimidated by the prospect of a dietary overhaul, let alone attempting to determine, reduce, and replace your trigger foods. Please don't feel discouraged. I'm here to help simplify the dietary changes that are usually needed in order to heal from or even reverse your autoimmune condition(s). Many have done so with wonderful results, and that's my hope for you. Once you experience freedom from symptoms by removing your food triggers and adding in nourishing foods and supplements, you may wonder why you haven't done this sooner.

To discover your optimal foods and shore up nutrient deficiencies, follow six simple steps:

Step 1: Take a food self-assessment.
Step 2: Eliminate SAD foods.
Step 3: Identify and eliminate your suspect foods.
Step 4: Add in nourishing foods.
Step 5: Supplement strategically.
Step 6: Create healthy food habits for life.

Step 1: Take a Food Self-Assessment

It can be hard to fathom the connection between mysterious symptoms and the foods you eat, but it can be enormously freeing once you can tell cause and effect. These are among the most frequently cited symptoms that diminish or vanish once SAD and suspect foods are removed:

- Extreme fatigue
- Digestive issues
- Body aches and pain
- Poor sleep
- Brain fog
- Hair loss
- Mood problems (anger, anxiety, or depression)
- Numbness or tingling
- Chronic skin conditions (rashes, acne, eczema, or psoriasis)
- Inability to lose or gain weight

Can you relate to any of these? If so, I'm excited for you to see how your food choices may be impacting your health. If none of these symptoms sound familiar, there's a good chance your diet is already dialed in; or perhaps your toxin bucket hasn't reached a tipping point. Now's a great time to get ahead of or address autoimmune issues by examining what you eat.

Consider the following statements and rate your responses from 0–3, where 0 = Never/doesn't apply/disagree, 1 = Occasionally, 2 = More often than not, 3 = Almost always

0 1 2 3   I eat gluten-containing grains or grains that may be contaminated with gluten (wheat, rye, barley, rice, corn, oats, sorghum, millet, and buckwheat).

0 1 2 3   I eat grains (quinoa, amaranth, rice, etc.).

0 1 2 3   I eat processed (packaged), fried, and/or fast foods.

0 1 2 3   I eat conventional animal dairy products.

0 1 2 3   I eat conventional animal meat or farmed fish.

0 1 2 3   I eat conventionally grown fruits and vegetables.

0 1 2 3   I eat vegetable oils like canola (rapeseed), corn, sunflower, safflower, and soybean oils.

0 1 2 3   I eat margarine or shortening.

0 1 2 3   I eat soy products.

0 1 2 3   I eat sugar (all types, including fructose, cane, honey, agave, maple syrup, etc.).

0 1 2 3   I use artificial sweeteners.

0 1 2 3   I drink unfiltered (tap) water.

0 1 2 3   I eat genetically modified (GMO) food.

0 1 2 3   I drink three or more alcoholic beverages a week.

Tally up your score: _____

FOOD KEY

0   Wow! You are a role model for food. Keep up the great habits for good!

1–6   Food may be a *possible* trigger for you if you have unwanted systems or autoimmune issues.

7–10 Food is a *likely* trigger for you if you have autoimmune issues and/or want to prevent them.

11+   Food is a *very likely* trigger for you to explore to reverse or prevent autoimmune conditions.

Whatever your score, the good news is that you're gaining awareness of a potential connection between food and unwanted symptoms. While intellectually understanding the link between food and how you feel is a good start, actually *experiencing* those connections firsthand can be transformative. There is abundant science connecting toxic foods and inflammation, a necessary precondition for most diseases, including autoimmune disorders. But there's also plentiful science linking nourishing foods with healing. Let's deal with the bad news first, and then we'll dig into the good stuff.

Step 2: Eliminate SAD Foods

The most common trigger foods are both inflammatory and toxic for *anyone*—and especially for those of us with a predisposition to autoimmune conditions. These foods promote inflammation and imbalances in gut flora (dysbiosis), damage the structural integrity of the intestines ("leaky gut") and the blood-brain barrier ("leaky brain"), create nutrient deficiencies, and cause mitochondrial dysfunction and immune system impairment. As we learned earlier in the chapter, anything that harms our guts also harms our immune system.

The hallmark of the standard American diet (SAD) is food or food-like substances that have been chemically altered or manufactured in some way to extend shelf life, not to support healthy human life. Processed foods, found in most packaged products and fast foods, contain highly processed oils, artificial and corn-based sweeteners, refined grains, chemical preservatives and additives, and highly processed white table salt. Processed foods are not created to promote health; they're created for convenience and profit. Sadly, they promote inflammation, raise blood sugar, promote insulin resistance and obesity, and can lead to cancer and autoimmunity.

These toxic "foods" and food-like substances have no place in a healthy diet. I hope that once you understand the effects of these toxic foods on your body, you will decide to reject them roundly. To achieve vibrant health, you must bid farewell to toxic "foods" and embrace the nourishing foods that help you thrive. When you begin, you'll quickly realize that eating for health, unlike typical restrictive diets, is all about abundance over deprivation: you'll replace the short list of harmful, SAD foods below with a long list of nourishing foods; you'll swap corn- and gluten-based junk food with new, healthy options that you may never have considered; and you'll overhaul your weekly eating habits to include more nutrient-dense and flavorful foods than ever before. Sound good? Then let's take a look at the biggest baddies.

TOP TOXIC SAD FOODS

Gluten. Gluten is the number-one autoimmune food trigger and has been implicated in at least fifty-five diseases in a review paper by the *New England Journal of Medicine*.[2] Research shows it creates a leaky gut in *anyone* who eats it. Gluten is not just one but *twenty-three thousand* different storage proteins found in *all* grains. While most research and testing is focused on one single gluten protein, alpha gliadin, until more and better testing is available, it may be prudent for people with autoimmune susceptibility to avoid all grains. Gluten can be as difficult to digest as human hair, which makes it highly inflammatory, but also ideal in baking, thanks to its gluey properties. American super-wheat, bred for its superior glueyness, may be the most indigestible gluten.

Recommendation: One hundred percent compliance with gluten removal is required for anyone who wants to heal from or prevent autoimmune conditions.

Caution: This is not a pass to eat products labeled "gluten-free." These packaged foods often contain sugar, preservatives, additives, and chemicals, and supply high levels of carbohydrates that promote blood sugar imbalances, insulin resistance, and obesity, which is a major contributor to the onset and progression of autoimmune diseases.

Processed Fats and Oils. Most vegetable oils are highly processed, inflammatory fats. They are produced using toxic chemicals like hexane and bleach, contain a high ratio of inflammatory omega-6 to omega-3 fats, oxidize (go rancid) quickly, and produce toxic byproducts when heated, creating disease-promoting free radicals, linked to heart disease, cancer, obesity, and autoimmune conditions. The following oils, and fast foods produced with these oils, are linked to many illnesses: canola (rapeseed), corn, cottonseed, peanut, sunflower, safflower, and soybean oils, and partially hydrogenated (chemically hardened) vegetable oils (margarine and shortening).

Recommendation: Avoid *all* processed vegetable oils (except olive), avoid margarine and shortening, and avoid fast foods, which are made with these oils, *for good.* Opt instead for organic extra virgin olive oil, coconut oil, ghee (clarified butter, which is usually well-tolerated by people sensitive to dairy), and grass-fed butter (if you can handle dairy).

Sugars and Sweeteners. Excess sugar in *all* forms—glucose, sucrose, and fructose—harms the immune system and promotes inflammation, leaky gut, obesity, cancer, and autoimmunity. This includes anything with high fructose corn syrup (HFCS), agave, cane sugar, maple syrup, and honey. Even high glycemic (blood sugar-spiking) fruits like bananas and watermelon contribute to yeast overgrowth, gut microbe imbalance, obesity, diabetes, and autoimmune disorders. When choosing fruits and vegetables, opt for whole fruits and vegetables as opposed to the juice. Whole fruits and veggies contain fiber, which slows down the digestion of sugars, keeping the insulin system in balance; fruit juice, however, which doesn't contain fiber, is a fast path to high blood sugar.

Research has shown that artificial sweeteners like aspartame (the blue packet), saccharine (the pink packet) and sucralose (the yellow packet) may be toxic for humans. Sucralose, which is made with chlorine, is shown to reduce beneficial gut bacteria and alter human insulin levels. Aspartame, which contains formaldehyde, has been linked with the development of cancer. And all have been implicated in increased risk of excessive weight gain, type 2 diabetes, and cardiovascular disease.

Recommendation: Avoid processed sugar and artificial sweeteners for good. Minimize fruit consumption if you are dealing with blood sugar imbalances, insulin resistance, diabetes, or obesity. Use organic stevia as your primary sweetener; you may also consider lo han (monk fruit) or xylitol (sugar alcohol produced from birch wood—not corn).

Caution: Sugar alcohols can cause digestive distress in some people.

Dairy. Many people with celiac disease or gluten sensitivities are also sensitive to dairy, specifically to the dairy protein *casein*. Casein is a difficult protein to digest and inflammatory for many, causing leaky gut and triggering a heightened immune reaction that can lead to autoimmune disorders including type 1 diabetes, lupus, MS, and rheumatoid arthritis (RA). The A1 beta-casein type, common to Holstein cows, is particularly inflammatory.

Beyond casein, there are a number of problems with conventional cow dairy: Most non-organically raised dairy cows are fed genetically modified grains that are often sprayed with glyphosate (Roundup), treated with antibiotics, and given rBGH, a genetically modified bovine growth hormone. Conventional milk is then pasteurized—killing beneficial enzymes and probiotics—and homogenized, which creates harmful free radicals.

Recommendation: Avoid *conventional* cow dairy, *for good.* After taking a 30-Day Food Vacation, if you want to try dairy, consider raw, organic, A2 beta-casein varieties like Jersey cows. You may try goat or sheep milk—ideally fermented like kefir or yogurt—which tend to be better tolerated and more easily digested.

Food Additives and Chemicals. Many added chemicals—used to alter flavor, color, and texture and extend shelf life—are linked to cancer and autoimmune disease. This means anything with preservatives, artificial flavors, colorings and chemicals, including MSG (monosodium glutamate) and artificial sweeteners. Conventionally grown fruits and vegetables often contain pesticide residue, which may increase the risk for developing autoimmune diseases. Unfiltered tap water often contains toxic chemicals including fluoride, chlorine, chloramine, lead, pharmaceutical drugs and other substances known to interfere with immune function, disrupt hormones, cause obesity, and increase risk of cancer.

Recommendation: Avoid toxins in your food and water to the greatest extent possible. If cost is a concern when it comes to buying organic produce, check out the Environmental Working Group (www.ewg.org) Dirty Dozen and Clean Fifteen charts to determine which fruits and vegetables are most or least affected by pesticide residue. For pure water, make sure at the very least that you are filtering out fluoride and chlorine from your drinking and bathing water.

Conventionally Raised Animal Products. You are not only what *you* eat, but you're also *whatever you eat* ate. Conventionally raised animals are often mass-produced in concentrated animal feeding operations (CAFOs) in order to produce the fattest animals as fast as possible, often with antibiotics and hormones. If that isn't enough, they are fed grains that are usually genetically modified, laden with pesticides and herbicides (glyphosate), and spoiled by toxic mold. Yes, that's right; moldy grain causes greater weight gain, fattier meat, more tender meat, and mycotoxin-laden meat, the first three of which traditionally appeal to American consumers. But if you have an autoimmune disorder, beware! You may be extra sensitive to the mycotoxins, glyphosate, and GMO proteins in such meat products.

> **KEY CONCEPT:** *You are whatever what you eat ate. Feed lot animals, most poultry, and farmed fish eat corn and soy.*

Sadly, these animals also suffer from the added stress of confinement. But whatever your views on animal cruelty, the bottom line is that conventional meat provides less nutritional value than organic, grass-fed, or free-range meats. And while conventionally raised meat is cheaper and easier to find, the cost to the animals, the environment, and human health is high.

Recommendation: Avoid *conventionally raised* meat, poultry, dairy, and eggs, and *farmed* fish, which are often fed unnatural diets of corn and soy. Choose animal products with designations "100 percent grass-fed," "pastured," or "wild."

Corn. Corn is a grain that contains a type of gluten which resembles the gluten in wheat and can cause a cross-reaction in people sensitive to wheat gluten. That means your body mistakes corn gluten for wheat gluten and mounts a similar immune reaction that can lead to autoimmunity. Furthermore, corn is frequently contaminated with harmful mold toxins, and most corn produced today is genetically modified to *resist* being destroyed by glyphosate (Roundup Ready corn). Roundup Ready crops are frequently sprayed with Roundup before harvesting. Studies show glyphosate causes leaky gut and increases the risk of many diseases, including Parkinson's, cancer, and rheumatoid arthritis.[3]

Recommendation: Avoid conventionally grown corn for good. If you find you can tolerate corn following the 30-Day Food Vacation, make sure you opt for organic corn and minimize consumption if you are dealing with blood sugar imbalances, insulin resistance, diabetes, or obesity.

Soy. While legumes as a category are addressed in the suspect food list that follows, soy has numerous additional problems that make it a harmful food for many. Soy contains numerous naturally occurring toxins to ward off plant predators and which can have a hazardous effect in humans. Lectins can trigger inflammation and stimulate a hyperimmune response, which can lead to autoimmunity in susceptible people. Phytic acid binds to minerals, especially calcium, magnesium, iron, and zinc, rendering them less available to your cells; saponins, soyatoxin, trypsin inhibitors and oxalates can interfere with enzymes needed to digest protein. Soy also contains phytoestrogens (plant estrogens), which are both endocrine and thyroid disruptors, and may promote hormonally sensitive cancers. Finally, more than 90 percent of soy harvested in the United States today is genetically modified with glyphosate.

Recommendation: Avoid conventionally grown soy for good. If you find you can tolerate soy following the 30-Day Food Vacation, make sure you opt for organic and, ideally, *fermented* soy products, which are easier to digest, like tempeh, natto, and miso.

White Table Salt. Excess processed salt may be one of the environmental factors causing an increase in autoimmune diseases. White table salt is chemically processed to eliminate magnesium and trace minerals, and usually contains additives and preservatives. Mice fed a diet high in processed salt showed a dramatic increase in the number of pathogenic Th17 cells that cause inflammation and can contribute to autoimmune disorders.[4]

Recommendation: Avoid processed white table salt. Replace with refined or raw sea salt.

Step 3: Identify and Eliminate *Your* Suspect Foods

There's a saying that *one man's food is another man's poison.* When it comes to autoimmune disorders and food sensitivities, this old adage is spot-on. Gray-area foods, which we'll call "suspect" foods, can be harmless to many but harmful for some. These foods can do damage without causing obvious symptoms, which makes them particularly stealthy triggers.

ALLERGIES VS. SENSITIVITIES

You're likely familiar with food *allergies*: the immediate and potentially severe reactions some have to peanuts or shellfish that cause unmistakable symptoms like hives, swelling, and even anaphylaxis or death. Food allergies can be verified by laboratory testing that reveals elevated IgE (Immunoglobulin E) antibodies. I like to think of the "E" for "emergency."

Much more common are food *sensitivities,* which appear on lab tests as elevated IgG (Immunoglobulin G) antibodies. I call that one "good grief" for "gG." While food allergies trigger an immediate reaction, food *sensitivities* often produce delayed reactions, sometimes not occurring for hours or even a week! Because the cause and effect are not concurrent and are rarely obvious, people do not make the cause-and-effect connection and continue to eat those foods, thereby unknowingly triggering and perpetuating autoimmune symptoms.

How can you possibly connect a cause to an effect if you can't feel it for hours or days? It's very difficult unless you take suspect foods out of your diet for a while. Once you remove these foods for a long enough period of time, the immune system has a chance to settle down, symptoms subside, and, ideally, health is restored. It's usually when you add foods back in after taking a break that you have a stronger reaction.

Sometimes food sensitivities arise from foods we crave and eat the most—even if those foods are not considered toxic for most people—like eggs, tomatoes, chocolate, coffee, or nuts. This is where you will employ courage, determination, and commitment to your good health above everything else. It may be that your morning cup of coffee or that irresistible square of chocolate is a trigger for you. But don't despair: the well-being that comes from removing these foods lasts far longer than a caffeine or sugar high. And, furthermore, these suspect triggers may be temporary. Once you remove them for several months and heal your gut, you may be able to enjoy them again.

The process used to detect food sensitivities is commonly known as an *elimination diet*. Functional Medicine practitioners consider the elimination diet the gold standard for uncovering an individual's unique food triggers. The process is so beneficial I think it deserves a more positive name. After all, who wants to give things up? I prefer the more encouraging 30-Day Food Vacation. You can do just about anything for thirty days, and a vacation sounds so inviting. When you go on vacation, you rest and rejuvenate—and you often try new things.

And this vacation is actually the opposite of deprivation. A 30-Day Food Vacation may expose you to more foods than you knew existed. Have you ever counted the number of foods you eat each week? If you're following a typical American diet, you may be getting most of your nourishment from just one: corn.

Contemplate your weekly food choices. How often do you try new vegetables, fish, or meats? When was the last time you had a juicy lettuce-wrapped bison burger or a garlicky massaged kale salad? How about zucchini pasta with green harissa sauce or a rainbow of colorful roasted veggies? Would you be willing to try liver pâté or keto cardamom custard? (Find these recipes, and more, in Appendix A.) When you eliminate toxic SAD and suspect foods, there is an abundance of nourishing foods waiting for you. I promise.

SUSPECT FOODS TO REMOVE DURING YOUR 30-DAY FOOD VACATION

Cross-Reactive Foods. People sensitive to gluten must also consider taking a vacation from cross-reactive foods that the immune system mistakes for gluten. They include dairy, milk chocolate, millet, oats, rice, whey, and yeast.[5]

Recommendation: Eliminate all cross-reactive foods during your 30-Day Food Vacation.

Grains. *All* cereal grains—wheat, barley, rye, corn, millet, oats, sorghum, spelt, teff, rice, and wild rice—and pseudo grains— quinoa, buckwheat, and amaranth—contain different forms of gluten proteins which may be harmful to anyone sensitive to wheat gluten. Grains are high-glycemic carbohydrates that can spike blood sugar, paving the way for insulin and leptin resistance, diabetes, and obesity, each a risk factor for autoimmune conditions. Grains also contain toxic antinutrients—natural compounds that interfere with absorption of nutrients—that can contribute to the manifestation of chronic inflammation and autoimmune diseases by increasing intestinal permeability and initiating a pro-inflammatory immune response.[6, 7]

Recommendation: Eliminate *all* grains during your 30-Day Food Vacation and consider a permanent vacation from grains for optimal health. If you are able to tolerate and want to eat non-glutinous grains, try soaking and sprouting before cooking to optimize digestion and reduce the toxic antinutrient load.

Egg Whites. Egg whites contain lysozymes, which can act like a Trojan horse, penetrating the gut barrier and allowing other large protein molecules and bacteria like *E. coli* into the bloodstream, potentially setting off an immune system inflammatory reaction. In addition, egg white consumption may contribute to autoimmune disorders via a process of molecular mimicry that is similar to the issues with dietary lectins found in wheat, legumes and grains.[8]

Recommendation: Eliminate eggs during your 30-Day Food Vacation. If you end up reacting to egg whites, you may be able to enjoy egg yolks, which are super nourishing. Also, some people can tolerate duck eggs even if they react to chicken eggs.

Nightshades (*Solanaceae* family). Many who suffer from arthritis (osteo, psoriatic, or rheumatoid) or a rheumatic disorder such as lupus and other aches and pains have found that consuming foods from the nightshade family is in part to blame. Nightshades include tomatoes, potatoes (except sweet potatoes and yams), eggplant, paprika, peppers, all pepper-based hot sauces and spices, ashwagandha, and goji berries. The lectin, saponin, and/or capsaicin content in these foods are all implicated in causing leaky gut.

Recommendation: Eliminate nightshades during your 30-Day Food Vacation.

Tree Nuts and Seeds. Tree nuts, including almonds, Brazil nuts, cashews, hazelnuts, macadamia nuts, pecans, pistachios, and walnuts, are one of the top allergens and most common food sensitivities. People with autoimmune disorders are more likely to have a sensitivity or allergy to nuts and seeds.[9]

Recommendation: Eliminate tree nuts and seeds during your 30-Day Food Vacation. If you are able to tolerate them, consider soaking and sprouting organic nuts and seeds to optimize their digestion.

Legumes. Soybeans, lentils, peas, chickpeas, all beans, and peanuts are high in lectins, a naturally occurring toxin found in plants to ward off predators, which also have a hazardous effect in many humans. Lectins can trigger inflammation and stimulate a hyperimmune response, which can lead to autoimmunity in susceptible people.[10]

Recommendation: Eliminate legumes during your 30-Day Food Vacation; and eliminate peanuts, which are frequently contaminated with mold, for good. If you can tolerate legumes and want to include them in your diet, soaking and sprouting before cooking—or eating fermented varieties—will help you digest them better.

Pork and Processed Meats. Pigs are notorious scavengers, eating anything they can find, and they tend to harbor more toxins, including antibiotic-resistant bacteria and other unsavory contaminants. Processed meats are preserved by smoking, curing, or salting, and often contain chemicals like meat glue and preservatives called *nitrates*. Nitrates convert into nitrosamines in the body and are associated with an increased risk of diabetes and certain cancers.

Recommendation: Eliminate pork and processed meats during your 30-Day Food Vacation. If you decide to continue to eat pork, choose organic, uncured, nitrate-free, minimally processed products.

Fruit. Fructose, the simple sugar in fruit, can promote inflammation, insulin resistance, elevated triglycerides, abdominal obesity, and oxidative stress. It makes sense to minimize fruit intake if you are overweight, have insulin resistance, diabetes, or yeast infections.

Recommendation: Eliminate all fruits (including fruit juices, with the exception of small amounts of organic, unsweetened cranberry juice) except raspberries, blackberries, blueberries, coconut, avocado, and lemon during your 30-Day Food Vacation. After the 30-Day Food Vacation, consider minimizing fruit consumption until you resolve blood sugar imbalances, insulin resistance, diabetes, or obesity. If you want to jazz up your water, add a splash of unsweetened organic cranberry juice and/or lemon, and a few drops of stevia if desired.

Coffee and Caffeinated Foods and Beverages. While there are numerous health benefits associated with drinking coffee, there are also some concerns:

1. Some people are super sensitive to the effects of coffee. One gene in particular, CYP1A2, determines how quickly our bodies break down caffeine. "Fast metabolizers" are people whose bodies clear caffeine from their systems rapidly, allowing the antioxidants, polyphenols, and coffee's other healthful compounds to kick in without the unpleasant side effects of caffeine; whereas "slow metabolizers" take twice as long to metabolize caffeine and are especially sensitive to the jitters, nausea, anxiety, and insomnia-producing effects of caffeine. Two or more cups per day can increase risk of heart disease in slow caffeine metabolizers.

2. Coffee beans and roasted coffee—particularly *decaffeinated* coffee—may contain the harmful mycotoxins (mold byprod-

ucts) Aflatoxin B1 and Ochratoxin A, which are linked with immune system suppression and cancer.[11]

3. The protein in coffee cross-reacts with gluten, meaning people who are sensitive to gluten may also be sensitive to coffee.[12]

Recommendation: Eliminate both regular and decaffeinated coffee and all caffeinated teas and beverages during your 30-Day Food Vacation. Try a variety of herbal and decaffeinated teas. Organic roasted dandelion root tea is a healthy coffee substitute. If you find you can handle coffee, take care to select high-quality, organic brands like Purity or Bulletproof; and buy "water-processed" decaf, to minimize mold exposure.

Chocolate. Raw cacao—the main ingredient in chocolate—has many beneficial effects on immune health, cardiovascular health, nervous system diseases, aging, and cancer prevention. But, regardless of the numerous health benefits, a small percentage of people react to chocolate, some to the dairy in milk chocolate, some to the cacao itself, and some to the small amount of caffeine. For people who are sensitive to caffeine, chocolate might pose a problem because an ounce of dark chocolate contains about the same amount of caffeine as a cup of green tea.[13]

Recommendation: Eliminate all chocolate and cacao during your 30-Day Food Vacation and avoid milk chocolate *for good*. If you don't react on reintroducing dark chocolate, choose organic dark chocolate with more than 70 percent cacao solids to minimize sugar intake. Better yet, make your own raw cacao treats like chocolate "fat bombs" using coconut oil, coconut butter, raw cacao with a pinch of sea salt, and stevia. As for store-bought bars, you might find some made with stevia, like Lily's non-GMO dark chocolate, which is a good option to reduce your sugar intake.

Alcohol. While research shows alcohol in small quantities can be protective against heart disease and type 2 diabetes, studies also reveal alcohol's harmful effects, including elevated risk of cancers (breast, colon, and liver), suppression of the immune system, and increased intestinal permeability (leaky gut). A single bottle of beer may contain more than ten allergens, including preservatives, histamines, pesticides, wheat, gluten, yeast, and corn—which may be genetically modified.

Recommendation: Eliminate alcohol during your 30-Day Food Vacation, and consider minimizing or eliminating alcohol for good to protect your gut, brain, and immune system.

Yeast. Some people are sensitive to brewer's yeast, a single-celled fungus known as *Saccharomyces cerevisiae,* sometimes found in probiotics, soy sauce, vinegar, wine, and beer; others are sensitive to baker's yeasts (yeast used to make baked foods rise), yeast extracts (found in salad dressings, seasonings, and bouillon cubes) and fermented products like vinegar and aged cheeses. The protein in brewer's and baker's yeasts cross-reacts with gluten, meaning people who are sensitive to gluten may also be sensitive to brewer's and baker's yeasts. Others have a histamine intolerance and may react to high histamine levels present in fermented foods. On the other hand, nutritional yeast flakes, like Sari Foods' brand (nonfortified with added vitamins), are a delicious swap for parmesan cheese.

Recommendation: Eliminate brewer's and baker's yeasts during your 30-Day Food Vacation. If you have a histamine intolerance, follow a low-histamine diet and consider supplementing with diamine oxidase (DAO), an enzyme that helps break down histamine. Go ahead and try sprinkling nutritional yeast flakes on roasted vegetables or sautéed greens and use it to make your Juicy Bison Burgers (see recipe on page 283) more flavorful and tender.

Shellfish. Tropomyosin has been identified as the major allergen in the shellfish family and is responsible for the majority of shellfish allergies and delayed sensitivities.

Recommendation: Eliminate shellfish during your 30-Day Food Vacation.

The best way for you to figure out whether any of these SAD and suspect foods are a problem for you is to take a vacation from them for at least thirty days. The second-best way to identify your potential food sensitivities is through laboratory testing. While food sensitivity testing is not 100 percent reliable, it can be a good route for people who have already done an elimination diet and still cannot determine which, if any, foods are causing an immune burden leading to their symptoms. Laboratory testing options are covered in the sidebar on pages 46–47.

The 30-Day Food Vacation Overview

If you are suffering from autoimmune issues or have troubling symptoms like digestive problems, brain fog, headaches, fatigue, or aches and pains, then a 30-Day Food Vacation may be the most profound experiment you'll ever do. It was for me. And it was for Linda Clark, nutrition educator, too.

Healing with Food: Linda Clark's Story

Decades before she became an authority on healing with nutrition, Linda was herself a frustrated patient trying to make sense of a catalog of disturbing physical sensations that started out as small signs but later developed into debilitating symptoms, including memory issues, brain fog, dizziness, numbness, body aches, pains, and muscle spasms.

Because Linda grew up in a home filled with stress and smoke, the stage was pretty much set for the development of what would later be labeled multiple chemical sensitivities (MCS), fibromyalgia (FM), chronic fatigue syndrome (CFS), Hashimoto's thyroiditis, and celiac disease. By her late forties, Linda's health plummeted. After exhausting the confines of conventional medicine, Linda sought holistic solutions from a variety of natural resources.

In her healing quest, Linda learned about the elimination diet as a means to uncover her food triggers. It was excruciating for her to contemplate giving up her favorite foods. She loved and ate grains, cheese, and yogurt almost every day, and it also seemed unfathomable for her to eat meat again, since she had been a vegetarian for years. But Linda thought thirty days seemed doable, and so she decided to give it a try. Sure enough, within thirty days of removing her suspect foods, Linda's symptoms faded. When the thirty days were up, however, she immediately reverted to her old food habits, and her symptoms flooded back. Eventually, Linda's determination to get well overrode her vegetarian preferences, so she removed all grains, dairy, and sugar for good and started eating meat. As Linda transitioned to a nourishing Paleo diet, incorporating a variety of vegetables, healthy fats, and protein, her occasional brain fog lifted completely, her memory and energy improved, and residual aches and spasms vanished.

Linda's experience informs her philosophy that health is a daily choice. She now teaches others about healing with nutrition and how life can be full of healing moments. At her thriving practice in Sacramento, California, she offers some tough love to her clients: "You have to understand that you're going to need to change your life in order to heal. For me, it was a willingness to learn, be curious, and do whatever it takes to heal. That's the thing that I expect of all my clients. You may never get your old lifestyle back, but take heart that you'll live a new, more vibrant existence—one in which you choose health every day rather than suffer with disease."

Many experts observe that most, if not all, of their clients' symptoms disappear when trigger foods are eliminated for a long enough period. How long is that? It can vary. Some say three weeks is fine since it takes that long for antibodies to dissipate. You may choose to continue the Food Vacation until all your symptoms disappear, which may be ninety days or longer. Some of my clients feel so good after thirty days that they choose not to add suspect foods back in *ever*. Taking a vacation from suspect foods for a minimum of thirty days allows your body to begin calming the autoimmune response, healing the gut lining, reducing inflammation, and repairing damaged tissues that were targets of the autoimmune attack.

In addition to the primary goal of identifying trigger foods, the 30-Day Food Vacation gives your detoxification organs a break, allowing your body to clear and recover from whatever toxic burden may have accumulated. It's also an empowering experiment, so put on your own lab coat, and let's get started!

30-DAY FOOD VACATION ACTION STEPS

1. **Select thirty days** when you know you can take a vacation from suspected food triggers. During travel or over the holidays, for instance, may not be the best time to start.
2. **Shop ahead** for the wide variety of delicious, organic foods you will eat for thirty days:

- ✓ **Protein:** wild fish, pastured (ideally not corn or soy-fed) turkey, chicken, duck, 100 percent grass-fed beef, lamb, and wild game (bison, elk, venison, ostrich)
- ✓ **Protein powder:** grass-fed collagen peptides or bone broth protein powder
- ✓ **Veggies:** *all* organic vegetables (except nightshade family), including seaweed
- ✓ **Fats:** extra virgin olive oil, coconut oil, medium chain triglycerides (MCT) oil, avocado oil, flaxseed oil, and ghee (clarified butter)
- ✓ **Other fats:** avocados and olives
- ✓ **Fermented foods:** veggies (except nightshades), sauerkraut, kimchi, plain coconut yogurt, and coconut kefir
- ✓ **Low-glycemic fruits:** organic lemons, limes, berries, and coconut
- ✓ **Herbs & spices:** all organic (avoid cayenne pepper)
- ✓ **Pantry items:** organic raw apple cider vinegar, meat and bone broths, coconut flakes, coconut butter, stevia and/or lo han, and nutritional yeast flakes
- ✓ **Dairy replacement:** organic canned coconut milk—for pantry and fridge. Or make your own coconut milk (see p. 298 for recipe)
- ✓ **Tea:** organic, decaffeinated black, green, white, and herbal selections
- ✓ **Pure water:** half your body weight in ounces of spring or filtered water
- ✓ **Cran-water:** an added splash of unsweetened cranberry juice to water, or a squeeze of lemon, plus stevia as desired
- ✓ **Sweeteners:** stevia, lo han (monk fruit) or xylitol (from Birch wood, not corn)

3. **Plan ahead** with meal options (see 30-Day Food Vacation Recipes in Appendix A). For more 30-Day Food Vacation recipes, Google "Autoimmune Paleo Diet (AIP)" for recipes free of dairy, eggs, sugar, grains, chocolate, coffee, nuts, and nightshades.
4. **Remove from your kitchen/house/office/car** all the foods you will be taking a vacation from so you won't be tempted. Even the hidden stash.
5. **Take a vacation** from all SAD and suspect foods for thirty days—*no exceptions*, otherwise you won't have an accurate outcome, and that just means you'll have to do it again. Argh!

6. **Pay attention to how you feel and keep a food-symptom tracker** (see example in Appendix B). Monitor your digestion, elimination, energy, and sleep. If you feel better during the Food Vacation (i.e., more energy, better sleep, reduced symptoms, etc.), it means that something you commonly eat is likely causing you problems.

7. **After thirty days, reintroduce foods** *one at a time* in *small amounts* over a minimum of a two-day (forty-eight-hour) period. Get your food-symptom tracker (Appendix B) ready for the reintroduction phase.

8. **You may reintroduce foods in any order.** For example, if you want to try coffee first, have a *small cup*—like a quarter to a half cup of organic black coffee (no dairy, but you may have a little stevia) the morning of day thirty-one. Pay attention. How does it make you feel? Write it down. If you don't have a negative reaction, have another small cup by noon, and then stop for the day. Continue paying attention and noting any undesirable symptoms. If you feel fine, do the same thing on day thirty-two. Any food that clears the reintroduction phase can be kept in your diet. On day thirty-three, add another food and repeat the small dosing over two days. The whole reintroduction process will take about a month, so have patience; soon you'll be able to clearly identify which foods to eat and which to avoid—at least temporarily.

9. **If you experience any negative reactions** on reintroducing a food, stop eating the food immediately. You can try again the next day if you'd like to verify your reaction. If you react again, this is a clear message from your body that the food(s) is at the root of mysterious or autoimmune symptoms. At this point, it is recommended that you remove the offending food(s) for at least three months before reintroducing it. Any of these symptoms is an indication that your body is reacting to the food:
   - Unusual fatigue
   - GI symptoms: diarrhea or constipation, gas, bloating, abdominal pain, heartburn, reflux, or nausea
   - Headaches or brain fog
   - Dizziness or lightheadedness
   - Muscle or joint pain
   - Skin irritation: flushing, breakouts, itching, or a rash
   - Trouble falling or staying asleep

- Sinus congestion or runny nose
- Mood issues: anxiety, depression, or just feeling blue

10. **Well done!** If you completed the steps, even if the process wasn't perfect, congratulate yourself. Hopefully you have been able to isolate your food triggers and feel relief from prior, unwanted symptoms. Ideally, you feel more in control of your food choices and motivated to continue avoiding the foods that are causing you ill effects. You are well on your way to more vibrant health!

AFTER THE 30-DAY FOOD VACATION AND REINTRODUCTION PHASE

It's time to heal your gut. If you have food sensitivities and/or auto-immune symptoms, there is an almost certain chance that you also have a leaky gut and imbalanced gut microbiome. Healing will remain elusive unless and until you heal and seal your gut. Once you've completed your 30-Day Food Vacation, the following chapter, Heal Your Gut, will assist you in tending your gut garden.

Rotate your foods. Unfortunately, we often develop sensitivities to the foods we eat and crave the most. By taking breaks from our habitual foods—even our optimal foods—we reduce our immune system burden while expanding our nutrient variety. Rotating foods helps to break the habits and cravings that have led to food sensitivities in the first place and reduces the chance of developing new ones. Because it takes two weeks for antibody production to subside after eating a food your immune system reacts to, ideally, you should rotate foods every fourteen days. While that seems impractical for many of us, there are strategies you can employ to make your immune system happier:

- Eat with the seasons instead of buying the same produce year-round, and make fruit a rare treat instead of a daily habit.
- Opt for variety. Make a conscious effort to try new foods and aim to eat a rainbow of colorful vegetables.
- Plan meals and snacks. Stock your fridge, freezer, and pantry with a variety of grass-fed meats, pastured poultry, veggies, avocados, coconut products, and frozen berries. If you don't live close to a store that offers organic options, check out the mail order companies in Appendix F.

What about backsliding? We're all human, and sometimes even the best intentions are no match for our most ingrained (pun intended) routines. Let's say, like Linda, that you complete the elimination and reintroduction phases and feel better. In fact, you feel so much better, you don't see the harm in indulging your cravings for your favorite trigger foods just this once. Before you know it, you've backslid straight into your old habits and uncomfortable symptoms.

This scenario can happen to even the most disciplined among us, but if it happens to you, please go easy on yourself. After all, feeling guilty or discouraged might be worse than the trigger food itself! Instead, listen deeply to your body. The return of symptoms is your body's way of communicating with you. If you ignore subtle messages, symptoms may get louder until you finally decide to step away from your trigger foods.

Consider Food Sensitivity Testing

Sometimes a 30-Day Food Vacation misses culprit foods, and sometimes it's more efficient to just get tested. But there is an important consideration before you spend money on expensive food sensitivity testing: Many people with autoimmune conditions are unable to mount a proper antibody response (immunoglobulins IgA, IgG, IgM), meaning their immune systems may not be functioning well due to excess toxins, chronic stress, infections, etc. Too few immunoglobulins leave you at risk for infections, and too many indicate you may have an overactive immune system.

If you don't test your total immunoglobulin status first, food sensitivity testing may produce false positives or negatives, indicating erroneously and frustratingly that you have no sensitivities or that you are sensitive to everything. *Find out if you can mount a proper antibody response before ordering a food sensitivity test.* This preliminary blood test is called a *total immunoglobulins* (IgA, IgG, IgM) *panel.* You can order one from Quest through your doctor or online directly through LabsMD, DirectLabs, or Request A Test for sixty-two dollars to ninety-nine dollars.

While there are numerous food sensitivity tests available, here are three that I have personally used and recommend to clients:

Your imagination can assist you in this process. Envision your future free of pain and suffering. What are you doing? Who are you with? Who would you be without the shackles of unwanted and debilitating symptoms? Imprint that powerful image in your brain and use it as a positive emotional attractor to help you get back on track whenever facing your favorite, harmful foods. If it takes five or fifty tries, that's okay! As long as you're being kind to yourself, you're on the right track.

Once you have completed the 30-Day Food Vacation and/or testing and have identified your culprit foods, experts advise staying away from the culprit food(s) for three or six months depending upon the severity of the reaction. The key to healing food sensitivities is to heal your gut, which we'll delve into in the next chapter. You may need to take a permanent vacation from some foods. No one knows your body as well as you do, so

- ELISA/ACT Biotechnologies (EAB). EAB's midrange comprehensive panel costs about $600 and bundles 315 popular foods with many common chemicals, molds, additives, and toxins. The big benefit of ELISA/ACT is that it directly tests lymphocyte (immune system cells) response, as opposed to just antibody (IgG) response, which can be either protective or reactive.

- Cyrex Laboratories. If you can afford it—pricing is in the neighborhood of $1,200 and not covered by insurance—consider doing Cyrex's 10C—a bundle of three arrays, including a comprehensive gluten test; a test of twenty-four common cross-reactive foods; and a test of 180 commonly eaten cooked and raw foods, including common dietary components like food additives and colorings.

- Meridian Valley Lab. Meridian Valley's FoodSafe Basic Panel is the slimmest and most cost-effective of the three options, offering a ninety-four-food IgG panel plus a *Candida* screen for about $150.

listen carefully to your body and experiment as you feel is needed. Personally, I won't ever go back to eating gluten or dairy (except organic ghee, which is casein-free), and nine years after giving them up, I don't miss them—but I do cherish vibrant health!

Step 4: Add In Nourishing Foods

Years of research and expert interviews, along with my own personal experience, has led me to advocate a diet known alternately as "hunter-gatherer," "Stone Age," "ancestral," or "Paleolithic" ("Paleo") as the best framework for those seeking to reverse or prevent autoimmune conditions.

The Paleo diet is how our hunter-gatherer ancestors ate for the majority of human evolution, at least up until the Industrial Revolution and the advent of modern agriculture. It includes a wide variety of whole, unprocessed foods, liberal amounts of healthy fats, moderate amounts of animal protein, and a low to moderate amount of carbohydrates—the USRDA food pyramid turned on its head! The Paleo diet avoids modern inflammatory foods like processed foods, sugar, grains, and dairy.

According to Loren Cordain, Ph.D., author of *The Paleo Diet* and one of the world's leading experts on Paleolithic nutrition, "By severely reducing or eliminating these [modern processed] foods and replacing them with a more healthful cuisine, possessing nutrient qualities more in line with the foods our ancestors consumed, it is possible to improve health and reduce the risk of chronic disease."

Eliminating gluten and dairy was my first giant step in healing with food. Soon after, as I learned more about the health benefits of following a Paleo approach, I decided to forgo all grains and sugar. I didn't miss the starch, and my sweet tooth subsided. Instead of feeling deprived, I enjoy double the amount and variety of vegetables on my plate and learned to bake delicious desserts with nut and coconut flours and stevia. Lab work shows that my blood sugar and inflammation markers have all improved. In short, I've reduced my risk of chronic disease by eating more like a cavewoman.

I realize that's just a nice little anecdote. What about bigger studies? Emerging research reveals similar good news. Both human and animal studies show the Paleo diet confers superior health benefits compared to modern, grain-heavy diets.

One long-term study of obese postmenopausal women found the Paleo diet to deliver multiple improvements in health markers, including lower systolic blood pressure and LDL cholesterol, each of which correlates with reduced risk for metabolic syndrome diseases like type 2 diabetes, cancer, and autoimmunity.[14]

An animal study examined the health effects of a Paleo diet on pigs. After piglets were weaned, they were randomly assigned cereal-based swine feed or a Paleo diet consisting of meat, vegetables, fruit, and tubers. After fifteen months, the piglets were measured. The Paleo pigs showed improved health profiles with significantly lower markers of inflammation than the cereal pigs, including C-reactive protein (CRP), higher insulin sensitivity, and lower blood pressure. Even pigs, it seems, are not adapted for modern grain-based diets.[15]

KEY CONCEPT: *You can improve your health markers within days on a Paleo diet.*

A small study published in the journal *Diabetologia* found that a Paleo diet resulted in significantly improved glucose tolerance in people with heart disease and diabetes or prediabetes over twelve weeks compared to a Mediterranean one that allowed grains, legumes, sugar, and low-fat dairy.[16]

Another small study looked at the short-term effects of the Paleo diet. Nine healthy, nonobese volunteers transitioned from a typical Western diet to a Paleo diet for just ten days. Volunteers gave up grains, dairy, and legumes in favor of meat, vegetables, fruits, and nuts. All nine participants had improvements in all health measurements, including improved blood pressure and glucose levels, lowered LDL cholesterol, and increased insulin sensitivity. Results demonstrate that even going Paleo for a short time delivers powerful health benefits.[17]

In summary, the Paleo diet lowers the risk of chronic degenerative disease, including heart disease, diabetes, cancer, and autoimmune conditions. Specific, measurable improvements are noted in the following health markers:

- Reduced inflammation
- Improved blood sugar and insulin levels
- Normalized blood pressure
- Better fatty acid composition
- Steady, sustainable fat loss[18]

As a result of following a Paleo template, people often report signs of vibrant health, including:

- Better immune function
- Reduced pain associated with inflammation
- Increased and more stable energy levels
- Less daytime fatigue
- Improved sleep
- Greater mental clarity
- Better mood and attitude
- Improved digestion
- Less or no bloating and gas
- Fewer food sensitivities

While a Paleo approach overall presents many health benefits, there is an ongoing debate within the Paleo community as to exactly which foods fit the Paleo model. After all, it's hard to be 100 percent certain as to which precise foods our ancestors ate and in what amounts. Some Paleo advocates are firm that there is no place for dairy, honey, alcohol, added salt, or any grains in this diet. Others have a broader scope about what to include.

How a Paleo Template Helps Balance Blood Sugar

All carbohydrates—whether cookies, cantaloupe or kale—get converted into sugar in your bloodstream. Your pancreas secretes insulin to bring that sugar (glucose) out of the blood and into your cells for energy. When you eat too many starchy and/or sweet carbohydrates (e.g., high-glycemic load carbs), you store those carbs as excess fat, often in the belly; your cells become resistant to the constant surge of insulin; and that insulin resistance over time leads to prediabetes and/or diabetes and may lead to metabolic syndrome, heart disease, autoimmune conditions, dementia, cancer, and higher mortality risk. By eliminating grains, sugar, and processed foods, minimizing fruits, and favoring a Paleo template of vegetables, fish, meats, nuts, seeds, and occasional fruits, you lower your risk of autoimmune and other degenerative conditions and help to optimize beneficial genetic expression.

I believe *you* are in the best position to determine what's optimal for *you*. That's why I recommend a Paleo *template*—a framework that follows core principles of ancestral eating without being dogmatic. A Paleo template offers a more flexible and individualized approach without losing important health benefits. I encourage you to experiment and observe what works best for you rather than blindly following someone else's dictates.

Michael Pollan offers a simple and powerful food mantra: "Eat real food. Mostly plants. Not too much." I would add the word *organic* to emphasize the importance of avoiding harmful pesticides and other chemicals you don't want in your food. An organic Paleo template fits that bill. It's all about *simplifying* your dietary choices and going back to the most natural and biologically beneficial ingredients possible. Your Paleo template might consist of the following real, organic or wild foods. Be sure to customize based on the outcomes of your 30-Day Food Vacation.

OPTIMAL FOOD CHOICES

Optimal Protein. Grass-fed, pastured, and wild animal sources have a better fatty acid profile and higher levels of vitamins and other micronutrients. Wild, cold-water, or small fish are less likely to be contaminated with mercury.

MEAT
✔ Beef
✔ Lamb
✔ Organ meats (e.g., heart, liver, and sweetbreads)
✔ Wild game (e.g., bison, venison, elk, and ostrich)

FISH AND SEAFOOD
✔ Anchovies
✔ Bass
✔ Catfish
✔ Clams
✔ Cod
✔ Sablefish (black cod)
✔ Halibut
✔ Herring
✔ Mussels

- ✔ Oysters
- ✔ Pollock
- ✔ Wild Alaskan, Coho, or sockeye salmon
- ✔ Pacific sardines
- ✔ Wild shrimp

POULTRY AND EGGS (MAKE SURE TO SELECT "PASTURED" POULTRY)

And if you are sensitive to grains, corn, and/or soy, you will need to do more research to find poultry and eggs that are not fed a supplemental "vegetarian diet" which is code for grains, corn and/or soy.

- ✔ Chicken
- ✔ Cornish game hen
- ✔ Duck
- ✔ Turkey
- ✔ Whole, pastured duck and chicken eggs

OPTIMAL VEGETABLES

Non-starchy, aboveground leafy greens are nutrient-dense and have the least negative impact on blood sugar.

- ✔ Arugula
- ✔ Asparagus
- ✔ Beet greens
- ✔ Bok choy
- ✔ Broad beans
- ✔ Broccoli
- ✔ Broccolini
- ✔ Brussels sprouts
- ✔ Cabbage
- ✔ Cassava
- ✔ Cauliflower
- ✔ Celery
- ✔ Cilantro
- ✔ Chicory
- ✔ Chives
- ✔ Collard greens
- ✔ Coriander
- ✔ Cucumber
- ✔ Dandelion greens
- ✔ Endive
- ✔ Escarole
- ✔ Fennel
- ✔ Garlic
- ✔ Ginger root
- ✔ Green beans
- ✔ Green onions (scallions)
- ✔ Hearts of palm
- ✔ Jicama
- ✔ Kale
- ✔ Kohlrabi
- ✔ Lettuces
- ✔ Mushrooms
- ✔ Mustard greens
- ✔ Onions
- ✔ Parsley
- ✔ Peppers
- ✔ Purslane

- ✔ Radicchio
- ✔ Radish
- ✔ Spinach
- ✔ Sprouts (alfalfa, bean, broccoli, clover, sunflower, etc.)
- ✔ Summer squash
- ✔ Swiss chard
- ✔ Tomatoes
- ✔ Turnip greens
- ✔ Watercress
- ✔ Rutabaga
- ✔ Seaweed
- ✔ Shallots
- ✔ Snap beans
- ✔ Snow peas
- ✔ Zucchini

OPTIMAL OILS AND FATS

Consuming healthy oils and fats can help ease inflammation, strengthen bones, improve lung, liver, and brain function, improve cardiovascular risk factors, modulate nervous system function, and strengthen immune system function. *Note: Rancidity is a huge concern with oils. Look at the harvest and bottling dates and make sure you are consuming the oil as close to those dates as possible.*

OILS

While high-heat cooking is inflammatory and should be minimized, some oils do better at high heat, and some should be

Organic Foods Are Nutritionally Superior

Organic produce has up to 60 percent more antioxidants—protection against autoimmune disease and cancer—and up to one hundred times lower pesticide residue than conventionally farmed produce.[19] Pasture-raised (100 percent grass-fed) animals roam and eat freely in their natural habitat and offer health benefits that conventionally raised, grain-fed animals do not, including less total fat, more good fats—omega-3 fatty acids and conjugated linoleic acid (CLA)—and more antioxidant vitamins like vitamin E and beta carotene. If you have access to a farmer's market or a local farm, get your produce, eggs, and meats there. And, for optimal freshness and nutrient density, plant a garden, even a pot of organic herbs in your kitchen window. For those super motivated to grow their own food in a limited space, consider a 4 Foot Farm: bit.ly/2HcdQuk.

avoided altogether. As a rule, saturated fats like grass-fed ghee, avocado and coconut oils have higher smoke points and less risk of harm at high heat, whereas polyunsaturated oils like olive, flax, and walnut oils should be avoided for high-heat cooking and should only be added after cooking for flavor. A healthy tip: always choose oils stored in glass bottles, as plastic can leach into oil.

Best oils for high-heat cooking (with smoke points in degrees Fahrenheit):

- ✔ Grass-fed ghee (clarified butter—OK for people sensitive to dairy) (450)
- ✔ Grass-fed butter (if you can tolerate cow dairy) (350)
- ✔ Lard or tallow from pastured animals (370)
- ✔ Coconut oil (350), organic, virgin, cold-pressed and unrefined
- ✔ Avocado oil (520), expeller-pressed and refined
- ✔ Macadamia oil (390)
- ✔ Hazelnut oil (430)

Use polyunsaturated oils *after cooking only*:

- ✔ Olive oil—cold-pressed, unfiltered extra virgin (EVOO); ideally California or US-estate bottled. Note that European countries can claim it's olive oil if it's only 51 percent olive oil.
- ✔ Walnut oil.
- ✔ Sesame oil.
- ✔ Red palm oil—virgin, unrefined (*not "palm kernel"*) oil. Note: Red palm oil should be consumed in moderation and not used as a staple oil due to its high carotene levels, which in excess has an antioxidant destabilizing effect.
- ✔ Pumpkin, flax, and hemp seed oils.
- ✔ MCT (medium chain triglycerides) oil—ideally C8 type. MCT oil is the optimal fuel for fat-burning efficiency and overall the best oil for the money. Note: While some say cooking with MCT oils (320) is fine, it's an expensive oil, and I prefer using it as a raw addition to coffee, tea, coconut yogurt, and smoothies.

FATS

- ✔ Grass-fed pastured meats (lard from 100 percent grass-fed animals may be used for cooking).

✔ Omega-3 fats from krill oil and small, fatty fish like anchovies and sardines.

✔ Organic, pastured egg yolks, raw or freshly and lightly cooked. Note: Don't cook yolks to hardness, which is an inflammatory state, and don't store in the refrigerator for extended periods. The black surface that forms on older hard-boiled egg yolks is from oxidized fats.

✔ Coconut butter (a.k.a. manna) is delicious and filling by the spoonful!

TREE NUTS AND SEEDS (ideally organic, soaked, and dehydrated or sprouted)

To ensure their survival, nuts and seeds contain toxic plant protectants like phytates and enzyme inhibitors, which are harmful for human digestion in raw form. Soak nuts and seeds for eight hours in filtered water with two tablespoons sea salt; rinse, and then thoroughly dry (twelve to twenty-four hours) in a single layer on the lowest possible setting in an oven at 115 degrees or in a dehydrator until crunchy.

✔ Nuts: pecans, almonds, walnuts, macadamia, and Brazil nuts (last two don't require soaking).

✔ Seeds: chia, flax, hemp, sesame, sunflower, and pumpkin. (If you can, find sprouted varieties of seeds for optimal digestion; home-soaked chia and flax seeds work best for egg replacers or smoothies since they become slimy when soaked.)

GUT-HEALING FOODS

Regular consumption of cultured foods introduces beneficial microbes into the digestive tract to aid digestion and detoxification, provide enzymes, vitamins, and minerals, and boost immunity. While kombucha, beer, and wine are fermented, they contain yeasts instead of bacteria and may adversely affect the microbiome. Further, kombucha and wine often contain too much sugar, so caution is advised.

✔ Fermented vegetables: sauerkraut (fermented cabbage), kimchi (Korean dish of fermented raw veggies usually including cabbage)

✔ Fermented dairy: unsweetened coconut or goat kefir or yogurt

    ✓ Nourishing animal foods: collagen, gelatin, meat broth (simmered a few hours), stock (simmered four to six hours) or bone broth (simmered eight to twenty-four+ hours)

OPTIMAL FRUITS

Opt for fruits with lowest impact on blood sugar.

    ✓ Avocados

    ✓ Olives

    ✓ Berries: all varieties, ensure organic to avoid pesticides

    ✓ Citrus: lemons and limes

    ✓ Coconut: flakes, meat, oil, and butter (a.k.a. manna)

OPTIMAL "MILKS"

Non-animal "milk" alternatives abound. Avoid soy and rice (rice may contain arsenic), and instead opt for organic coconut and other nut or seed milk products with minimal other ingredients and *no* added sugar.

    ✓ Coconut milk: organic, unsweetened and full-fat (see recipe on p. 298)

    ✓ Nut milk: unsweetened almond, hazelnut, macadamia, cashew, or other nut milk. (Consider homemade to avoid additives like carrageenan.)

    ✓ Seed milk: unsweetened hemp, pumpkin, or flax milk.

    ✓ Animal dairy: If you can tolerate animal milk, opt for organic, raw, full-fat cow (from A2 Jersey or Guernsey cows), goat, or sheep.

OPTIMAL HERBS, SPICES, AND SALT

Ounce per ounce, herbs and spices are some of the most potent anti-inflammatories. Use fresh when possible and use often and liberally:

    ✓ Allspice

    ✓ Apple pie spice mixture

    ✓ Basil

    ✓ Cayenne pepper (if you can tolerate nightshades)

    ✓ Cinnamon

    ✓ Cloves

- ✔ Coriander
- ✔ Cumin
- ✔ Curry
- ✔ Garlic
- ✔ Ginger
- ✔ Italian spice seasoning
- ✔ Marjoram
- ✔ Mint
- ✔ Nutmeg
- ✔ Oregano
- ✔ Parsley
- ✔ Pumpkin pie spice
- ✔ Rosemary
- ✔ Saffron
- ✔ Sage
- ✔ Tarragon
- ✔ Thyme
- ✔ Turmeric
- ✔ Vanilla

SALT:

Unrefined and minimally processed sea salt products offer higher trace mineral content than refined white table salt; but they may also include trace amounts of naturally occurring metals like lead, uranium, thorium, plutonium, and mercury. Best unrefined options include:

- ✔ Celtic gray
- ✔ Himalayan pink
- ✔ Real Salt from Utah salt beds

To avoid all trace minerals and metals, opt for *refined* (white) sea salt, which keeps the majority of magnesium that is naturally rich in ocean water.

OPTIMAL SWEETENERS:

Use only those sweeteners that do not raise blood sugar or insulin.

- ✔ Organic stevia. (You may need to experiment with different brands to find one you enjoy.)

✔ Lo han guo (also spelled luo han kuo or just lo han), a sugar made from monk fruit.

✔ Xylitol (a sugar alcohol made from birch wood). Avoid sugar alcohols made from corn. Head's up: some people experience tummy distress like gas or loose stools from sugar alcohols.

OPTIMAL BEVERAGES

✔ Drink antioxidant-rich, unsweetened beverages. If you prefer flavored waters, add lemon, cucumber, or a splash of unsweetened cranberry juice.

✔ Water: spring or filtered.

✔ Veggie juice: green veggies with *no fruits added.*

✔ Teas: organic green, white, black, and herbal.

✔ Coffee: organic. Note: To limit mold exposure, choose European coffees or consider Purity or Bulletproof brand coffees, which are tested for toxins and mold.

OPTIMAL DESSERTS

Chocolate is a health food for most people—as long as it's 70 percent or more cacao fat. If you did not react to chocolate during the reintroduction phase, enjoy dark chocolate or raw cacao, but avoid milk chocolate.

✔ Opt for more than 70 percent dark chocolate.

✔ Lily's brand makes a non-GMO 70 percent dark chocolate, stevia-sweetened bar.

OCCASIONAL FOODS

Higher-carbohydrate foods cause blood sugar to spike, leading to belly fat and risk of diabetes, dementia, autoimmune disorders, and cancer. Minimize or ideally eliminate these foods to optimize health.

OCCASIONAL PROTEIN

Pork: Make sure you choose Animal Welfare Approved, Humanely Raised, or USDA-certified organic labeling for all pork products. Choose traditionally prepared (i.e., marinated or uncured, nitrite and nitrate-free) bacon, ham, prosciutto, and sausages.

OCCASIONAL VEGETABLE CHOICES

Consider smaller portions of these higher-carbohydrate veggies to accompany leafy greens and nourishing fats:

- Artichokes
- Beets
- Carrots
- Eggplant
- Okra
- Parsnips
- Plantains
- Potatoes
- Sweet potatoes
- Taro
- Turnip
- Winter squash (butternut, pumpkin, spaghetti)
- Yams
- Yucca

OCCASIONAL FRUIT CHOICES

Moderately high glycemic index fruits may cause insulin surges, which can lead to fat storage and diabetes in sensitive people.

- Apples
- Apricots
- Cherries
- Grapefruit
- Kiwi
- Melons
- Nectarines
- Oranges
- Peaches
- Pears
- Plums
- Tangerines

HIGHER-GLYCEMIC FRUIT CHOICES

Eat only if you have no weight, blood sugar, or insulin issues:

- Bananas
- Dates

✔ Figs
✔ Grapes
✔ Mango
✔ Papaya
✔ Watermelon

Step 5: Supplement Strategically

The era of nutrient supplements to promote health and reduce illness is here to stay... There is overwhelming evidence of immunological enhancement following such an intervention.
—JOURNAL OF THE AMERICAN MEDICAL
ASSOCIATION (JAMA), 1997

Ideally, there would be no such thing as nutrient deficiencies; we'd get all we need from eating nourishing foods. Unfortunately, we live in the modern world where a combination of toxic environmental factors, like SAD foods, mineral-deficient topsoil, chronic stress, and excess toxins, deplete our vitamin and mineral levels. A recent study of sixteen thousand Americans by the National Center for Health Statistics found that 94 percent of Americans are deficient in vitamin D, 88 percent in vitamin E, and 52 percent in magnesium—all essential nutrients needed for health and chronic disease prevention.[20]

It is thought that chronic disease is due in large part to a combination of excess toxins and nutrient deficiencies. If you're dealing with an autoimmune disorder or want to prevent one, then you must address both sides of that equation: *minimize toxins and shore up nutrient deficiencies.* To restore balance, it's vital to both eat nourishing foods *and* take high-quality supplements, as needed. The idea is to build up and maintain your nutrient reserves to assist the healing process.

Functional Medicine has a catchy refrain: *test, don't guess!* When it comes to supplements, this is an area where it can pay to get the data. An integrative or holistic practitioner can order the right tests to check your nutrient levels and recommend specific supplements. Many practitioners offer a cash or "easy pay" price for Genova lab tests, which is often greatly reduced from the insurance or list price that you would pay by going direct. And practitioners are trained to interpret test results and guide you in choosing optimal supplements. Or, you can order your own tests online through companies like www.directlabs.com or www.mymedlab.com. Heads up on ordering your own labs: 1. It's usually costlier, since practitioners can negotiate better bulk pricing, and 2. interpreting results on your own can prove difficult. Two good options to ask your practitioner about or consider ordering for yourself include:

ION Profile by Genova Diagnostics. The ION Profile uses both blood and urine to measure over 125 key nutrient biomarkers and ratios that can help identify nutritional shortfalls that may be a root cause of complex chronic conditions. The ION Profile evaluates organic acids, fat-soluble vitamins, coenzyme Q10, homocysteine, oxidative stress markers, nutrient and toxic elements, fatty acids, and amino acids.

NutrEval by Genova Diagnostics. NutrEval is Genova's most comprehensive nutritional evaluation and is designed to assist with management of symptoms related to nutritional and digestive insufficiencies. This profile assesses numerous metabolic pathways and synthesizes this complex biochemistry into actionable treatment options. The nutritional profile includes: antioxidants, B vitamins, minerals, essential fatty acids (EFAs), digestive support, and even select genetic markers.

This is not an area to skimp on, nor is it an area that replaces nourishing food. Poor quality supplements may at best provide no benefit, and at worst, may harm you. Some people are sensitive to fillers, dyes, and additives like magnesium stearate, titanium dioxide, silicon dioxide, corn, or soy. You will pay more for high-quality supplements, so view supplementation as an essential investment in your long-term health.

GENERAL AUTOIMMUNE HEALING & PREVENTION SUPPLEMENTS

People with autoimmune conditions may be even *more* deficient in many key micronutrients. Generally recommended autoimmune supplements help to balance and strengthen the immune system, calm inflammation, promote a balanced microbiome, and support natural detoxification and energy production. I get it, though, it's easy for costs to add up fast with supplements. So, if you're only going to pick three, take a good multivitamin, vitamin D3 (with K2), and magnesium. You can get your probiotics from fermented foods like sauerkraut and kimchi and your prebiotics from a variety of vegetables. Two strategies I've found helpful are to "pulse" and to "rotate" supplements. Pulsing means to take for a time, and then take a break—like five days on, two days off, or one week off per month. Rotating has more to do with brands. Try one brand for one to three months, and then try another one for a while. The idea is to assist your body, not to create a crutch.

Always check with your physician or trusted health care provider before beginning a supplementation protocol, especially if you are pregnant or taking prescription medication.

- ✔ **Hypoallergenic multivitamin (with coenzymated B vitamins and minerals)** is like an insurance policy; it helps to fill gaps in your nutrition with a baseline of vitamins and minerals. A multivitamin is a good starting point, but most (with the exception of Empowerment Formula and Pure's Nutrient 950) do not include sufficient quantities of needed nutrients, so you may want to consider adding the other vitamins listed below. Make sure to find brands that are free of fillers and folic acid (oxidized synthetic compound). Good brands include Pure Encapsulations' Nutrient 950, Klaire Labs, Thorne, Designs for Health, and Empowerment Formula Essential Super Nutrient Complex.

    Dose: Follow directions on bottle and usually take twice a day, with food.

    Caution: Avoid multivitamins made with soy, corn, gluten, fillers, or folic acid.

- ✔ **Probiotics** (beneficial bacteria) help support a balanced microbiome by reducing overgrowth of gut pathogens, supporting nutrient absorption, and building immune function and tolerance. We'll explore more in the Gut chapter; in the meantime, consider taking a good quality broad-spectrum probiotic with several different strains of both *Lactobacillus* and *Bifidobacterium,* including *lactis, longum,* and *bifidum;* and *Lactobacillus acidophilus* (*L. acidophilus*), including the *plantarum* and DDS-1 strains. Top quality brands will cost more (figure fifty to sixty dollars for a thirty-day supply) but are professional grade without fillers or allergens: The Gut Insti-

tute's BIFIDO/MAXIMUS, Ortho Molecular Products' Ortho Bi-
otic 100, Transformation Enzymes' 42.5, and Custom Probiotics.
Excellent complements to regular probiotics to add or rotate include soil-based, spore-forming (*bacillus subtilis*) (e.g., Microbiome
Labs' MegaSporeBiotic), and yeast-based (*Saccharomyces boulardii*
or *S. boulardii*) organisms.

Dose: one to two capsules 50B CFU (colony forming units) per
day. Some work best away from food and others with meals. Follow directions on bottle.

Notes: It may take some time to discover which probiotic is best
for you. Have patience and experiment. Also, there is no rule on
rotating probiotics, but you
may benefit from introducing
different strains every few
months or even taking a few
brands at the same time, like a
broad-spectrum type plus a
soil- or yeast-based probiotic.
Many probiotics today are

KEY CONCEPT: *Probiotics
eat prebiotics. Said
another way, prebiotics
feed probiotics.*

shelf stable, meaning they don't require refrigeration. Steve Fowkes,
my biochemistry mentor, also points out that sometimes stomach
acidity kills off certain probiotic strains, making them less viable.
You can try to activate your favorite probiotic for a few hours in
one tablespoon of warm (body temperature) growth medium like
coconut milk or bone broth, then swallow it on an empty stomach,
followed by twelve to twenty ounces of body-temperature pure
water. The extreme dilution of the growing bugs can fake out the
protein-sensing systems of the stomach and allow the probiotic
quick passage into the intestine, for a dramatically higher probiotic
implantation.

Caution: In rare cases, probiotics may pose some risk for people with weakened immune systems, such as those infected with
the AIDS virus or for people undergoing chemotherapy. Some
people are sensitive to any yeast-based organism; if you are in this
camp, avoid *S. boulardii*, at least for now.

✔ **Prebiotics** (fiber that probiotics like to eat) feed your good gut bacteria. Examples of good prebiotic fibers include inulin (from

chicory root), acacia fiber, larch tree arabinogalactans, and fructooligosaccharides (FOS)—oligosaccharides that occur naturally in plants such as onion, chicory, garlic, asparagus, banana, artichoke, and soluble dietary fiber. Look for and rotate organic varieties. Some good brands include Klaire Labs' Biotagen (capsules), Heather's Tummy Fiber Organic Acacia Senegal (powder), Hyperbiotics Prebiotic (powder), and Pure Encapsulations Arabinogalactan (capsules).

Dose: Follow directions on bottle.

Note: Ramp up prebiotics slowly and back down if you get gas, pain, or bloating.

✔ **Vitamin D3** (25-hydroxyvitamin D3)—the "sunshine vitamin"—is actually a prohormone proven to increase your immune defenses in a major way. Vitamin D is commonly very low in people with autoimmune conditions, and low vitamin D is even predictive of some autoimmune conditions including MS, RA, and type 1 diabetes (read more about vitamin D in the Hormones chapter). You can get your level with a simple blood test. Optimal levels of vitamin D for preventing and reversing chronic disease appear to be between 70 and 100 ng/ml, with normal maintenance levels between 50 and 80 ng/ml. While it may be ideal to raise your D levels from twenty minutes of daily sun exposure, most of us do not get nearly enough sun—due to sunscreen and/or lack of sunshine—and need to supplement with D3. Vitamin D increases your need for vitamin K2, but they should be taken at separate times for best results.

Dose: To calculate daily needed vitamin D3 IUs, use a simple formula: If your current level is 30 ng/ml and you'd like to get it to 80 ng/ml, subtract your current level from your goal: 80 − 30 = 50. Multiply the difference by 100 to get your daily value, in this case 50 x 100 = 5,000 IU vitamin D3 per day. Take D3 in the morning with food and take K2 in the evening with food. It may take six months to a year to reach your goal. Remember to retest a few times a year to monitor your levels.

✔ **K2** (MK-7 form) works synergistically with D3 and helps to reduce and prevent inflammation in the body and move calcium into your bones. Even so, K2 and D3 can be taken on the same day but should not be taken at the same time.

Dose: 100–200 mcg per day with dinner (amounts correlate with 5,000 or 10,000 IU vitamin D3).

✔ **Omega-3 essential fatty acids (EFAs)** decrease inflammation, support brain health and cognitive function, and help protect against cancer, heart disease and Alzheimer's. Take supplemental omega-3 EFAs and eat more omega-3–rich fish like wild salmon, anchovies, and sardines. Look for a high-quality, refrigerated oil from wild salmon, anchovies, or krill that has been tested for metal and has been verified metal-free, like OmegaBrite, Nordic Naturals, Green Pasture, and Dr. Mercola.

Dose: 1,000–2,000 mg of EPA and DHA twice per day with food; plus 200 mg vitamin E as mixed tocopherols if fish oil supplement or multivitamin does not contain 200 mg vitamin E.

Note: To get to 2,000–4,000 mg total of combined EPA and DHA per day, you may need to take more than the recommended dose on the bottle.

Caution: All oils are at risk for rancidity (spoilage) due to oxidization. Purchase high-quality supplements and minimize their exposure to air, heat, and light. Keep refrigerated, ideally in glass containers, and toss if fish oils smell or taste fishy. Omega-3 fatty acids may increase the effects of blood-thinning medications.

Steve Fowkes cautions that while fish oils are highly anti-inflammatory and offer huge clinical benefits, they also pose a burden on the antioxidant defense system, which tends to be weak in people with autoimmune conditions. As you recover, you may want to halve your daily dose of omega-3s.

✔ **Glutathione (GSH)**, the body's most important antioxidant, helps to strengthen liver and immune function, neutralize free radicals, and bind to and excrete toxins out of cells. Unfortunately, glutathione production declines steadily after age forty as metabolic rate declines; if you have an autoimmune condition, you're probably even more deficient. Furthermore, half the population is genetically unable to produce sufficient quantities and would benefit from supplementing with glutathione directly. If you're in pretty good health, a good option to boost your own glutathione production is to take the glutathione precursor N-acetylcysteine (NAC). If you're dealing with health challenges and/or chronic stress, you are likely deficient in glutathione and may benefit even more by taking *liposomal* glutathione, a more bioavailable form than oral glutathione capsules. I personally take NAC and liposomal glutathione to maintain good health.

NAC dose: 200–600 mg twice a day on an empty stomach.

Note: If you have GI symptoms, reduce your dose.

Caution: Avoid NAC if you have a stomach ulcer or organ transplant; also, speak with your doctor if you are on antibiotics or undergoing cancer treatments.

Liposomal glutathione dose: 100 mg reduced glutathione as two pumps or one teaspoon twice per day on an empty stomach. Hold in the mouth for thirty seconds to initiate absorption in the capillaries under the tongue. Look for high-quality brands in glass bottles like Quicksilver Scientific or Designs for Health.

Note: Keep liposomal glutathione refrigerated and take along with vitamins C and E to keep glutathione at optimal levels.

✔ **Vitamin B complex** is a group of eight vitamins, including vitamin B1 (thiamin); vitamin B2 (riboflavin); vitamin B3 (niacin); vitamin B5 (pantothenic acid); vitamin B6 (pyridoxine); vitamin B7 (biotin); vitamin B9 (folate); and vitamin B12 (cobalamin). B vitamins are critical for energy production, the maintenance of your nervous system, detoxification, and healthy adrenal function. Deficiencies in B vitamins can cause fatigue, muscle weakness, anemia, heart issues, immune system problems, headaches, insomnia, irritability, other cognitive losses, and even birth defects. Many people—especially those suffering from autoimmune issues—have methylation issues too (an elaborate and essential process involved with gene expression) and require a methylated form of B vitamins. To determine whether or not you have methylation issues, consider ordering a basic genetic test from 23andMe and

> **KEY CONCEPT:** *Sufficient doses of high-quality supplements are extremely helpful in the healing equation.*

then uploading the raw data for interpretation to MTHFR Support, LiveWello, or Genetic Genie.

Since B12 is primarily obtained from animal protein, vegans and vegetarians may be especially deficient. Good brands include: Life Extension, Doctor's Best, Country Life, and Pure Encapsulations.

Dose: Typically, one to two capsules of enzymatically active complete B complex by early afternoon with food.

Note: B vitamins may cause mild stomach upset or flushing (niacin); both are temporary and may disappear as your body adjusts.

Caution: Consult your doctor before taking B complex if you have diabetes, liver disease, or pernicious anemia (vitamin B12 deficiency).

✔ **Magnesium** is a mineral that plays a role in more than three hundred different biochemical reactions in the body, including energy production, heart health, and nervous system and blood sugar regulation. It has been estimated that up to 70 percent of Americans are deficient, and it's been observed that magnesium deficiency creates inflammation, which promotes autoimmunity.[21, 22]

Dose: Start with about 400 mg magnesium (one capsule) with or without food, ideally at bedtime, and increase one capsule each day, up to 2,000 mg per day. Preferred types include malate, glycinate, ascorbate, and threonate. Natural Calm is a widely available magnesium citrate powder that contains organic stevia.

Note: All types of magnesium have laxative effects, which can be helpful for people who are constipated. To find your ideal dose, start with a low dose (one 400 mg capsule) and increase one capsule a day until you experience loosening of your stool, then reduce by one capsule.

Caution: Avoid the glutamate or aspartate forms of magnesium due to excitotoxicity risks. People with impaired kidney function or hyperparathyroidism, or those taking antibiotics or diabetes medications, should consult their doctor before taking magnesium. Magnesium citrate may decrease absorption of some antibiotics and will decrease thyroid hormone if taken at the same time.

✔ **Polyphenols** are naturally occurring, often-colorful antioxidants found in plant products like tea, coffee, grape skins, fruit peel, cacao, nuts, seeds, and plant leaves, stems, and bark. Polyphenols neutralize tissue-damaging free radicals and protect against oxidative damage (think cellular rust) caused by aging, chronic illness, and toxins. A good strategy is to rotate superstar polyphenols like green tea extract (ECGC), resveratrol (found in skin of red grapes), pycnogenol (pine bark), quercetin (found in many foods, including red onion), curcumin (turmeric root), and grape seed extract, and to take along with vitamin C (l-ascorbic acid or buffered forms).

Dose: Consider a low-dose blend of multiple polyphenols (organic or wildcrafted) or rotate high-dose individual polyphenols. Follow directions on bottles and take with food for best absorption.

✔ **Mitochondrial support.** Remember those tiny but mighty power plants in all of your cells? People with autoimmune conditions typically suffer from significant fatigue, in large part due to mitochondrial dysfunction. Consider taking a rotation of supplements proven to reduce fatigue and even restore mitochondrial function, including: acetyl-l-carnitine (ALCAR), alpha-lipoic acid (ALA), PQQ (polyquinoline quinone), CoQ10 (coenzyme Q10) and D-ribose. There is no harm in taking all of these at once, and in fact, there is often an even more beneficial, synergistic effect—like ALCAR plus ALA and PQQ plus CoQ10. If you're sensitive, you may prefer to add supplements one at a time to gauge any reactions. Give the supplements up to twelve weeks for optimal effects.

DOSES:

- **Alpha-lipoic acid (ALA):** 200 to 600 mg per day on an empty stomach. Consider taking the R-lipoic acid form, which is more bioavailable.

   Note: Rarely reported side effects in humans include skin rashes and gastrointestinal distress.

   Caution: ALA may lower levels of thyroid hormone T3 and increase levels of TSH. ALA may lower blood glucose levels, so insulin-dependent diabetics should consult their doctor before taking.

- **Acetyl-l-carnitine (ALCAR):** Take 500 mg twice a day for six weeks, then 500 mg per day for six weeks (and it can often simply be stopped after the first six weeks).

    Note: Rarely reported side effects with more than 2,000 mg per day include nausea or other gastrointestinal distress.

    Caution: ALCAR can inhibit the activity of thyroid hormones.

- **PQQ:** 20 to 40 mg per day with or without food.

    Note: No negative side effects have been reported, which means more research is needed.

- **Coenzyme Q10 (CoQ10):** Take 400 mg per day of ubiquinol form with food for six weeks, then 200 mg per day for six more weeks.

    Note: Rare but mild side effects can include headache, rash, gastrointestinal distress.

    Caution: CoQ10 might make blood-thinning drugs less effective.

- **D-Ribose:** 5 g three times per day for six weeks, then 5 g twice a day for six more weeks.

    Notes: D-ribose is usually made from corn, so look for a non-corn brand, like Life Extension. If you have dysbiosis, D-ribose may produce gas, in which case, lower dose or discontinue.

    Caution: D-ribose may lower blood glucose levels, so insulin-dependent diabetics should consult their doctor before taking.

Step 6: Create Healthy Food Habits *for Life*

Hopefully by now you have a better understanding of which foods may be harming you and which ones nourish you. The Paleo template minus your suspect foods is your optimal food plan, at least for the time being. Once you've eliminated your suspect foods for at least three months, your immune system will calm down and you'll have time to heal and seal your gut. Your optimal food plan is not a "diet"; it's a way of life. To integrate new healthy habits, it's helpful to have a few rules of thumb:

1. **Take a permanent vacation from SAD foods** and beverages.
2. **Use glass and stainless steel** for food and water storage—at home and on the road.
3. **Budget more for organic food,** which is a long-term investment in your health.
4. **Shop mostly at the periphery of grocery stores,** where you'll find fresh produce, meats, and fish.
5. **Cook at home** and get your kids and/or partner to help.
6. **For optimal blood sugar balance,** compose your plate with two-thirds mostly above-ground vegetables, one-third healthy protein, and liberal amounts of good fats.
7. **Frequent local farmer's markets** and consider joining a CSA (community-supported agriculture) for weekly deliveries of seasonal vegetables, meats, eggs, and raw dairy (if you can tolerate it).
8. **Select a rainbow of colorful produce**—in season, organic, and locally grown.

Consider Ketosis … with Cautions

If you're up on recent health and diet trends, chances are good that you've at least heard of the ketogenic (or just "keto") diet. While it may seem like the latest fad diet, it's actually the way we've been eating for the past 200,000 years—with the exception of the last one hundred years, thanks to the advent of modern agriculture. Our biology is built for feast and famine cycles, not for 24/7 feasting and snacking. Until recent history, we feasted when food was available, and we stored it as fat to draw down on for longer periods of famine.

Turns out that the keto diet, partnered with periodic fasting, enables us to mimic ancestral feast-famine cycles. By emphasizing healthy fats, moderating protein intake, and restricting carbs (roughly 70 percent fat, 25 percent protein, and 5 percent carbs), hunger is greatly reduced, calorie intake goes down, energy soars, brain function improves, inflammation is lowered, and insulin resistance can even be reversed.

Research shows that a ketogenic diet may be especially beneficial for people with neurological conditions including epilepsy or other seizure disorders, MS,

9. **Plant a garden**, even in pots or small containers on your kitchen window.

10. **Eat slowly and chew your food** thoroughly to optimize digestion.

11. **Replace white table salt** with high-mineral-content options like pink Himalayan or gray Celtic salt.

12. **Rotate foods and try new foods**, like organ meats, wild game, and homemade bone broth.

No matter your autoimmune status, it's never too late to change your food, begin to rehabilitate your cells for optimal wellness, and reclaim the vibrant good health that is your birthright. I know the prospect of a dietary overhaul is intimidating, but once you experience the beneficial effects, adapting to food and lifestyle changes only becomes easier.

While there is no guarantee that changing your food will reverse or prevent autoimmune conditions, I'm willing to bet that by making healthier choices you will tilt toward better health. And as you feel better, you'll have more energy to make even more wellness improvements, and that's a

Parkinson's, and Alzheimer's; for people with type 2 diabetes or insulin resistance; and for people who are overweight or obese. As with almost anything that sounds too good to be true, there are cautions. Thanks to The Paleo Mom, Sarah Ballantyne, Ph.D., for sharing these red flags: the ketogenic diet may disrupt liver, kidney, and thyroid function; it may mess with the balance of your microbiome; it can create hormonal imbalances; and it may increase cardiovascular risk factors and lower bone mineral density.

Bottom line, before diving into a high-fat, very low-carb, ketogenic diet, work with your trusted health care provider to determine whether or not you are a good keto candidate. You will want to closely monitor your blood sugar levels, kidney, liver, and thyroid function, and markers of inflammation to make sure you stay out of the harm zone. For many people, dipping in and out of ketosis periodically, like a few times per week or four times per year, may be ideal to derive the greatest benefits while avoiding the biggest pitfalls. Explore keto resources in Appendix F.

positive upward spiral. Starting is the hardest part, but just by reading this chapter, you've already begun! When you're ready, return to the Food chapter to work your way through each step in the Healing Foods Toolkit.

Summary: Top Five Healing Food Actions

1. **Eliminate SAD foods:** processed foods, sugar, grains, and dairy.
2. **Identify and eliminate your suspect foods** from a 30-Day Food Vacation and/or testing.
3. **Add in nourishing foods** and consider a Paleo-template diet.
4. **Supplement strategically** with a baseline supplement regime.
5. **Cook at home** to control food quality and cooking methods.

CHAPTER 2

Heal Your Gut

The gut is the seat of all health.
—Vincent Pedre, integrative MD and author of *Happy Gut*

More than 2,500 years ago, Hippocrates, now known as the father of modern medicine, wisely observed that "all disease begins in the gut." Today, we are finally catching up in our understanding of why the gut plays such a central role in both health and disease. And not a moment too soon. The past few hundred years have been hugely disruptive to our gut's natural function. As we'll uncover in the following pages, the collective effects of our modern diet, frequent use of antibiotics, and oversanitation may be the biggest contributors to the steep increase of autoimmune conditions. With this knowledge, we can take the reins of our health back in our own hands in large part by healing our guts.

Since the late nineteenth century, when Louis Pasteur popularized the "germ theory" as the cause of disease, Western medicine adopted the belief that microbes are a primary reason we get sick. Germ theory views microbes as evil perpetrators of disease and humans as passive targets at the mercy of the microbes. Long after Pasteur was reported to have recanted his support of germ theory on his deathbed—agreeing, instead, with physiologist Claude Bernard's claim that "the microbe is nothing; the terrain is everything"—Pasteur's original view about microbes is still entrenched as official advice and has us sanitizing everything and taking antibiotics at the first sign of a bug.

While antibiotics have had a profoundly beneficial impact on society, helping to wipe out many infectious (also known as *communicable* or *contagious*) diseases like malaria, rheumatic fever, and tuberculosis, it is only more recently understood that the collateral damage done by overuse of antibiotics may be one of the greatest threats to our health and well-being. As we have brought the scourge of infectious diseases under control, we are now facing an upsurge of autoimmune conditions.

Could it be that our overuse of antibiotics is contributing to the autoimmune epidemic? In the past ten years, scientists have made giant leaps forward in understanding the gut's role in health and disease. Emerging research reveals that the microbiome—the vast ecosystem of microbes in our gut—is a powerful ally and perhaps our greatest defense against autoimmune conditions.

Scientists have also discovered that the use of antibiotics often has an adverse effect on the microbiome, harming both beneficial and harmful bacteria alike. It gets worse when the damaged microbiome transforms our gut lining from a protective barrier into a broken fence, the latter potentially leading to autoimmune problems. Because it takes decades for doctors to put research into practice, it's critical that you understand how your gut governs your health and do what you can *today* to influence its optimal function.

Defining the "Gut"

You may be wondering, what is the "gut," anyway? The gut can sometimes be shorthand for your whole digestive system, but when people refer to the "gut" in terms of health and disease, they are usually referring to the *intestines*, both small and large. The large intestine is often called the *colon*.

Justin and Erica Sonnenburg, a husband and wife Ph.D. scientist team and coauthors of *The Good Gut*, offer a colorful description of the small intestine as a "flexible passageway, approximately twenty-two to twenty-three feet long, an inch in diameter, and piled like a plate of spaghetti in the middle of our body." You read that right. Over twenty feet long, the small intestine is anything but small. Stretched flat, the small intestine could cover a doubles tennis court! That's because it has some big jobs. Tucked into the lining of your small intestine are thousands of tiny finger-like projections called *villi* (pronounced VIL-eye) resembling shag carpeting. These villi increase the surface area for absorbing nutrients. And, it's the home of your immune system, which defends and protects you from unwanted invaders, most of which are things you eat and pass through your digestive system.

Bottom line: the lining of your small intestine is arguably the most important barrier between you and the outside world. Maintaining the integrity of this barrier, you'll soon see, is crucial for maintaining your health and well-being.

Conversely, your large intestine, also known as your *colon*, is only about five feet long. The large intestine earns its name thanks to its wide four-inch diameter. It also has a huge role in maintaining your health, as it hosts the largest microbiome in your body, a vast ecosystem of microbes made up of mostly beneficial bacteria, fungi, parasites, and bacteriophages—viruses that infect bacteria but are harmless to humans.

But There's Nothing Wrong with My Gut!

Wait a minute, you may protest. You don't have an inflammatory bowel disorder like irritable bowel syndrome (IBS), Crohn's disease, or colitis. You don't even have problems with your digestion. So why do you need to heal your gut? The short answer is that if you have mysterious or unwanted symptoms anywhere in your body, you also have gut issues, whether or not you can feel it in your gut. Turns out, Hippocrates was right: the primary reasons for which we seek out a specialist are actually downstream symptoms of issues that arise in the gut. If you have autoimmune issues and/or any number of the symptoms below, chances are highly likely that you have gut issues too:

- Allergies
- Alzheimer's
- Anxiety
- Arthritis
- Asthma
- Attention issues (ADD/ADHD)
- Autism
- Brain fog
- Cancer

- Celiac disease
- Chronic aches or pains
- Chronic fatigue
- Dementia
- Depression
- Food cravings (especially sugar and carbs)
- Food sensitivities
- Fungal infections
- Gastrointestinal (GI) issues (abdominal discomfort, bloating, constipation, diarrhea, gas, GERD [gastro-esophageal reflux disease], etc.)
- Headaches or migraines
- Insomnia
- Inflammatory bowel disease (IBD), colitis, Crohn's, or irritable bowel syndrome (IBS)
- Joint pain
- Lowered immunity (chronic colds, flu, or other infections)
- Memory problems
- Mood problems
- Mouth sores
- Sensory issues (numbness, tingling, tightness, etc.)
- Sinus conditions
- Skin conditions (acne, eczema, hives, jock itch, psoriasis, rosacea, unexplained rashes, etc.)
- Schizophrenia
- Weight loss resistance

It may take years of environmental assaults to the gut before our system finally breaks down, but given time, our health usually suffers wherever our genetic weakness lies. For me, that was MS; for others, the weak link might be Hashimoto's thyroiditis, lupus, heart disease, rheumatoid arthritis, cancer, or even Alzheimer's.

Why Didn't My Doctor Tell Me This?

The sad fact is that your doctor may not know the gut's significant role in your health. Scientific evidence connecting the gut with a wide range of chronic health issues is fairly recent and still emerging; and, medical text-books (and medical education) typically lag behind science by a few decades. If your physician went through traditional medical school, he or she learned to diagnose problems specific to a body part and offer medication that may provide short-term relief for that specific issue. Modern health care still divvies us up by body parts. For joint pain, you go to a rheumatologist, for issues with your brain or central nervous system, you see a neurologist, and for thyroid or other hormone problems, you go to an endocrinologist. If you have digestive problems, your doctor will refer you to a gastroenterologist.

A major problem with this siloed approach is that it doesn't match the reality of who we are: complex beings with interrelated and interdependent systems. The gut is deeply connected to other systems in the body, like a central networked hub that controls or influences much of your health and well-being. For example, about seventy-five percent of your immune system is located in the gut; and autoimmune conditions are immune system problems, not body part problems.

KEY CONCEPT: *If you have mysterious or unwanted symptoms anywhere in your body, chances are you also have gut issues, whether or not you can feel it.*

You may be worried, thinking about the food you've eaten or the stress that's impacted your life, but don't despair! Whether you've consumed SAD foods for decades, dealt with loads of stress, or taken more than a few courses of antibiotics, you have the power to address the bacterial composition and integrity of your gut; and that, in turn, will help shift your health back to balance and vibrancy.

In this chapter, we'll explore the many ways we damage our guts, how that can lead to autoimmune problems, and how we might take a page from ancestral cultures that have managed to avoid our modern autoimmune issues altogether. For inspiration and motivation, you'll read a story of a Functional Medicine doctor who, after dealing with breast cancer and an autoimmune diagnosis, returned to good health by healing her gut. Then, in the Gut Healing Toolkit, I'll guide you through time-tested steps to heal and seal your gut.

Some Important Facts About Your Gut

- Your gut, small and large intestines combined, is a thirty-foot inner tube. Only when nutrients are absorbed into your bloodstream do they move into your body.
- Your gut lining, called the *epithelial layer*, is only one cell thick—much thinner than your eyelid, and much more vulnerable.
- The gut—also known as the *enteric nervous system* (ENS)—is sometimes called the *second brain*, since it contains around one hundred million neurons, which often operate independently of the brain in your head.
- Approximately 90 percent to 95 percent of serotonin, the "feel-good" neurotransmitter and signaling mechanism, is produced in the gastrointestinal tract—and only 5 percent to 10 percent in your brain.
- About 75 percent of your immune cells reside in the gut, so the gut is truly the center of your immune system.
- Laid out flat, the surface area of a healthy gut measures about the size of a doubles tennis court—about three thousand square feet!
- Your gut houses your largest microbiome, an ecosystem of an estimated hundred trillion microbes—good, bad and neutral—normally composed of up to one thousand species and weighing up to five pounds.
- Merely twenty-three thousand genes make up the human genome, whereas the microbiome contains approximately *eight million* genes. Those microbial genes often fill functional gaps that your own DNA leaves open.
- There are roughly ten times more microscopic organisms in your gastrointestinal system than there are human cells in your whole body. From a numbers perspective, *you're more bacteria than human*!
- And, while human DNA remains unchangeable, it only represents 1 percent of total DNA. The other *99 percent of your DNA is microbial and modifiable.*

What's at the Root of Gut Problems?

Mounting research reveals causal connections between gut imbalances and chronic disease of many types, not just disorders of the gut or brain. Imbalances in gut flora and intestinal permeability have far-reaching consequences and have been implicated in virtually all autoimmune conditions as well as asthma, autism, anxiety, cancer, depression, diabetes, heart disease, HIV, non-alcoholic fatty liver disease, and obesity.[1]

For physicians willing to consider the research, these findings have been astonishing—and have naturally led to seeking increased understanding of what is creating these disease-producing imbalances in the hopes of addressing the root causes. World-renowned neurologist and *New York Times* bestselling author David Perlmutter, MD, shares the importance of this shift:

> I have to say that as a neurologist, we were taught to stay focused on the brain, because that's where we thought the "money" was. The reality is that the brain is highly influenced by the gut. And this has relevance for every neurodegenerative condition. So, we now understand the mechanism that's leading to Alzheimer's, Lou Gehrig's disease, multiple sclerosis, Parkinson's, autism, ADHD, etc. And in one word that is inflammation, which has its genesis in the gut. I would submit that all of the so-called treatments that I had been schooled in, and that neurologists still continue to pursue, are not looking at the fire. They're looking only at the smoke. Meaning they are squarely focused on dealing with symptoms that occur downstream because inflammation has done its dirty deed.

As Dr. Perlmutter notes, the invisible enemy present in almost every disease process is *inflammation*. That's a mysterious-sounding concept, but it's actually a normal function that happens in response to an injury, like when you cut your finger, scrape your shin, get bitten by an insect, or break a bone.

In a healthy person, inflammation acts as your immune system's short-term (acute), emergency response to the site of injury. You've seen inflammation in action when you hit your thumb with a hammer or get bitten by a mosquito: The area of injury warms, turns red, and swells. If there is an infection, the invading white blood cells may produce pus. These are sure signs that inflammation—your immune system's repair team—is hard at work. But when it becomes long-lasting (chronic), inflammation can turn into a big, body-wide problem.

Normally, with an acute injury, your emergency crew does its thing, attends to and resolves the injury. Inflammation subsides, and then healing happens. But with repeated or long-lasting injuries—like a steady diet of inflammatory foods (e.g., sugar, gluten, or pesticide-laden produce), regularly taking pain meds, a sustained course of antibiotics, being stressed out much of the time, not getting enough sleep, or getting too much or not enough exercise—your immune system gets overwhelmed and repair processes slow or shut down. That's when inflammation moves from being a localized, short-term benefit to a systemic (body-wide) and long-term problem. Unlike the red and throbbing stubbed toe, you can't see or feel systemic inflammation until symptoms surface. Even then, it's hard to tell that your aching knee, brain fog, or even extra weight has anything to do with inflammation—let alone your gut.

> **KEY CONCEPT:** *Chronic inflammation defers healing. Put simply, when you're inflamed, you don't heal.*

Chronic inflammation happens when sources of inflammation are continuously or frequently present. And where in the body is ground zero for widespread inflammation? You guessed it. *The gut!*

What Creates Inflammation?

The inflammation that harms your gut may be caused by many environmental factors, not just SAD foods. Sometimes these factors cause issues in isolation, but often inflammation is a result of a combination of triggers. For me, the inflammatory combo was a SAD diet that centered on gluten and sugar, plus high levels of mercury and chronic stress. For other people it could be some combination of dairy reactivity, an especially serious case of infectious mononucleosis, and/or living in a house contaminated by black mold. Even childhood trauma can trigger inflammation and set the stage for autoimmune disorders decades later. And let's not forget medical treatments, like antibiotics for infections or mercury-amalgam fillings for cavities. Consider this partial but long list of inflammatory root causes:

- Acute or chronic stress
- Antibiotics, antacids, and prescription medications
- Birth control pills
- Chemotherapy and radiation
- Concussion
- Excessive alcohol or caffeine consumption
- Excessive electromagnetic frequencies (EMFs)
- GMO (genetically modified organism) foods
- Heavy metals
- Infections
- Oxidative stress (poor antioxidant defenses, low cellular energy, intracellular damage)
- Pain relievers
- Poor sleep
- Smoking
- Soda (both regular and diet)
- SAD foods: sugar, artificial sweeteners, gluten, dairy, grains, processed oils
- Toxins: pesticides, herbicides (glyphosate), bacterial byproducts (endotoxins), fungal toxins (mycotoxins)
- Unresolved emotional trauma

To understand how these inflammatory factors harm the gut, we have to peek under the hood at the two elements in your gut that play leading and interconnected roles in keeping you healthy or making you sick: your microbiome and the lining of your gut.

The Mighty Microbiome

Microbes have been present on Earth for more than 3.5 billion years and humans only about two hundred thousand. And consider that there are more microbes currently living on your hand than there are people on the planet! But even though these little guys are invisible to the human eye, they are highly evolved, and scientists are just beginning to understand them and their multiple, critical roles.

Humans have at least eight microbiomes in us and on us. Smaller microbiomes are found on skin and in damp, dark places like the mouth, ears, nose, lungs, belly button, and genitals. Our largest microbiome is housed in our large intestine (the colon). That's the one we'll focus on here.

Passed from mother to baby at birth and during breastfeeding, and from the environment to the child who plays in the dirt, the microbiome is actively cultivated by our biology for our benefit. In a healthy person, the microbiome is comprised of wide diversity, maybe one thousand different species of bacteria, each of which can have multiple strains.

Alessio Fasano, MD, renowned pediatric gastroenterologist and research scientist, has said that a healthy microbiome is like a big, diverse neighborhood where people of many races and nationalities get along, or at least coexist. Trouble starts when one race or nationality dominates and basically rules the roost to the detriment of others, who get marginalized or squeezed out of the neighborhood entirely.

We'll explore more about what can go wrong when the microbiome becomes imbalanced, but first, let's look at a well-functioning microbiome. When there is harmony in your microbial ecosystem, it helps you function in a mutually beneficial or symbiotic way. You house and feed the microbes, and in return, they fulfill a long list of important functions that you often couldn't do on your own, including:

- Influencing the immune system response, helping to distinguish friend from foe
- Modulating inflammation, helping the gut lining to heal
- Supporting digestion, helping to assimilate nutrients
- Making neurotransmitters and vitamins
- Regulating hormones
- Helping to eliminate toxins
- Controlling appetite and metabolism
- Influencing mood
- Regulating gene expression

It turns out that these microscopic companions play another critical role when it comes to health or disease: *they help maintain the integrity of the lining of the gut,* which you'll see is the gateway to good health or the down-ward spiral toward autoimmune conditions.

The Battlefront of Health or Autoimmune Disorders

We already know that about 75 percent of our immune system is located in the gut. More specifically, the majority of your immune system cells live in the *lining* of your gut, and there's good reason for that. The long, hollow tube that is your digestive system may be inside you, but it's also intelligently and selectively sealed off from you. Its protective barrier ensures unwanted pathogens—bad bugs, toxins, and waste—don't get into the general circulation of your bloodstream. Having immune cells right in the gut lining gives them a front-row position to monitor and decide which incoming molecules are potential threats and must be destroyed, and which are good guys, like the broken-down nutrients from digested food, which can be safely absorbed and used to promote health and well-being.

In an interview, Dr. Fasano spoke to the significance of the location of the immune system: "It seems to me that evolution has dictated that this is precisely where the battle between health and disease begins in humans and why our immune system is set up ready on that battlefront."

What's crazy to me is that this battlefront between health and disease is only *one cell thick*! To visualize it, imagine the single-cell barrier as a brick wall where each brick represents a cell. Where the cells touch each other, there are tight junctions where the mortar would be. These tight junctions are not hard and static like mortar or grout. They are dynamic gatekeepers, opening and closing by the adjacent cellular responses to your environment: food, drugs, toxins, or even stress. When the tight junctions are working properly, they're like effective security gates: good guys are allowed in; bad guys get stopped. Homeostasis, or harmony, is maintained as long as the intercellular gates are working properly.

But what happens if the gates get stuck open? That's the bazillion-dollar question, because this is precisely how and where autoimmune conditions begin. We learned a little about what it means to have a leaky gut in the Food chapter, but let's take a closer look and examine this problem in relation to inflammation. When those tight junctions become damaged or inflamed, it's like you've broken the remote control to the gate and now anyone can enter. When the gates are damaged and stuck in "open sesame"

mode, the gut becomes porous or leaky, and large, undigested food particles, microbes, toxins, and digestive waste slip past the guards and float
freely in your body where they're not supposed to be. Technically, this state
is called *intestinal hyperpermeability*, but most people call it "leaky gut syndrome" or just "leaky gut" for short.

When something leaks through that shouldn't, it causes the immune
system to react. The immune system's first line of defense is inflammation,
which defers the natural healing of
the gut lining in favor of killing the
invader. This is quite necessary
when the invader is a harmful bacterium, but not so much if the
invader is a gluten protein fragment
from your sandwich. The resulting
rise of inflammation at the gut lining impairs gut healing, which
increases the leaking, which increases the inflammation—and on

KEY CONCEPT: *SAD foods,
food sensitivities, chronic
stress, infections, and
toxins are inflammatory
and can keep your gut
flora imbalanced and
gut lining leaky.*

and on in a vicious cycle. After months or years of such 24/7 inflammation,
the leaky gut deteriorates to the point that the immune system starts to
overreact, cross-react, and misreact.

As the lining of your gut breaks down, so does the balance of microorganisms that line your digestive tract. The bacterial composition can shift
from being predominantly symbiotic (mutually beneficial) and health-
promoting to being predominantly destructive with overgrowth of certain
types of bacteria, yeast, and even parasites that can further break down
your digestive tract lining and continuously weaken your immune system.
Imbalance in the bacterial composition is called *dysbiosis*, from ancient
Greek, meaning "bad way of life," which is the opposite of *symbiosis*, meaning "living together."

Poor Gut Health and the Autoimmune Connection

Once food particles or toxins enter the bloodstream, the immune system
mobilizes by creating reactive antibodies (bullets) to kill off the antigens
(potentially harmful invaders). In a healthy response, the antibodies do

their job, neutralizing the threats, and then the immune system relaxes. And, given that cells of the gut lining normally repair themselves every three days in an optimal environment, the gut barrier is restored to its protective function pretty fast. But with repeated exposure to inflammatory elements, like SAD foods or ongoing stress, etc., the immune system's repair processes may get delayed, become inefficient, lose ground, and eventually become overwhelmed.

KEY CONCEPT: *Gluten looks like your own tissue at a molecular level.*

For someone susceptible to autoimmune conditions, when the invaders are destroyed, the immune system stays revved up, and excess antibodies continue scouting like soldiers eager for another fight. A domino effect of downstream problems ensues, including increased food sensitivities and, as inflammation builds over time, the advent of autoimmune conditions.

We already considered how the similar structure of thyroid cells and circulating gluten molecules can confuse your immune system and leave you vulnerable to Hashimoto's thyroiditis, depending on your genetic predisposition. Likewise, if you have the genetic propensity for MS, the antibodies will attack the myelin sheath, and in rheumatoid arthritis (RA), the joints, and so on. This mistaken identity is known as *molecular mimicry*, a primary way the immune system initiates and perpetuates the autoimmune attack.

Emerging science is demonstrating compelling links between declining gut health—dysbiosis and/or leaky gut—and the advent of autoimmune disorders:

- Increased intestinal permeability has been observed in the development of type 1 diabetes.[2]
- Women with lupus, an autoimmune condition that affects women nine times more often than men, may have higher levels of disease-causing *Lachnospiraceae* (a type of *Clostridia*) and lower health-promoting *Lactobacillus* than a healthy population.[3]
- Researchers have found that people with MS have dysbiosis, including significant changes in the abundance of species, namely a reduction of anti-inflammatory *Bacteroidetes* and *Clostridia* species, compared to healthy individuals.[4]

- Compared to a healthy control group, people with Alzheimer's had much higher levels of bacterial waste—both lipopolysaccharides (LPS) and an *E. coli* protein—which is indicative of a leaky gut.[5]

Before we jump straight to solutions in the Gut Healing Toolkit, it helps to have a bird's eye view of how the autoimmune problem may be directly related to modern life.

What in the World Is Going Wrong?

On a macro level, we know autoimmune conditions are escalating at an un-precedented rate, particularly within "civilized" Western countries, and scientists are trying to figure out why. One of the leading hypotheses is that our microbiomes have been altered in dramatic and often devastating ways since the modern era, after World War II, with the advent of processed foods and mass use of antibiotics.

The Sonnenburgs, who wrote *The Good Gut*, are studying changes in the microbiome over time to understand the connection between gut health and chronic disease. What they have found so far is shocking: the

---

The Downside of Low-Fiber Diets

- Traditional hunter-gatherer cultures eat approximately 100 to 150 grams of fiber per day.
- The USRDA recommends Americans eat thirty-five grams of fiber per day.
- The average American actually eats only ten to fifteen grams of fiber per day.

Guess what happens when you don't eat enough fiber? *Your gut microbes start eating you!* More specifically, they resort to eating the mucus layer of your gut lining. And as they gnaw though the mucus layer, your immune system triggers an inflammatory response because the gut lining is under attack.

total volume and composition of modern-day microbiomes compared to hunter-gatherer microbiomes are drastically shrinking, and in subsequent generations, may even become extinct. To visualize the difference, imagine our ancestral microbiome as a lush rain forest teeming with a wide variety of plants and wildlife; now imagine the typical Western microbiome as a cleared field with sparse crops and few animals.

The big reason for this deforestation of our microbiomes appears to be the modern quest for convenience and cleanliness. The SAD or Western diet has stripped the fiber from our food; our impatience to wait out the course of a common cold has us demanding antibiotics from our doctors; the rise in caesarean sections (C-sections) has deprived more newborns of the vitally important flora from their mothers' birth canals; and finally, in our quest for cleanliness, we have become super quick to sanitize ourselves, washing and wiping away microbes, 99 percent of which are harmless and may even be helpful.

The implications of this loss of microbial diversity and numbers is catastrophic for our health and well-being.

Harmed Gut Leads to Crohn's: Jill Carnahan's Story

What follows is a story that illustrates the connection between missing microbes and the advent of autoimmune conditions. While elements of modern life may wreak havoc on our microbiomes, it's enormously hopeful to know that you can often course-correct, in large part by healing your gut.

Jill Carnahan, MD, is a Functional Medicine doctor who today has a thriving practice in Boulder, Colorado. But fifteen years ago, her life was anything but thriving. At twenty-five, when Jill was newly married and enjoying the intensity of her third year of medical school, the unthinkable happened: she found a lump in her breast that turned out to be carcinoma, an invasive form of breast cancer. Jill did what most people would do and followed the standard treatment: several surgeries and multiple rounds of chemo and radiation.

Jill went into remission and was eager to move on with her life, but the treatment left her sick, weak, and underweight. Her gut was "just not right" anymore, and she endured months of loose stools, bleeding, and pain. Finally, she saw a gastroenterologist who diagnosed her with Crohn's disease, an autoimmune disorder of the lower part of the gut. The gastroenterologist presented a grim diagnosis. Jill was told her Crohn's was incurable; for the rest of her life, she would need to be on medication: specifically, steroids and powerful immune-suppressing drugs.

Jill instinctively knew that food would help her heal, but when she asked what type of diet she should try, the doctor said, "Diet has nothing to do with this." Jill decided then and there to take her health into her own hands.

She soon stumbled upon the book *Breaking the Vicious Cycle: Intestinal Health Through Diet* by Elaine Gottschall, a biologist who had been a mother on a mission to find a cure for her daughter's severe ulcerative colitis (UC), an inflammatory bowel autoimmune condition. Gottschall's daughter was treated by Sidney V. Haas, MD, whose Specific Carbohydrate Diet (SCD) requires the elimination of grains, starches, dairy, and sugar—simple carbohydrates that feed bad gut bacteria. After following the diet, Gottschall's daughter was completely symptom-free in just two years.

Inspired by Gottschall's story, Jill, too, embarked on the Specific Carbohydrate Diet. Within two weeks, her gut pain and inflammation calmed down enough to relieve her Crohn's symptoms. After five years of following this food plan, Jill considered herself cured of both breast cancer and Crohn's; but it would take another ten years for her to completely rehabilitate her gut and recover from the toxic chemo drugs.

Looking back, Jill is sure that the chemo altered her gut microbiome, creating a prime setup for the Crohn's. Studies confirm that beneficial microbes are missing and pathological ones flourishing in patients who develop Crohn's disease. The greater the pathological organisms, the more severe the symptoms. Studies also show that, as with pesticides, chemotherapy agents disrupt the normal balance of the microbiome and create a leaky gut.[6, 7]

While you might not be dealing with a situation quite as dire as a cancer diagnosis and chemotherapy, even *stress* can be problematic. While it may be easier to imagine the connection between toxic chemicals and a messed-up microbiome, research shows that ongoing or traumatic stress can have a similar toxic effect on your gut.

I bet you've seen the connection between stress and your immune system from experiences in your own life. After a rough few weeks at work or dealing with a sick child, you're more susceptible to a cold. Similarly, albeit with more dire consequences, stressful or shocking events often precede the advent of autoimmune conditions and flare-ups. But scientists have only recently learned the mechanisms. The evidence is in: There are definite connections between stress, dysbiosis, and leaky gut. Scientists have demonstrated that stressful events can affect changes in composition, diversity, and number of gut microorganisms, leading to greater numbers of potentially harmful bacteria. One study shows that psychological stress can cause a decrease in protective species, while other studies have found that short-term psychological stress, like anticipating an electric shock or being nervous about public speaking, increases small intestinal permeability.[8, 9, 10]

Wherever You Are, There Is Hope

No matter where you are on your healing journey—newly diagnosed, a veteran on the healing path, or simply wanting to stay healthy—it's never too late to nurture your gut health. No matter how high the deck seems to be stacked against you from years of SAD foods, multiple courses of antibiotics, or a lifetime of stress, there are new levels of healing you can reach when you tend to your microbial garden and work to seal your gut lining.

Like Jill, if you've already undergone a microbiome-destroying procedure, such as chemotherapy, or even a few courses of antibiotics, you must double your efforts to rebuild a balanced microbiome. And, if you've faced a lifetime of chronic stress, like me and many others with autoimmune conditions, it's vitally important that you prioritize gut healing.

The action plan that follows is the result of personal experience, research, and guidance from multiple autoimmune experts who, like Jill, have healed themselves from autoimmune disorders.

Gut Healing Toolkit

Integrative gastroenterologist and author of *The Microbiome Solution*, Robynne Chutkan, MD, offers a catchy yet powerful mantra to guide us back to health: "Live dirty, eat clean." Bottom line, we need to remove things that harm the gut and add in things that nourish it. In the Food chapter, we learned which foods are toxic and which are nourishing, and how to figure out which foods are right for you. In the coming pages, I'll share the best ways to learn more about your gut's needs, how to introduce more good bacteria into your microbiome, and how to maintain balance once you've achieved optimal gut health.

It's important to have realistic expectations on how long it might take to heal your gut. It can take anywhere from a month to six months or even longer, depending on multiple factors like how many courses of antibiotics you've taken, how much inflammation is present, whether or not you have gut infections, and how disciplined you are in removing ongoing sources of inflammation. To optimize your gut health, follow four steps and consider the extra step if appropriate for you:

Step 1: Take a gut health self-assessment.
Step 2: Get the data.
Step 3: Follow the 5R Gut Restoration Program.
Step 4: Live dirtier.
Extra Step: Consider "big guns" in gut healing.

Step 1: Take a Gut Health Self-Assessment

Consider the following statements. If you don't know an answer, just skip it. Rate your responses as 0 or 1, where 0 means "no" or "never" and 1 means "yes" or at least "sometimes":

0 1 My mother was given antibiotics while pregnant with me.
0 1 I was born by C-section.
0 1 I was bottle-fed as an infant.
0 1 I had numerous ear, nose, and/or throat infections for which I was given multiple courses of antibiotics.

0 1 I frequently use hand sanitizers.

0 1 I have food allergies or sensitivities.

0 1 My skin itches after I eat certain foods.

0 1 I am overweight (ten or more pounds).

0 1 I have blood sugar imbalances: insulin resistance or type 2 diabetes.

0 1 I crave sweets or processed carbs.

0 1 I've taken steroids, acid blockers, or nonsteroidal anti-inflammatory pain meds for longer than a week.

0 1 I am on or have been on the birth control pill.

0 1 I have ongoing gastrointestinal issues: constipation, diarrhea, nausea, abdominal pain, acid reflux, or GERD.

0 1 I suffer from an inflammatory bowel disease: ulcerative colitis (UC) or Crohn's disease.

0 1 I have irritable bowel syndrome (IBS).

0 1 I often feel bloated, gassy, cramping, pain, or general tummy distress after eating.

0 1 I've been diagnosed with an autoimmune condition.

0 1 I suffer from mood disorders: anxiety or depression.

0 1 I have brain fog, headaches, migraines, or memory issues.

Please list any other relevant signs or symptom(s):

1 _____

1 _____

Tally up your score: _____

GUT ASSESSMENT KEY:

0 Fantastic! You may be among the very few with a super healthy gut. Keep up the great work!

1–4 Not bad! You may have mild gut issues or autoimmune symptoms. Now's a great time to get ahead of health issues by tending to your gut.

5–9 Gut health is clearly a priority for you. Take heart in knowing you're not alone. Many people have healed in part or fully from many chronic illnesses by prioritizing gut healing!

10+ Okay, so your gut may need extra loving care. Consider taking the Extra Step on page 107 and have patience with the process.

Step 2: Get the Data

If you have an autoimmune condition or suspect you may, there is a very good chance you have an imbalance of gut bacteria (dysbiosis) and a leaky gut. It can be useful to get a baseline on your gut status so you can measure healing progress over time; and it can be important to learn which, if any, pathogens—like yeast, parasites, or other infections—are present so you can take the right action. This is a complicated arena, so I encourage you to work with a functional, integrative, or naturopathic doctor who has experience treating people with autoimmune conditions and who can help you order the best tests for your needs, interpret results, and guide you back to health.

Three favorite comprehensive stool tests are Genova Diagnostics' (GDX) GI Effects comprehensive stool profile; Doctor's Data's (DD) Comprehensive Stool Analysis; and Viome's RNA sequencing, which provides identification and quantification of *all* living microorganisms in your gut down to the species and strain level. Prices for comprehensive stool kits can range from $289 to $653, based on number of samples required.

If you'd rather go it alone, there are several direct-to-consumer options that will ship you test kits, analyze your results, and provide the results to you directly, while guaranteeing privacy:

- www.mymedlab.com
- www.directlabs.com
- www.mylabsforlife.com
- www.viome.com

You can also test for a leaky gut. Two of the more advanced tests available today are Vibrant Wellness's Wheat Zoomer and Cyrex Laboratories' Intestinal Antigenic Permeability Screen, also known as Cyrex Array 2. To order either test, you must go through a practitioner who has an account set up with the lab. Note that insurance is not likely to cover these tests. Cost: about $295.

Step 3: Follow the 5R Gut Restoration Program

The 5R program is a foundational gut-healing plan created by the Institute for Functional Medicine to help you restore gut balance and function.

Small Intestinal Bacterial Overgrowth (SIBO)

If you have symptoms like abdominal pain, nausea, gas, diarrhea, acid reflux, and GERD, you may have small intestinal bacterial overgrowth, or SIBO (SEE-bow). SIBO is not a pathogen per se, but rather an overgrowth of normal bacteria normally found in your large intestine that have migrated upstream into your small intestine, where they don't belong. Once in the small intestine, these bacteria feed off the carbohydrates you eat, proliferate, and ferment methane and hydrogen gases, leading to intestinal distress. A functional, integrative, or naturopathic practitioner will be able to assist you in diagnosing and treating SIBO.

Whether you choose to get tested or not, you can get started on the next step, 5R Gut Restoration, right away.

Many who follow it experience dramatic improvements in symptoms, and sometimes, complete resolution, as I did.

1. **Remove** the "bad stuff." The first step is to identify and remove the things that are harming your gut. That means eliminating the inflammatory foods we discussed in chapter 1, minimizing use of medications (if possible and under medical guidance), clearing any gut infections that may be present, and reducing stress. Use this list to take inventory on what to remove and for healthy swaps or strategies:

   - **SAD foods:** Processed foods and chemicals prevalent in the Western diet have been shown to harm the microbiome and cause leaky gut. Additionally, remove any suspect foods you have identified from the 30-Day Food Vacation (page 36).

     Heathy swap: Follow a Paleo-template food plan (page 49) emphasizing a variety of vegetables, moderate amounts of organic or wild sources of protein, and ample nourishing fats, like olive or coconut oil, olives, nuts and seeds (if you don't react), and avocado.

   - **Medications:** Bottom line, medications—whether prescription or over-the-counter—often harm the gut and are, ironically, a top trigger for autoimmune conditions. Non-steroidal anti-inflammatories (NSAIDs) like ibuprofen, naproxen, and acetaminophen have been shown to damage the gut lining in both short-term and long-term use.

Healthy swaps: Curcumin, a spice from the turmeric root, has been shown to be as effective in reducing pain and inflammation-related symptoms as NSAIDs. The recommended dosage of turmeric powder is 400 to 600 mg capsules three times per day. *Boswellia serrata* resin (Frankincense) is another powerful anti-inflammatory. Recommended dosage is 300 to 500 mg two or three times per day of an extract standardized to contain 30 percent to 40 percent Boswellic acids. One study demonstrated that a combination of Boswellia and curcumin showed superior efficacy and tolerability compared with diclofenac, an NSAID used for treating pain, arthritis, and migraines.[11]

- **Antibiotics:** Antibiotics are a major microbiome disrupter, so proceed with great caution, and if you must take a round of antibiotics, supplement with high doses of probiotics (see Step 3 below). The more you use antibiotics, the greater the damage to your microbiome, and the greater your risk of developing antibiotic resistance, which may leave you unprotected in the event of a major infection.

  KEY CONCEPT: *Save your use of antibiotics for extreme or potentially life-threatening infections.*

  Healthy swap: Herbal antimicrobials have been shown to be as effective as some antibiotics—without the gut-harming effects. Consider natural antibiotics like silver, oil of oregano, or monolaurin, which is derived from coconuts. (See Infection-Clearing Toolkit on page 125 for details.)[12]

- **Antacids:** Prolonged use of proton pump inhibitors (PPIs), one of the most commonly prescribed antacid medications in the United States, reduces microbial diversity, setting the stage for a potentially deadly *Clostridium difficile* infection (CDI).[13]

Healthy swap: Did you know that most "acid tummy" is actually an indication of *too little* stomach acid rather than too much? You'll want to work with your doctor to wean off acid blockers; and you may want to experiment with taking a little apple cider vinegar or digestive bitters before meals and/or hydrochloric acid (HCl) with pepsin when consuming protein-rich meals. (Read on for more information about HCl.)

- **Gut infections:** One of the main causes of widespread inflammation is low-grade bacterial, viral, and fungal infections in the gut.

  Healthy strategy: Work with a healthcare practitioner who, through comprehensive stool testing, can help you identify and clear up these underlying problems with herbal antimicrobials, antifungals, and other nontoxic treatments.

- **Excess stress:** Both acute and chronic stress are linked with gut dysbiosis and leaky gut, promoting increased levels of inflammatory chemicals, including IL-6 and lipopolysaccharides (LPS).[14]

  Healthy strategy: Do what you can to eliminate or minimize sources of stress in your life and read the Emotional Well-Being Toolkit (page 198) for stress-reducing strategies.

Which gut-harming elements can you remove or minimize, and what swaps and healthy strategies will you try?

2. **Replace** digestive secretions. The second step in the 5R program is to replace, or replenish, digestive juices that may be compromised by diet, medications, stress, dysbiosis, and even aging.

   ✔ **Digestive enzymes:** If you suffer from gas, bloating, minor abdominal pain, nausea, heartburn, SIBO, and/or occasional constipation, your enzyme production may be low. Consider taking digestive enzymes to help you break down food while your gut heals. Look for brands that include enzymes that address all of the macronutrients: protease (breaks down protein), amylase (breaks down carbohydrates), and lipase (breaks down fats).

   Dose: Take one or two digestive enzymes with meals.

Caution: If you have pineapple (bromelain) or papaya (papain) allergies, you should avoid enzymes with those ingredients.

✔ **Hydrochloric acid (HCL or HCl):** If you have trouble digesting meat or fat, or have bloating, gas, indigestion, food sensitivities, acid reflux, or heartburn, you may need *more* stomach acid, not less. Many people over the age of thirty lack sufficient stomach acid, which is a condition called hypochlorhydria, estimated to affect half the population.

Dose: Start with one 650 mg HCL with pepsin capsule at the beginning of a meal, and if you don't experience any GI discomfort like warmth or burning, you may need *more* HCL. Ramp up the number of capsules per meal until you feel the slightest discomfort/warmth, and then back off one capsule. Some people require 5,000 mg HCL with pepsin per meal. Over time, as your gut heals, you may be able to reduce and then go off HCL.

Caution: Do not use HCL if you are taking corticosteroids (e.g., prednisone), aspirin, or NSAIDs. In combination with HCL, these drugs can further damage the gut lining, increasing the risk of gastric bleeding or ulcers.

✔ **Bile Acids:** Your gallbladder stores bile produced by your liver and releases it into the digestive tract as needed to emulsify (make digestible) the fat you consume. If you have poor bile production or sluggish bile flow, you may become deficient in fat-soluble vitamins and essential fatty acids, and you may develop poor cholesterol metabolism and even weight problems. Signs that you may have a sluggish gallbladder include: bloating, burping, or reflux after eating; stomach cramps after eating or pain in your right upper abdomen; inflammatory bowel disease (IBD); a history of gallstones or gallbladder surgery/removal; or taking cholesterol-lowering meds.

Dose: Try one 100 to 500 mg ox bile capsule before meals.

Note: If you don't have a gallbladder, bile acids are essential to help you digest fats.

3. **Reinoculate** your gut garden. The third step is to "seed" and then "feed" your microbiome with beneficial gut bacteria to restore balance, abundance, and diversity of species.

"SEED" WITH PROBIOTICS: FOOD AND SUPPLEMENTS

Probiotics, which literally mean "for life," are the seeds of new, beneficial bacteria, and include two primary species: *Bifidobacteria* and *Lactobacillus*. Probiotics from fermented foods and supplements are not likely to take up permanent residence in our microbiomes; however, they *do* interact positively with the microbiome and host immune system as they pass through. So, we should think of probiotics as healthy placeholders for the replenishment of beneficial bacterial, crowding out pathogens that might otherwise take up residence.

> **KEY CONCEPT:** *Your microbiome is a reflection of your macroenvironment.* Get outside!

✔ **Get outside!**

According to triple board-certified MD and gut expert Zach Bush, our microbiome mimics our macroenvironment. We've become so separate from nature with our busy, modern lives that we must make it a priority to get back into nature as often as possible. Whether you're hiking, surfing, walking barefoot on the grass (pesticide-free, of course), playing in a park, or weeding in your garden, you'll be soaking up the macrobiome, which can help repopulate the microbiomes of your skin and nasal passages, which can slowly repopulate your body.

✔ **Eat fermented foods regularly.** The best way to edge out pathogens is to eat fermented foods with live cultures (beneficial bugs) regularly, like sauerkraut, pickles, kimchi (and other fermented vegetables), kefir, and yogurt. If you are avoiding cow dairy, you might try goat or coconut yogurt and kefir. Make sure you choose unsweetened and, ideally, organic and raw varieties (often found at farmer's markets) and add stevia if needed. According to Dr. Mercola, *fermented foods may contain one hundred times more probiotics than probiotic supplements.*[15]

Caution: Sometimes you can have a healing crisis (meaning the bad bugs are getting crowded out a little quickly and releasing their toxins) when adding fermented foods, so start with a teaspoon—even the juice of the sauerkraut—and gradually increase.

✔ **Take quality probiotics daily.** The next best way to introduce beneficial bacteria is to take probiotic supplements, especially if you must take antibiotics. Consider these criteria when choosing a probiotic:
- A USP (United States Pharmacopeia) symbol on the bottle is a sign that the product has been verified by an independent third party to contain what the bottle says it contains.
- High diversity, also known as multiple strains, has been shown to do a better job at reducing pathogens than single strains.[16]
- Potency matters, so take at least 50B or more CFUs (colony forming units) per day.
- *Saccharomyces boulardii*, a powerful yeast-based probiotic, often recommended for use with antibiotics, has also been proven effective in treating and preventing GI infections including *Clostridium difficile* and *Helicobacter pylori*, and the GI-related autoimmune conditions Crohn's disease, ulcerative colitis (UC), and irritable bowel syndrome (IBS).[17]
- Types that colonize the gut more successfully include *Lactobacillus plantarum, Lactobacillus rhamnosus GG,* and *Lactobacillus reuteri DSM.*[18, 19]
- Newer forms of probiotics that are gaining in popularity due to their reported effectiveness include soil-based (e.g., Primal Defense HSO Formula and CoreBiotic) and spore-based organisms (SBOs) (e\.g., MegaSporeBiotic.)[20]

If you scored a five or more on the gut assessment, you might consider eating fermented foods *and* taking supplemental probiotics.

Dose: One to two capsules 50B CFU twice per day. Some work best away from food and others with meals. Follow directions on bottle.

Note: It may take some time to discover which probiotic is best for you. Have patience and experiment. There's no rule on rotating probiotics, but you may benefit from introducing different strains every few months.

Caution: In rare cases, probiotics may pose some risk for people with weakened immune systems, such as those infected with the AIDS virus or people undergoing chemotherapy.

✔ **"Feed" with *Prebiotics: Eat More Fiber!*** Prebiotics are simply fiber that makes its way, undigested, to your large intestine (colon), where it feeds your beneficial bacteria. In other words, *probiotics eat prebiotics.* This may be the single most important step you can take in restoring your gut health: feeding the beneficial bacteria that already live in your gut with a wide variety of fiber from different types of vegetables. Remember, if you are not feeding your beneficial bacteria, they will resort to eating *you*—the mucus layer of your gut lining, that is!

You'll find the best sources of prebiotics in your local farmer's market, your garden, or an organic produce section, and the best types of prebiotics are a wide variety of colorful, local, seasonal vegetables. Excellent prebiotic vegetables include dandelion greens, asparagus, artichokes, avocado, cabbage, root vegetables (jicama, garlic, leeks, onion), flax, hemp and chia seeds, and psyllium husk. By eating many different types of seasonal produce raw or lightly cooked, you are feeding a broader diversity of good bacteria, and that's a good insurance policy for the health of your microbiome and you.

Other good sources of prebiotics are powders including acacia fiber, chicory root, raw Jerusalem artichoke, baobab fruit, inulin, larch, and fructooligosaccharides (FOS), which you can add to smoothies and yogurt or mix into kefir or water. Combine and rotate prebiotic powders to feed as many types of beneficial bacteria as possible.

Dose: Aim for 40 to 50 grams of fiber from various sources per day.

Caution: If you currently suffer from SIBO and/or dysbiosis, too much fiber too soon can make your gut feel temporarily worse. Once you resolve the imbalance(s), you will be able to tolerate adding fiber. Just ramp up fiber intake slowly to avoid too much fermentation (gas) as your gut gets used to the new amounts.

4. **Repair** your gut lining. The good news is that the cells of the intestinal lining replace themselves every three to six days. This means that, given proper support, your gut can repair itself pretty quickly. The strategy here is to continue Step 1 by strictly avoiding inflammatory elements like SAD foods plus any additional food triggers you've identified, minimizing medications, reducing stress, and adding targeted supplements and nourishing foods that help repair your damaged lining.

FOODS AND SUPPLEMENTS TO SEAL A LEAKY GUT

There are a plethora of foods and nutrients that can assist in sealing a leaky gut. While there's no harm in adding *all* of these foods and supplements at once—except maybe to your budget—see if you can add several to assist in repairing your gut lining:

✔ **Meat broth, stock and bone broth, collagen, and gelatin powder** have been staples in gut healing protocols for generations for good reason. They strengthen the mucus layer of the gut lining; they contain amino acids proline and glycine which are essential building blocks of the mucosal gut lining; and they promote tissue repair. Make or buy broth from 100 percent grass-fed, pasture-raised animals, and select 100 percent grass-fed collagen, gelatin, or bone broth powders.

Strategies: Sip a cup of broth two to three times a day, and/or use two to four tablespoons collagen, gelatin, or bone broth powder per day in smoothies, soups, stews, curries, or pudding. If you drink coffee (organic, of course), try adding collagen powder to get some protein and minimize its irritating effects on your gut.

Note: People who have histamine issues might consider shorter-cooked meat broth or stock instead of bone broth (one to four hours versus 8+ hours).

✔ **Coconut oil and MCT oil** contain medium-chain triglycerides (MCTs) that help the body reduce inflammation, burn fat, and heal the gut lining. Coconut oil is also rich in lauric acid, a powerful antimicrobial agent that kills off harmful bacteria and yeast.

Strategies: Use two to four tablespoons of extra virgin, unrefined coconut oil (or non-GMO MCT oil, which is more concentrated and does not have coconut flavor) daily in smoothies, fat bombs (see Recipes in Appendix A), tea, or coffee. Consider using coconut oil and ghee as your primary oils for cooking, and use MCT oil for drizzling on food after cooking.

Caution: Start slowly with MCT oil, as in one half to one teaspoon a day, and ramp up slowly to avoid tummy distress. If you experience mouth or throat irritation, stop using MCT oil and try coconut oil instead.

✔ **Ghee** is simply clarified butter without the allergens, lactose, and casein, which means it's generally safe for people who are sensitive to cow dairy. Ghee is nutrient-dense in vitamins A, D, E, and K, and rich in short- and medium-chain fatty acids and butyrate—anti-inflammatory fats that have been shown to help heal leaky gut.

Strategies: Use organic ghee from 100 percent grass-fed cows as you would butter and consider making organic tea or coffee with one to two tablespoons ghee (salt-free, of course). Google *Bulletproof coffee* for recipes.

✔ **Restore**, a lignite (fossil soil) extract supplement containing trace minerals and amino acids, has been shown in lab testing to help heal the gut lining *in a matter of minutes and hours*, as opposed to the months it may take other supplements to work.[21] Restore's carbon-based redox molecules from ancient fossilized soil help restore the communication network between bacteria in the gut, mitochondria, and cells in the body.

Dose: one teaspoon three times a day.

✔ **Colostrum**, a momma mammal's premilk, is a concentrated source of protein, growth factors, and antibodies essential for early development of newborns. Bovine (cow) colostrum has also been clinically proven to prevent and heal leaky gut in human trials.[22]

Dose: Use 100 percent New Zealand colostrum, which meets highest purity standards of 100 percent grass-fed cows without hormones, steroids, or antibiotics, uses flash pasteurization with low heat, and undergoes rigorous testing. Take one teaspoon powder (or four capsules) colostrum on an empty stomach, twice a day, thirty minutes before breakfast and before bed.

Cautions: If you have an IgE allergy to cow's milk, you may also be allergic to bovine colostrum. However, many people sensitive to lactose and/or casein (IgG) are able to tolerate colostrum, which contains only small amounts of lactose and casein. Bovine colostrum contains insulin growth factor (IGF-1), which has been found to correlate with the risk of prostate and breast cancers.

✔ **Zinc** has been shown to have a protective effect on the gut lining, and zinc deficiency has been shown to have a "catastrophic and aggravating effect" by inducing barrier leakage and perpetuating disease processes.[23] Well-absorbable forms include zinc monomethionine, carnosine, and picolinate.

To determine your zinc dosing needs, do a DIY zinc taste test: Put a tablespoon of liquid zinc (a concentration of one gram per liter or a zinc lozenge) in your mouth and hold for thirty seconds without swallowing (zinc can cause nausea without food), then spit it out. A) If you didn't really taste anything, you may be very deficient in zinc. B) If you get a slight taste, you may have low zinc levels. C) If you get a distinct taste that builds over time, you may be moderately low in zinc. D) If you get an immediate strong, metallic taste, your zinc levels are fine, and no to low supplementation is recommended.

Dose: A) 90 mg zinc plus 3 mg copper; B) 60 mg zinc plus 2 mg copper; or C) 30 mg of zinc plus 1 mg copper per day depending on your DIY test results, with food to avoid nausea. Low-dose zinc: 5 to 10 mg with each meal may be more effective at binding tight junction gaps than one single 30 mg dose.

Notes: Taking zinc without copper may create a copper deficiency, so be sure to take 1 mg of copper for every 30 mg zinc. Stress and/or toxin exposure increase the need for zinc.

Caution: Zinc on an empty stomach may cause nausea, so take with food.

✔ **Vitamin A** (retinoic acid or retinyl palmitate) is a critical factor in both regulating immune function and repairing and maintaining tissues including the gut lining. Animal sources of vitamin A, including oily fish and liver, are considered the most bioavailable. Consider taking cod liver oil capsules to get vitamins A and D3 plus omega-3 fatty acids. Good brands include Green Pasture, Nordic Naturals, and Carlson Labs.

Dose: For cod liver oil, the Weston A. Price Foundation suggests adults and children over twelve take one teaspoon or ten capsules per day, providing 9,500 IU vitamin A and 1,950 IU vitamin D. Or take 5,000 to 10,000 IU/day of vitamin A from mixed carotenoids and retinyl palmitate.

Caution: All oils are at risk for rancidity (spoilage) due to oxidization (exposure to air). Purchase high-quality supplements and minimize their exposure to air, heat, and light. Keep refrigerated, ideally in glass containers, and toss if cod liver oil or fish oils smell or taste fishy.

✔ **Omega-3 essential fatty acids** (EFAs) decrease inflammation, support brain and cognitive function, and help protect against cancer, heart disease, and Alzheimer's. Take supplemental omega-3 EFAs and eat more omega-3–rich fish like wild salmon and sardines. Look for a high-quality, refrigerated oil from wild salmon or krill that is free of metals, like OmegaBrite, Nordic Naturals, Green Pasture, and Dr. Mercola.

Dose: 2,000 to 3,000 mg of EPA and DHA combined in divided doses daily (i.e., half at breakfast and half with dinner) with food and vitamin E (if supplement does not contain vitamin E).

Note: To get to 2,000 to 3,000 mg of combined EPA plus DHA, you may need to take more than the recommended dose on the bottle.

Caution: All oils are at risk for rancidity (spoilage) due to oxidization. Purchase high-quality supplements and minimize their exposure to air, heat, and light. Keep refrigerated, ideally in glass containers, and toss if cod liver oil or fish oils smell or taste fishy. Omega-3 fatty acids may increase the effects of blood thinning medications.

✔ **Vitamin E** (mixed tocopherols) helps heal and reduce scar tissue of the intestinal mucosa. Consider taking a balance of all eight vitamin E compounds—called *mixed tocopherols*—in a single formula if your multivitamin does not contain vitamin E.

Dose: 200 mg per day mixed tocopherols form with food.

Caution: People with bleeding disorders, cancer, or heart conditions should consult their health practitioners before using vitamin E.

✔ **L-glutamine** is the most abundant amino acid in the bloodstream and a preferred fuel source for repairing and regenerating cells of the gut lining, and for increasing intestinal secretory IgA ("sigA"), the first line of defense in protecting gut immune function.[24]

Dose: Start slowly with 2.5 to 5 grams of l-glutamine powder twice a day between meals.

Caution: L-glutamine is a precursor to glutamate and aspartate, excitatory amino acids, which may cause anxiety in some people. For people with liver or kidney issues, consider supplementing with alpha-ketoglutarate (AKG) form, which converts to glutamine, as an ammonia-lessening strategy.

✔ **Quercetin**, a noncitrus bioflavonoid found in many fruits and vegetables, notably onions, enhances intestinal gut barrier function through the assembly and expression of tight junction proteins—those vital gut lining gatekeepers.[25] Quercetin may work even better in synergy with other polyphenols like vitamin C, resveratrol, and ECGC (an anti-cancer compound found in green tea), so feel free to mix and match.

Dose: 2,000 mg daily in divided doses with food.

✓ **GI UltraMAX Pro**, a relatively new-to-the-scene powder by Mother Earth Labs, Inc., offers a comprehensive blend of gut-healing elements, including some elements listed above: colostrum, glutamine, and quercetin, plus numerous additional nourishing elements like prebiotic fibers, medicinal mushrooms, adaptogens, and phospholipids.

Dose: one scoop to four ounces of liquid, shaken or stirred well into four ounces of liquid and immediately followed by eight ounces of water, in the afternoon or evening, between meals. www.motherearthlabs.com/product/gi-ultramax/

5. **Rebalance.** Once you're underway with the first four steps, it's time to focus on creating nourishing and supportive habits that promote optimal, ongoing gut health. Relaxing is crucial in gut restoration. Find at least one mind-body practice you can do for about twenty minutes each day to release stress and build more resilience. For relaxation-promoting strategies, see the Emotional Well-Being Toolkit on page 198. Below are some suggestions to help you create the right gut-healing lifestyle environment for good.

MIND YOUR FOOD ENVIRONMENT

It turns out that it's not just *what* you eat that matters for optimal digestion and health. *Where, when, how, and with whom you eat matters greatly, too.* Consider these tips to establishing a better eating environment.

✓ **Cook at home most of the time**, so you have greater control over ingredients and cooking methods.

✓ **Chew, chew, chew!** Ancient Chinese medicine wisdom says, "Drink your food and eat your drink." That's because digestion starts in your mouth, and chewing food long enough signals your stomach to produce the right enzymes in advance. See if you can chew each bite forty times before swallowing.

✓ **Eat in a calm state.** Studies show that eating while stressed interferes with digestion. That means dinnertime is not a time for stressful topics or violent TV shows.

✓ **Consider eating your biggest meal before three p.m.**, when you are most active.

✔ **Finish eating at least three hours before bed** so that while you sleep, your body can focus on rest and repair, not digestion.

✔ **Try intermittent fasting (IF).** Going twelve to twenty hours without eating any calories gives your digestive organs a break, reduces inflammation, helps strengthen the gut barrier, and helps move you into the metabolically beneficial state of fat burning, rather than sugar burning. Consider stopping eating by six or seven p.m. and break your fast at nine or ten a.m. for a fifteen-hour fast. Once that's comfortable, see if you can increase the fasting time to eighteen or even twenty-four hours. If that becomes doable, you might even consider a five-day water fast, which offers powerful healing benefits. Check out the fasting resources in Appendix F.

Step 4: Live Dirtier

Taking a page from integrative gastroenterologist Dr. Chutkan, find a way to live a little dirtier and embrace microbes rather than sanitizing them away. Scientific evidence is mounting that exposure to environmental microbes like soil-based organisms may help protect us from autoimmune disorders. Here are some tips to live dirtier:

✔ **Ease way up on the hand sanitizer**—unless you are in a place where pathogenic microbes may be more prevalent, like a hospital or doctor's office.

✔ **Plant a garden**, even a small one in pots in your kitchen. Consider the 4 Foot Farm if you are inspired to produce your own toxin-free produce: www.playtheplanet.org/thegreatlibrary/wp-content/uploads/sites/4/2016/03/The-4-Foot-Farm-Blueprint.pdf

✔ **Subscribe to a CSA** (community supported agriculture) box from your local farmer.

✔ **Leave a little dirt on your produce**—if it was grown organically.

✔ **Consider getting a pet**, and don't fret so much about washing your hands before eating.

✔ **Get outside**, go barefoot, play in nature, soak up some sun.

✔ **Open your windows** and let fresh air into your home.

✔ **Shower less** to nourish your skin microbiome.

EXTRA STEP: CONSIDER "BIG GUNS" FOR GUT HEALTH

If you have taken many courses of antibiotics, had chemotherapy, or are not able to balance your microbiome with the standard 5R program, you may be a good candidate for the following prescription-strength tools:

✔ **Ultra-strength probiotics.** Your microbiome contains 100 *trillion* microbes, so adding a mere 50B CFU probiotic per day is barely a drop in the bucket. That said, you want to make sure you're adding beneficial microbes without the addition of allergenic ingredients like corn, dairy, gluten, strep, fillers, or maltodextrin,

---

Promising Microbiome Treatment: Fecal Microbiota Transplantation (FMT)

Fecal microbiota transplantation, also known as stool transplantation, is a procedure in which stool from a healthy donor is placed into another person's colon. While ingesting (or inserting) someone else's poop may sound gross, emerging research is demonstrating that FMT may be one of the most effective treatments in restoring microbial balance. For example, FMT has been shown to be more than 90 percent effective at resolving *Clostridium difficile* (*C-diff*) infections, dramatically superior to the 30 percent to 40 percent effectiveness of antibiotic therapy. Early research also offers evidence that the transplantation of an optimized microbiota induces clinical remission in ulcerative colitis.[26, 27, 28]

Despite these promising results and growing interest in FMT for treating other autoimmune disorders, the Food and Drug Administration (FDA) has decided that fecal microbiota is considered both a "drug and a biological product," and today the procedure is limited to patients with recurrent *Clostridium difficile* infections. It is evident that better understanding of and oversight for this emerging and potentially risky treatment is needed. Concerns about FMT include transferring a predisposition to obesity and potentially transferring unwanted infectious organisms and other environmental contaminants.

For more information on FMT and to find a doctor near you or a clinical trial, refer to www.OpenBiome.org.

which can each harm the microbiome. Quality brands with high potency strains and allergen-free ingredients include:

- ✔ The Gut Institute's BIFIDO/MAXIMUS: The 200B CFU probiotic supports people with histamine, D-lactate, gut dysbiosis, and *Candida* overgrowth issues.
- ✔ General Biotics' Equilibrium: Time-release formula contains 115 interdependent strains.
- ✔ Bio-Botanical Research, Inc.'s Proflora4R includes soil-based probiotics plus co-factors, quercetin, marshmallow root, and aloe vera.
- ✔ Enviromedica will be coming out with a new formulation, so stay tuned.

Now that we know that a healthy gut is vital for good health, and that our microbes are way more helpful than harmful, we must live in a way that nurtures and supports them. And, as with food choices, it doesn't mean we have to revert to cave living, but it does mean we need to become way more conscious of our modern lifestyle choices, especially the foods we eat, the medications we take (or choose not to take), how we deal with stress, and how much dirt we can live with.

Summary: Top Five Gut-Healing Actions

1. **Get a comprehensive stool test** to get a snapshot of your microbial composition.
2. **Minimize medications** to avoid harming your microbiome and gut lining.
3. **Consider digestive enzymes** to help you better digest and absorb nutrients.
4. **Get outside often** to benefit from nature's macrobiome.
5. **Aim to eat forty to fifty grams of fiber—*prebiotics*—per day** to feed your good gut bugs.

CHAPTER 3

Clear Infections

It's not the bug, it's the terrain.
—MARIE MATHESON, ND,
chronic disease and infections expert

Many experts believe that *if you have an autoimmune condition, you almost certainly have an infection, too.* Growing scientific evidence indicates that chronic infections from bacteria, viruses, parasites, and fungi are a big contributing factor in the development and exacerbation of autoimmune conditions. Holistic practitioners report that they almost always discover at least one infection—hidden or evident—that either precedes the initial autoimmune attack (e.g., mononucleosis, aka Epstein-Barr virus or EBV) or shows up opportunistically when the immune system is weakened (e.g., a yeast infection, aka *Candida albicans*). In either scenario, an infection can make a bad situation worse, stressing an already overworked immune system and exacerbating or perpetuating autoimmune conditions.

Despite the fact that scientists identified the link between infections and autoimmune disease more than a century ago, the standard of care for autoimmune conditions still doesn't include testing for infections—or treating them. This is a grave error, because as you'll learn in this chapter, when infections are identified and properly treated—ideally, as early as possible—autoimmune conditions are more likely to improve, sometimes radically, and even completely. Adding insult to injury, current treatment for people with autoimmune conditions often includes immunosuppressive medications that do as they suggest: *suppress* the immune system! While this may be an appropriate short-term approach, it is not a viable long-term strategy and may set the stage for additional opportunistic infections to emerge, which can worsen autoimmune conditions and impede your chances of healing. When it comes to addressing infections, you need a *robust and intelligent* immune system, not a weakened one.

Consider the following compelling evidence of the close relationship between infections and autoimmune disorders:

- One study found that 70 percent of patients with chronic fatigue syndrome had an active human herpesvirus (HHV-6) infection, in contrast to 20 percent of healthy controls.[1]
- In a test of 114 people, a bacterium named *Prevotella copri* was present in the gut of 75 percent of people with rheumatoid arthritis (RA) as compared to only 21 percent of healthy control subjects.[2]
- One study found a fortyfold viral load increase of EBV, commonly known as *mononucleosis* or *mono*, in people with lupus when compared to healthy controls.[3]
- A study looking at the prevalence of antibodies (evidence of exposure) to *Yersinia enterocolitica* (YE), a foodborne infection, was fourteen times higher in people with Hashimoto's thyroiditis than in control groups.[4]
- A longitudinal study reports the strongest known risk factor for MS is infection with EBV. Compared with healthy controls, the hazard of developing MS is approximately fifteenfold higher among individuals infected with EBV in childhood, and about thirtyfold higher among those infected with EBV in adolescence or later in life.[5]

Not only is evidence piling up linking infections and autoimmune conditions, but scientists are now able to artificially induce autoimmune conditions in mice by using infective microbes. What's more, scientists have been able to arrest and even *reverse* autoimmune conditions in mice models, which suggests that *if you address the infection, you can potentially reverse the autoimmune condition.* Humans are obviously not the same as mice, but this is a bit of supporting evidence for the value of treating infections as a core part of our overall strategy for recovering from autoimmune conditions.

The Infection Paradox: Friend and Foe

Our bodies encounter infections regularly throughout our lifetime; we are constantly fighting off, living with, and even *benefiting* from microbes like viruses, bacteria, fungi, and parasites.

Most of the time, we are not even aware of infectious microbes, since our immune system fends them off naturally. Sometimes we experience an acute infection—something self-limiting that lasts a few days or weeks, like a urinary tract infection (UTI), strep throat, the common cold, or flu. Other infections will definitely get our attention, like an outbreak of oral (type 1) or genital (type 2) herpes, the chicken pox (varicella-zoster virus or VZV), or a bout of mono (caused by the Epstein-Barr virus or herpesvirus 4).

While we tend to think of all infections as bad, certain infectious microbes actually offer *beneficial* effects and may even be essential for developing both a balanced immune system and microbiome. While it's not clear exactly how it works, viral infections at a young age may prime our immune system, providing immunization against infections and preventing immune overreactions like allergies and even autoimmune conditions later in life. Not long ago, before the chicken pox vaccine was available, parents brought their children to "pox parties" to expose them to the highly contagious varicella zoster virus that causes the red, itchy, blistery rash. Most kids got the chicken pox before age twenty, and that gave them immunity from getting it as an adult, which could be much worse. Studies confirm that having other childhood viruses, like the measles, is protective against potential allergies and autoimmune conditions like psoriasis and juvenile rheumatoid arthritis (JRA).

And if you can get past the gross factor, scientists have discovered that parasitic worms known as *helminths*, like hookworms and whipworms, or the worms' eggs, can be a viable *treatment strategy* for autoimmune conditions including MS, inflammatory bowel disease (IBD), celiac disease, Crohn's disease, and asthma.

According to Moises Velasquez-Manoff, author of the thought-provoking book *An Epidemic of Absence*, a big reason for the explosion of autoimmune conditions in the United States over the past fifty years is the disappearance of parasites, thanks in large part to improvements in sanitation. Velasquez-Manoff asserts that the absence of microbes like parasites has caused our immune systems to become unbalanced, increasing our vulnerability to autoimmune and other inflammatory disorders. Research is confirming this "hygiene hypothesis," that there is such a thing as too much cleanliness. Preliminary studies offer strong evidence that infection with helminths can improve autoimmune symptoms and even decrease gluten sensitivity.

Bottom line: It's early innings in our understanding of the various roles and functions of bacteria, viruses, yeasts, and parasites, so best to keep an open mind about our microbial companions.

And yet, according to many holistic or integrative practitioners who treat autoimmune conditions, if you don't get better after addressing food triggers, correcting nutrient deficiencies, and healing your gut, it's time to test for hidden infections—and treat them.

In this chapter, we'll explore the connections between infections and autoimmune conditions, and learn about people who developed an autoimmune condition largely due to an infection, and who healed by strengthening their immune systems and/or directly addressing the infection. The Infection-Clearing Toolkit offers steps you can take to address infections if you already have an autoimmune condition and want to optimize your health.

Infections and Autoimmune Conditions

While we have naturally coadapted to live symbiotically with many microorganisms, including bacteria, viruses, yeast, and even parasites, when we have an overabundance, an imbalance, or an invasion of microorganisms not normally found in the body, we call that an infection. Infections vary in their intensity, duration, and life cycle. Some come and go, some remain permanently, and others can reactivate and become a big burden on the immune system. If you have an autoimmune condition, any type of infection can be burdensome, but the hidden ones are the toughest to treat and recover from. Here's a quick reference guide to the different types of infections:

- **Active:** An infection is currently producing symptoms; for example, when cold sores are present, the herpesvirus 1 is active.
- **Acute:** Short duration, lasting several days to a few weeks, like a cold or flu, which comes on fast, spreads quickly, and then clears completely.
- **Chronic or persistent:** Long duration, lasting weeks or months.
- **Stealth/hidden:** Many microbes, especially bacteria, have various strategies to evade attack by the immune system and protect them-

selves from antibiotic treatment. Mycoplasma, *Chlamydia pneumoniae*, and Lyme *Borrelia burgdorferi* hide in cells, deep tissues, and organs, and behind thick mucus layers they produce called *biofilms*.

- **Latent:** The infectious organism is hidden, inactive, or dormant, often not causing obvious damage or showing clinical signs of reactivation; for example, for most people, the herpesviruses remain mostly quiet and hidden in a latent or dormant state. In the latent state, the immune system is not stimulated to respond.
- **Opportunistic:** When the immune system is weakened, some latent or new infections emerge or take hold.
- **Reactivated:** A latent virus can shift from a dormant state to an active one, especially during or following stressful periods. Reactivated viruses like EBV can be a heavy load for the immune system.

The infections most commonly associated with autoimmune disorders include:

- Any of more than eight types of **herpesviruses**, including **EBV** (viral infection)
- **Mycoplasmas** (bacterial infection)
- *Chlamydophila pneumoniae* (also known as Chlamydia or *C. pneumoniae*, a bacterial infection)
- **Lyme disease** spirochetes and coinfections (bacterial infections)
- **Gastrointestinal (GI) infections** including *Helicobacter pylori* (*H. Pylori*), *Candida albicans*, and small intestine bacterial overgrowth (SIBO)
- **Oral infections** like gingivitis (gum inflammation), periodontitis (gum disease), and cavitations (infections in jawbones following tooth extraction or root canals)

Pages 114–15 list some infections frequently associated with the most common autoimmune disorders. If you have been diagnosed with an autoimmune condition, use this chart to be proactive with your health. Conventional doctors may not be aware of the connections between infections and autoimmune conditions, so you may need to encourage your doctor to test for the noted infections; or it may be a good opportunity to find and work with a practitioner who is skilled in this arena. If your

AUTOIMMUNE DISORDER / COMMONLY LINKED INFECTIONS

Alopecia	Lyme *Borrelia burgdorferi* (Lyme *Bb*)
ALS	Lyme *Bb*
Alzheimer's	Lyme *Bb*, *Helicobacter pylori* (*H. Pylori*), *Chlamydia pneumoniae* (*Cpn*), cytomegalovirus (CMV), human herpesvirus (HHV-1), *Porphyromonas gingivalis* (*P. gingivalis*) and other oral infections
Ankylosing spondylitis (AS)	*Klebsiella pneumoniae*
Atherosclerosis	*Cpn*, *H. pylori*, CMV, and periodontal (gum) infections
Alopecia areata	EBV, also called HH4 (human herpesvirus 4), *H. pylori*
Celiac disease	Adenovirus, enterovirus, Hepatitis C virus (HCV), rotavirus, and reovirus
Crohn's disease	*Yersinia enterocolitica (Yersinia)*, *Campylobacter (C. jejuni)*, *Escherichia coli (E. coli)*
Inflammatory bowel disease (IBD)	EBV, *Klebsiella pneumoniae*, *Candida albicans*, and small intestinal bacterial overgrowth (SIBO)
Graves' disease	*H. pylori*, EBV, *Yersinia*, HHV-6 and -7, parvovirus B19 (B19), *Enterobacter*, *Campylobacter jejuni (C. jejuni)*
Guillain-Barré syndrome	EBV, CMV, *C. jejuni*
Hashimoto's thyroiditis	*Yersinia*, EBV, HHV-6, *H. pylori*, B19, SIBO, HCV, Lyme *Bb*, *Blastocystis hominis* (protozoal parasite) and *Candida albicans*
Lupus	*Ureaplasma urealyticum* (UU) and *Mycoplasma hominis* (*M. hominis*), EBV, CMV, B19, HCV
Multiple sclerosis (MS)	Lyme *Bb*, EBV, HHV-6, rubella, influenza virus, human papillomavirus (HPV), *Cpn*, and measles virus

AUTOIMMUNE DISORDER / COMMONLY LINKED INFECTIONS

Myalgic encephalomyelitis/ chronic fatigue syndrome/ fibromyalgia syndrome	Lyme *Bb*, mycoplasma, HHV6, EBV, CMV
Myasthenia gravis	HCV, HHV-1
Myocarditis	CB3, CMV, *Cpn*
Polymyalgia rheumatica (PMR)	Influenza virus, *Cpn*
Psoriasis	*Streptococcus pyogenes (S. pyogenes)*, latent tuberculosis infection (LTBI)
Rheumatoid arthritis (RA)	Lyme *Bb*, EBV, HCV, *E. coli, Citrobacter, Klebsiella, Proteus*, B19, mycoplasma infection
Sjögren's syndrome	EBV
Type 1 diabetes mellitus (T1DM)	Coxsackievirus B4, CMV, mumps virus, and rubella virus
Vitiligo	HCV, CMV

autoimmune condition is not listed, do your own research by searching online for "[your autoimmune condition] and infections" to learn which specific infections may be linked to your autoimmune condition.

While infections are extremely common throughout our lifetime, they only occasionally lead to an autoimmune disorder. For example, more than 90 percent of Americans have some form of the herpesviruses, but only 20 percent of us will develop an autoimmune condition. The Centers for Disease Control and Prevention (CDC) report that:

- Nearly 100 percent of Americans are infected with human herpesvirus 6 (HHV-6) by the time they are three years old.
- Over 95 percent of Americans are infected by VZV, which causes chicken pox, at some time in their life.
- Of adults in the United States, 95 percent have been infected with EBV—herpesvirus 4.
- More than half of adults in the United States have been infected with CMV.
- Two-thirds of all adults under fifty have herpes type 1.[6]

So, if infections are common but autoimmune conditions less so, why are some people grievously affected and others remain unscathed?

Little-Known Lyme Facts

According to the CDC, Lyme disease is the fastest-growing vector-borne (biting insect) infectious disease in the United States. The CDC reports that more than 300,000 new cases develop each year in the United States—more than one and a half times more cases than breast cancer and six times higher than HIV/AIDS. If you have aches, pain, or swelling in large joints like knees, elbows, or shoulders, debilitating fatigue, decreased short-term memory, dizziness, facial palsy (drooping on one side), shooting pains, numbness and tingling, severe headaches, or an autoimmune condition, consider getting tested for Lyme and coinfections.

- Lyme was first discovered in 1975 in Lyme, Connecticut, by Wilhelm Burgdorfer.
- Fewer than 50 percent of people who develop Lyme disease recall a tick bite, and only about 20 percent of people develop the hallmark bull's-eye Lyme rash known as *erythema migrans* (EM).
- Lyme is not just carried by ticks. You can get a Lyme infection from biting insects like mosquitos, deerflies, and horseflies; and evidence suggests that Lyme can be sexually transmitted or passed from mother to the fetus through the placenta.[7]
- Acute Lyme symptoms feel like the flu and include fever, malaise, fatigue, and generalized achiness.
- It is estimated that 40 percent of those diagnosed and treated early for Lyme remain ill after treatment—a condition known as chronic or persistent Lyme or post-treatment Lyme disease (PTLD)—an autoimmune condition.[8]
- Lyme is known as "the great imitator," as it has been reported to mimic more than 300 other diseases, including those that affect the joints, like lupus, osteoarthritis, and rheumatoid arthritis; those that affect the heart, like Lyme carditis and heart block; and those that cause neurodegeneration, like ALS (amyotrophic lateral sclerosis), Alzheimer's, MS, and Parkinson's disease.

The Pathway to Problems:
A Malfunctioning Immune System

Our immune system is our armed forces, responsible for protecting us from harmful invaders. When it functions properly, we are resilient against infections like the common cold and even Lyme disease. But with inflammatory lifestyle factors like a diet of simple carbohydrates, sugar, and refined grains, poor sleep, minimal movement, excess stress, and environmental toxins, our immune systems get run down and don't operate optimally. In short, our modern lifestyles are burdening our immune systems, making us more prone to immune dysfunction, infections, and autoimmune conditions.

A malfunctioning immune system is fertile ground for infections. You may have noticed that a particularly stressful time can be the perfect opportunity for an infection to take up residence or reactivate and wreak havoc on your body. And once your immune system mounts a reaction to the infection, it produces a huge amount of inflammation, which we've already learned creates a prime environment for autoimmune conditions to emerge or worsen.

As mentioned in my story (and to be more fully described in the Toxins chapter), we each carry a body burden. Whether you can withstand more or fewer additional toxic assaults depends on how full or empty your "toxin bucket" is. A person with a moderately filled bucket who has genetic detoxification weaknesses is closer to the tipping point than a person with a moderately filled bucket who can readily process and excrete toxins. And a person with a fully loaded bucket may be one infection away from developing an autoimmune condition.

Women are more vulnerable to the consequences of infections

KEY CONCEPT: *Chronic inflammation causes the immune system to stay reactive all the time.*

than men. Women's bodies mount a faster and stronger immune-system attack to clear infections—and the resulting inflammation that floods their systems increases their risk of autoimmune troubles. Beyond gender, the following factors weaken immunity, and in combination, increase the risk of infections and autoimmune conditions in predisposed people:

- Inflammation: Sources of inflammation include environmental toxins, SAD foods, nutrient deficiencies, poor sleep, lack of exercise, chronic stress and, of course, infections.
- Insulin resistance: People who are insulin resistant, prediabetic, or diabetic are more prone to infections.
- Imbalanced hormones: Hormonal events like puberty, pregnancy, perimenopause, menopause, thyroid dysfunction, estrogen dominance, and insulin resistance contribute to body burden.
- Hypometabolism: Aging, underactive thyroid, and/or a heavy toxic load can cause a slow (hypo) metabolism which weakens your immune response, lowers your core body temperature, and makes you more vulnerable to all types of infections.
- A malfunctioning immune system is party time for infectious microbes: stealthy or dormant infections like mycoplasma bacteria, herpesviruses, or sequestered Lyme spirochetes often opportunistically emerge from hiding and reactivate when the immune system falters. When our toxin buckets are filled, any big stressor or shock to the system can be the last drop that sets off an autoimmune cascade.

Common Flu Precipitates Chronic Disease: Dr. Jacob Teitelbaum's Story

Sometimes a common, acute infection, like the influenza virus or mono, is the last straw. Dr. Jacob Teitelbaum's story is a cautionary tale about how the impact of emotional stress on the immune system can lay the groundwork for a devastating infection. Dr. Teitelbaum was a people-pleaser for decades, creating a heavy body burden of chronic stress. Chronic stress in turn set up the perfect environment for a viral infection to wreak havoc, causing Jacob's bucket to finally overflow, triggering a cascade of chronic illness.

Jacob is the child of Auschwitz concentration camp survivors whose families suffered tremendous loss during Hitler's reign. After the war, Jacob's parents immigrated to the United States and made their home in Cleveland, Ohio, where Jacob was raised in the dark shadow of his mother's recent trauma. Although his parents provided a loving home, Jacob felt the weight of his mother's expectations for perfection. As part of her mission to fight Hitler's attempt to eradicate the Jews and replenish the six million Jews who had been killed, Jacob's mother required him to be a righteous, high-achieving Jewish boy. But Jacob's identity didn't always align with his mother's vision for her child. Highly empathetic, Jacob deeply felt the emotional wrath of his mother's terrible concentration camp experiences whenever he failed to meet her desires. It's not surprising that after paying his way through college and completing his coursework in a little over two years, Jacob went on to medical school to become a doctor as quickly as possible.

It was during medical school that Jacob's health plummeted—not because of the demands of the program, but because ongoing family pressures took an insurmountable toll. During his second year, two of Jacob's cousins decided to marry Catholics—an unforgivable sin, according to his mother and uncle, who insisted the grandchildren be raised Jewish. Because Jacob was the family peacemaker, relatives implored him to convince the cousins to cancel their weddings.

The stress and responsibility pushed Jacob over the edge, and he developed what he calls the "drop-dead flu," which may have actually been a severe mononucleosis infection. He struggled to complete his coursework, but the fatigue and brain fog became so debilitating, he finally heeded the advice of a caring professor who told him there was a time to push forward and a time to pause and regroup. This intense "flu" lingered for months, triggering an escalating collection of painful and mysterious symptoms that would later be identified as chronic fatigue syndrome (CFS), fibromyalgia syndrome (FMS), and myofascial pain syndrome (MPS), abbreviated together as CFS/FMS/MPS. Unable to work, Jacob had to drop out of school and ended up homeless. While most people might consider being homeless and jobless a high-stress situation, in fact, Jacob was actually able to reduce his stress and gain profound healing benefits. It was during this time that Jacob felt the freedom to explore a variety of healing modalities. He describes it as if the universe had stamped

"Holistic Homeless Medical School" on his park bench; healers of many backgrounds came and taught him the bits and pieces of what he needed to learn to recover his health and happiness.

Central to his healing journey was addressing his primary trigger: *chronic stress*. Jacob found that the key to reducing his stress was simply to do more of what he enjoyed and less of what he didn't. His health and happiness increased as he discovered and followed his bliss. As he embraced new passions for natural healing, his overworked adrenal glands healed, and his immune system finally restored. In turn, his symptoms faded or vanished, and Jacob returned to medical school with renewed vitality and a personal mission to help the six million people worldwide affected by CFS/FMS/MPS.

How Infections Lead to an Autoimmune Attack

Dr. Nikolas Hedberg, a board-certified chiropractic internist who specializes in the infection–autoimmune disease connection, describes the most common way infections cause our immune systems to mistakenly attack our own tissue:

> One of the most common triggers for Hashimoto's thyroiditis is an infection with *Yersinia enterocolitica*, bacteria normally found in contaminated food or water. Most people infected with *Yersinia* may have gastrointestinal distress that feels like food poisoning or diarrhea, and then the infection clears on its own pretty fast. But in some people, *Yersinia* sets up shop in the lining of the gut and multiplies. The immune system kicks in, tags the *Yersinia* protein surface sequences, and starts producing antibodies to attack those sequences. But, it turns out that the *Yersinia* have the same molecular protein sequence as thyroid tissue, so when the immune system goes after the *Yersinia*, it also attacks the thyroid. Molecular mimicry means that your immune system is not only making antibodies against an infection, but it's also making antibodies against your own tissue that looks just like the infection.

Molecular mimicry may occur whenever foreign proteins like infections, toxins, or even foods share a similar or identical structure to human tissue. The molecular structure of gluten happens to resemble myelin protein, which is the tissue targeted in multiple sclerosis; the molecular structure of *Streptococcus pyogenes,* which causes the fairly common strep infection, looks like the heart tissue myosin and can lead to autoimmune heart disease; and many viruses, including Coxsackie B, rubella, and herpesviruses, mimic pancreatic islet cells and can result in type 1 diabetes.

Sometimes a common infection may be the trigger for autoimmune troubles that arise years, or even decades, later. We've long known about the connection between poor oral health like gingivitis (bacterial infection in gums) and increased risk of heart disease, but it may be news to you that infections in your mouth can also lead to autoimmune conditions like rheumatoid arthritis (RA).

Oral Infection Leads to Rheumatoid Arthritis: The Story of Aristo Vojdani's Mother

In this story, autoimmunologist Aristo Vojdani, Ph.D., describes the likely trigger for his mother's rheumatoid arthritis, from which she suffered for more than forty-seven years. Looking back, Dr. Vojdani recalls that when he was a teenager, his mother visited the dentist frequently due to recurring toothaches and swollen gums caused by gingivitis. After multiple extractions and dentures, his mother began to suffer from severe joint issues.

Witness to his mother's steep physical decline following the dental procedures, Dr. Vojdani questioned her doctors about the cause. He intuited a connection between the oral infections and her increasing arthritis symptoms, but her physicians "didn't know" or chalked it up to "bad genes." During his Ph.D. program, Dr. Vojdani began to study the cause and effect relationship between infection and autoimmune disease, eventually revealing the most likely source of his mother's RA.

He relates what probably occurred:

My mother did not take the best care of her teeth and by the time she was in her forties, she had to have teeth removed and eventually dentures put in. During the two years she had dental procedures, she also had gingivitis—an active bacterial infection in her gums like *Porphyromonas gingivalis or Streptococcus sanguinis*. Either of these bacterial strains release a toxin. When the dentist removed her teeth, the barriers were broken, and the bacterial toxins got into her blood immediately. She started making antibodies against the toxins and, because of the molecular similarity between the toxin and her joints, her immune cells started attacking her joints. Within five years, she started having joint pain from osteoarthritis. Within a few more years she had to have knee replacement surgery, and within ten years, she developed complete rheumatoid arthritis, which caused her hands to become very painful and deformed.

Reflecting on his mother's experience, Dr. Vojdani believes her cascade of ill health could have been prevented had the dentist treated the gum infection with penicillin, the antibiotic of choice at the time, prior to any surgery. Unfortunately, Mrs. Vojdani never recovered from the RA. The painful experience of watching her health decline was a major catalyst for Dr. Vojdani to study immunology and to eventually develop lab tests that provide early detection of immune system irregularities that might help others prevent autoimmune conditions like his mother's.

A Vicious Cycle: Infections →
Lowered Resistance → *More* Infections

The relationship between infections and autoimmune diseases is often described as "multifaceted and multidirectional," involving a multitude of complex actions and reactions in the body. Although infections may trigger disease, many infections likely occur and persist due to the illness itself, setting up a vicious cycle of inflammation, infection, lowered immunity, and more illness. Compounding that, infections are opportunistic and often travel together; many people with autoimmune conditions eventually discover that they have multiple bacterial, viral, parasitic, and/or fungal infections. And adding insult to injury, people suffering from multiple infections are more prone to mold illness or chronic inflammatory response syndrome (CIRS), a state of systemic inflammation brought on by exposure to toxic organisms produced by water-damaged buildings and amplified by excessive exposure to electromagnetic frequencies (EMF).

You may live and function pretty well for years or decades with a load of chronic infections like multiple herpesviruses, *Candida,* and Lyme. But all it takes is one hit or stressful event to tip the bucket, triggering symptoms or full-blown illness.

Chronic Infections at the Root of Hashimoto's: Toréa Rodriguez's Story

While thriving as a busy executive, long-distance cyclist, and professional pilot, Toréa Rodriguez unknowingly harbored a host of infections for years, until three extremely stressful back-to-back events preceded a diagnosis of Hashimoto's thyroiditis.

Raised by a single, "hippy mom" in laid-back Colorado, Torea's personality and love of science led her to get a BS in biochemistry followed by a career as a rising executive in Silicon Valley. But over time, Toréa grew to hate "cubicle life." When a girlfriend from Alaska took her flying, Toréa was hooked and signed up for flying lessons on the spot. Certain of her new path, she tore through the certifications and was soon able to quit her tech job. When she wasn't piloting charter flights, Toréa could be found riding her road bike about 150 miles a week. Life was high-flying, until a quick succession of stressful events knocked her down to earth.

When she was thirty-eight years old, Toréa was forced to make a rapid, emergency descent midflight. While somewhat routine and ultimately successful, this intense experience lingered and was the first of several traumatic events that year: a few months later her mother died unexpectedly, and shortly thereafter, Toréa was in a serious bicycle accident that left her with an excruciating set of injuries, including a dislocated shoulder, bruised spleen, and multiple, painful hematomas.

After she healed physically, Toréa still felt profoundly tired. She'd sleep for fourteen hours and wake unrefreshed. Also, her hair was thinning, she was cold most of the time, and she was gaining weight. Tests revealed she had Hashimoto's thyroiditis, and her endocrinologist prescribed a synthetic thyroid medication. On meds, Toréa would swing from hypo- to hyperthyroid and back again, never settling into the "sweet spot." And she wasn't feeling better. This was a precarious time for a pilot who needed to pass regular medical examinations. When she asked the endocrinologist what he could do to help her pass, he offered to irradiate and remove her thyroid. For Toréa, this was a step too far, and she decided to find a better approach.

Her research led her to Chris Kresser, LAc, Functional Medicine and ancestral nutrition expert and health educator, who became her personal practitioner. Toréa agreed to try a Paleo-template diet, swapping her grain-heavy vegetarian diet for more vegetables and even some meat, fish, and chicken. Within a month, she was amazed by how much better she felt—the fatigue lifted, her hair loss subsided, and she even lost a little weight—but test results indicated she was far from healed.

Further lab work revealed that Toréa had adrenal dysfunction, a clear sign of toxic, chronic stress; her cortisol was so low, Chris was concerned she was a few steps away from another autoimmune diagnosis: Addison's disease, which causes the adrenal glands to produce too little cortisol. But even after working with a therapist and giving up her beloved adrenaline-boosting activities, cycling and piloting, Toréa still felt off. She and Kresser continued to dig deeper into possible root causes.

A stool test revealed that Toréa was dealing with a trio of gut infections—H. Pylori, clostridium, and giardia—likely in her system for years. It would take multiple rounds and a rotation of herbal antibiotics, including oil of oregano, berberine, mastic gum, monolaurin, and Biocidin, a broad-spectrum antimicrobial botanical, for Toréa to finally rid herself of the gut infections. Again, things greatly improved, but Toréa still suffered from debilitating multiday headaches.

Determined to return to her former full vitality, Toréa continued testing and discovered she had two final infections to fight: a chronic sinus infection and a reactivated Epstein-Barr virus—the latter, perhaps the stealth root cause of her Hashimoto's. From Dr. Aviva Romm's book *Botanical Medicine for Women's Health*, Toréa learned that herpes viruses often respond to a combination of lemon balm, echinacea, and St. John's wort. Her sinus infection—called MARCoNS (Multiple Antibiotic Resistant Coagulase Negative Staphylococci), an antibiotic-resistant staph usually caused by mold exposure, persistent Lyme disease, or biotoxin illness—she treated with Biocidin-saline nasal spray.

Both treatments worked, her sinus infection cleared, headaches vanished, and in 2014, five years from the beginning of her autoimmune journey, Toréa went back to school to get certified as a Functional Diagnostic Nutrition Practitioner. These days, her adrenaline rush comes from "geeking out on the biochemistry" and helping people who suffer from autoimmune conditions return to vibrant health, like she did.

To maintain her health, Toréa manages her stress levels and continues to take a small amount of compounded T3 and T4 thyroid medication to support her thyroid function, as well as the lemon balm, echinacea, and St. John's wort combo to keep the EBV as quiet as possible.

If, like Toréa, you have an autoimmune condition and are still suffering from symptoms after addressing food triggers, correcting nutrient deficiencies, and healing your gut, it's time to dig deeper and address hidden infections. Sometimes, as Toréa found, the return to good health takes unwavering determination, dogged detective work, and the patience to allow the natural remedies to work. In the toolkit, we'll consider infection root causes, examine proven strategies and treatments, and discuss the importance of collaborating with an experienced practitioner.

Infection-Clearing Toolkit

It may be tempting to think that eliminating an infection will resolve your autoimmune condition, but attacking the infection alone does not address the underlying reasons that your immune system was unable to fend off the infection in the first place. Consider the examples of Dr. Teitelbaum and Toréa Rodriguez. Had they just used microbe-killing strategies without addressing the underlying reasons they got so sick in the first place, they would not have created the conditions for complete healing. A cancer diagnosis provides a good analogy. If you choose chemotherapy to kill cancer cells without addressing the root cause of *why* you got the cancer in the first place, there's a good chance the cancer will return, often with a vengeance.

According to Lee Cowden, MD, board-certified cardiologist, integrative health educator, and founder of the Cowden Protocol to treat Lyme disease, *the key to recovery from infections is to strengthen the resistance of the host.*

> **KEY CONCEPT:** *The goal of infection clearing is less about killing bugs and more about optimizing immune function so the immune system can keep infections at bay.*

Strengthening resistance means getting your immune system in good fighting shape. That entails addressing all of F.I.G.H.T.S.—eating optimal foods, healing your gut, minimizing toxins and stress, balancing your hormones, and addressing infections, as naturally and holistically as possible. This comprehensive mind-body-spirit strategy reduces inflammation, revs your metabolism, and optimizes your immune system—making your body an inhospitable place for infections and a welcome environment for optimal health. By improving your defenses with healthy lifestyle practices, you will be making it easier and more efficient to clear infections.

You don't need to do the steps in sequence; if you're eager to get going, I encourage you to begin Steps 1 through 4 while finding and beginning to work with an experienced practitioner. To reduce your burden of infections, follow all five steps; and if you require extra help, consider the extra step.

Step 1: Take an infections self-assessment.
Step 2: Get the data.
Step 3: Raise your metabolism.
Step 4: Unburden your immune system.
Step 5: Consider herbal antimicrobials.
Extra Step: Explore "Big Guns" to clear stubborn infections.

Step 1: Take an Infections Self-Assessment

If you have an autoimmune condition, there is a high likelihood that you also have one or more infections, too, whether they triggered the condition or set up shop later. The purpose of an infections self-assessment is to help you gain awareness about past and present infections that may be burdening your immune system. Consider the following statements. If you don't know an answer, just skip it. Rate your responses as 0 or 1, where 0 means "no" or "never" and 1 means "yes," "at least once," or "sometimes":

0 1   I have been bitten by a tick.
0 1   I've had the mumps, measles, chicken pox, or mono.
0 1   I have or have had yeast infections.
0 1   I have or have had oral infections including gingivitis, periodontal disease, or infected root canals/dental implants.
0 1   My gums bleed when I brush them.
0 1   I have or have had chronic sinus infections.
0 1   I've taken multiple rounds or an extended course (four weeks or longer) of antibiotics.
0 1   I have a sexually transmitted disease (STD) like herpes.
0 1   I get or used to get cold sores.
0 1   I have had travelers' diarrhea.
0 1   I have or have had other GI infections: bacteria, fungus, parasites.
0 1   I get more than three colds per year.
0 1   My lymph nodes are sore or swollen.
0 1   I run a fever a lot of the time.
0 1   I have one or more autoimmune conditions.

Please list any other relevant infection signs or symptom(s):

1   _____

1   _____

Total: _____

INFECTIONS ASSESSMENT KEY:

0   Incredible! You may be among the very few unburdened by infections. Keep on the prevention path.

1   If you answered yes to any of the statements and/or have an autoimmune condition, please consider working with a practitioner who can order and interpret the right tests and then offer a custom treatment plan for you.

Extra If you have an oral infection (e.g. gingivitis), root canal, dental im-
       plant, extracted wisdom teeth, chronic Lyme disease, asthma,
       autoimmune liver disease, celiac, Crohn's, MS, type 1 diabetes (T1D),
       ulcerative colitis (UC), or other stubborn infections, be sure to check
       out the Big Guns considerations on page 136.

Step 2: Get the Data

Infections are a complicated arena, especially if you're dealing with
overlapping issues like heavy metals, Lyme disease, and mold illness. I
urge you to find and work with an experienced integrative, naturopathic,
or Functional Medicine practitioner who can help you order the right
tests, design and prioritize a comprehensive treatment plan, and support
you through the process. If you suspect Lyme and related coinfections,
find a Lyme-literate physician at LymeDisease.org (www.lymedisease
.org/find-lyme-literate-doctors) or the International Lyme and Associated Diseases Society (ilads.org/ilads_media/physician-referral). Lyme,
unfortunately, is a controversial arena, with many well-intentioned doctors simply not believing persistent Lyme is even possible. To make sure
you get the most accurate lab test results, consider more advanced Lyme
testing through DNA Connexions, IGeneX, Fry Laboratories, or Immunosciences Lab.

Many practitioners offer a free fifteen-minute phone consultation to
see if there is a good mutual fit. You might consider asking the following
questions:

- Do you have experience helping people reverse autoimmune
  conditions?
- Which infections do you typically see connected with [your au-
  toimmune condition(s)]?
- What type of lab tests do you use?
- How do you treat infections and autoimmunity?
- How long does it normally take for you to help a person address
  infections and reverse autoimmune conditions?

Keep these red flags in mind when considering a practitioner:

- If the practitioner doesn't have experience in helping people re-verse autoimmune conditions—or doesn't believe it's possible—my advice is to steer clear.
- If the practitioner doesn't typically see infections at the root of or alongside autoimmune disorders, that's a sign he may not be dig-ging deeply enough.
- If the practitioner only uses standard labs like LabCorp and Quest, he may not be able to help you get the best data available. Infec-tions testing is far from perfect, and there are lots of false negatives and positives.
- If the practitioner only prescribes antibiotics to get rid of infec-tions, regardless of how long the infection has been present, his toolkit may not be comprehensive enough.
- And if the practitioner claims it usually takes a month or two to address the infection and resolve an autoimmune condition, it sim-ply doesn't seem realistic.

Step 3: Raise Your Metabolism

People with autoimmune conditions typically suffer from a sluggish me-tabolism—a depleted energy state called *hypometabolism*. It's like your body's energy-producing mitochondria and thyroid (the "gas pedal gland") have both gone on strike; you feel tired, cold, and seem unable to lose weight. Being in a hypometabolic state not only decreases your vitality, it decreases the robustness of your immune system and makes you more vul-nerable to infections. To clear infections, you can assist your body in cranking up your natural energy production.

To assess whether or not you are hypometabolic, take your tempera-ture over the next five days. Keep a good old-fashioned mercury thermometer right by your bed; shake it down the night before and then place it under your tongue for five minutes or in your armpit for ten min-utes as soon as you wake up. Note and write down your temperature. If your temperature is lower than 98.0°F (37°C) five mornings in a row, you may be hypometabolic. Your goal is to raise your temperature closer to 98.0°F (37°C) on waking.

To rev up your metabolism, give these strategies a try:

✔ **Breathe deeply, slowly and intentionally** several times per day. Conscious breathing is one of the easiest and most deceptively simple ways to raise your metabolism and relax at the same time.

Give it a try: Take ten conscious breaths with a 1-4-2 ratio. For example, inhale for four seconds, hold for sixteen seconds, and exhale for eight seconds. Find cues to remember to breathe: for example, when you wake up, while you're walking, or before you go to sleep. Do three rounds of ten breaths a few times per day. For more info on breathing to boost your metabolism, check out Pam Grout's *Jumpstart Your Metabolism: How To Lose Weight By Changing The Way You Breathe.*

✔ **Use red lights** from when the sun goes down until you wake up. Standard artificial lights emit a blue wave spectrum, which, if you are exposed to in the evening and early morning, suppresses melatonin, harming your circadian rhythm and keeping you in a hypometabolic state.[9]

Give it a try: Replace your bedside lamp with a red LED bulb from Amazon for five to ten dollars and get a red night-light for bathroom use; install the free light-dimming software F.lux on your electronic devices, wear "blue blocker" glasses at home in the evening, and make it a ritual to get some morning sun soon after waking.

✔ **Dip into ketosis periodically.** The ketogenic diet, a high-fat, moderate-protein, low-carb diet (roughly 70 percent fat, 25 percent protein, and 5 percent carbs) helps to lower inflammation, reverse insulin resistance, improve brain function and energy levels, and even detoxify you from heavy metals. When you seriously restrict your carbohydrate consumption, as in about twenty to fifty grams of net carbs (carbohydrates minus fiber) per day, and get most of your calories from healthy fats—coconut oil, MCT oil, ghee, avocado, nuts and seeds, you'll soon lose your cravings for carbs and improve your health in many ways.

Give it a try: Check out CharlieFoundation.org, KetoDiet App.com, and Mark Sisson's book *The Keto Reset Diet: Reboot Your Metabolism in 21 Days and Burn Fat Forever* to help you take the step from Paleo to keto. Verify your keto status with urine keto strips from your local drugstore and aim for ketones of 0.5–3.0 mmol/L. Before you go keto, review the Consider Ketosis cautions on page 70.

✔ **Practice intermittent fasting.** Studies confirm that going without food periodically has numerous health benefits, like improving insulin sensitivity, boosting metabolism and energy levels, and reducing the risk of and even helping to reverse diabetes, cardiovascular disease, cancer, autoimmune conditions, and Alzheimer's.[10]

Give it a try: To ease into it, allow fifteen hours between dinner and breakfast (that means zero calories) a few times per week. Or try skipping dinner a few times a week and just eat breakfast and lunch. As you get used to it, experiment with longer fasts, like eighteen, twenty, or twenty-four hours, or even periodic five-day water fasts for even greater benefits.

✔ **Exercise**, especially these three types, can have both short- and long-term effects on your metabolism: 1. Resistance training with heavy weights produces active muscle tissue, which is more metabolically active than fat, helping you burn more calories even at rest. 2. High intensity interval training (HIIT) and high intensity interval *resistance* training (HIRT), like fast circuits at the gym, are efficient ways to rev up your metabolism. 3. Moderate cardio in a fasted state, for example, first thing in the morning, has been shown to offer superior metabolic effects than exercising after eating.[11]

Give it a try: If you are able, do Dr. Izumi Tabata's super-efficient four-minute HIIT protocol: twenty seconds of all-out effort (e.g., sprint, high step, jumping jacks) and then rest for ten seconds. Repeat eight times, and you're done! You can find four- and twelve-minute Tabata workouts on YouTube.

✔ **Take cold showers** routinely to help boost your metabolism. Like fasting, cold water immersion has a hormetic effect—meaning a little bit of stress has a beneficial effect. Not only does cold water force your body to work harder to keep you warm, thereby burning more calories, it also activates healthy brown fat, which helps to eliminate harmful adipose (white) fat.

Give it a try: Alternate twenty seconds of hot and twenty seconds of cold water in the shower for a few minutes. Or if you have access to a body of cold water, like an unheated pool or a chilly stream, ocean, or lake, take a cold plunge every day if you can.

Per biochemist Steve Fowkes, if your body temperature isn't lower than normal (approximately 98°F), it's possible that you are running a low-level chronic fever because of inflammation and infection that can mask a low body temperature. So, it might be a good idea to reassess your body temperature periodically as you make progress toward clearing infections and inflammation.

Step 4: Unburden Your Immune System

Your immune system is your most powerful curative system—when it's working properly. A well-functioning immune system is balanced and resilient, fending off infections as needed, not overreacting to foods and other harmless environmental factors like pollen or attacking your own body in an autoimmune response. An underactive or poorly functioning immune system increases your susceptibility to disease, like colds, fungal infections, and cancer, while an overactive immune system produces too much inflammation in the body and is prone to hyperactive reactions like allergies and autoimmune conditions.

Years of chronic, low-level inflammation from a poor diet, ongoing stress, lack of (or too much) exercise, and a heavy load of environmental toxins causes your immune system to become imbalanced—tipping to under or overactive. The good news is that the body has an innate regenerative ability, and your immune system can be nudged toward balance within just days or weeks simply by removing sources of inflammation and adopting nourishing lifestyle habits:

✔ **Remove processed foods, sugar, and starchy carbs.** Microbes love sugar; your immune system does not. Studies show that sugar in all forms (glucose, fructose, and sucrose) suppresses immune function for five hours after eating it.[12] To make yourself inhospitable to infectious microbes and improve your immune function, stop eating sugar and feeding the microbes. A Paleo-template diet, which we looked at in depth in the Food chapter, is ideal for nourishing you and not infectious microbes.

✔ **Add immune-enhancing foods.** A wide body of scientific evidence shows that garlic and ginger offer powerful anti-inflammatory and antimicrobial properties—even against drug-resistant pathogens. Coconut oil has been shown to control the fungal pathogen *Candida albicans*. Curcumin, the yellow-orange pigment from the turmeric root, has been shown to modulate the immune system and improve autoimmune conditions, and fermented foods, like sauerkraut and kimchi, are antimicrobial and immune-enhancing. Consume these foods liberally to fight infection and support your immune system.[13, 14, 15, 16]

✔ **Supplement strategically.** More than 148 studies show that Vitamin C (also known as ascorbic acid) may alleviate or prevent infections caused by viruses, bacteria, and protozoa. Take 2,000 to 5,000 mg (ideally corn-free) vitamin C per day in divided doses, with or without food. Vitamin D3 has been shown to modulate the immune system and protect against autoimmune conditions; whereas low levels of vitamin D are associated with increased infection and autoimmune disorders. Get your D levels tested and aim for levels of 70 to 100 ng/ml to heal from or prevent autoimmune conditions with 5,000 to 10,000 IU vitamin D3 in the morning. D3 is most beneficial when taken the same day as vitamin K2 to help get calcium into the right places, like your bones, and not into the wrong places, like your arteries (check out the supplements section of the Healing Foods Toolkit on page 26 for more details). Test your D again within six months. Zinc is an essential element that supports immune function and infection resistance, and correcting zinc deficiencies may improve symptoms of autoimmune and other diseases. Take 30 mg zinc per day with food—either at one time or in divided doses; and take 2 mg copper to balance 30 mgs of zinc. Probiotics including *Lactobacillus*, *Bifidobacterium*, and *Saccharomyces* species have been found to have a beneficial, modulating effect on the immune system. Refer to the Gut chapter for detailed info on probiotics.

✔ **Get restorative sleep.** Fewer than six hours of sleep per night suppresses immune function, turns on inflammatory genes, and increases risk of obesity, type 2 diabetes, and cardiovascular disease (CVD). The immune system functions best when you get enough sleep. Eight or more hours may be ideal for anyone with a chronic health condition.

✔ **Move more.** They say "sitting is the new smoking," and science is backing that up. A review of eighteen studies found that those who sat for the longest periods of time were twice as likely to have diabetes or heart disease and had a greater risk of death compared to those who sat the least.[17] Moderate daily exercise, as in forty minutes of walking most days, reduces systemic inflammation and incidence of upper-respiratory illness (URI).[18] Because sitting for two hours can undo twenty minutes of exercise benefits, make sure you stand and move throughout the day, even if it means using a reminder app like Time Out, Stand Up!, or Awareness.

✔ **Minimize stress.** Chronic stress, like living with chronic illness, caregiving for someone with dementia, or unemployment, has negative effects on almost all functional measures of the immune system. It makes sense to do what you can to eliminate unnecessary stressors and find healthy ways to relax, like soaking in a hot Epsom salts bath, laughing, and slow, conscious breathing, which has been proven to reduce stress and lower inflammation. Explore more relaxation strategies in the Emotional Well-Being Toolkit on page 198.

Step 5: Consider Herbal Antimicrobials

Once you've gotten the data about any underlying infection, you're on your way to healing. Herbal antimicrobials and coconut-based compounds are safe and effective for infections of all types and can be used in conjunction with antibiotics. Unlike antibiotics, herbal remedies do not disrupt the gut microbiome, and microbes rarely develop resistance to herbal medicine. Natural remedies with broad-spectrum, antimicrobial effects include:

- **Monolaurin.** A natural compound found in coconut oil, monolaurin has been shown to have antiviral, antibacterial, antiparasitic, and antifungal properties. A review of research on monolaurin indicates that it is an effective therapy against lipid (fat)-coated bacteria, including *H. pylori*, influenza, *Staphylococcus aureus* (*S.*

aureus), and *Streptococcus agalactiae*, and lipid-coated viruses including herpesviruses, influenza, HIV, and measles virus.[19]

- **Oregano extract (*Origanum vulgare*).** Oil of Mediterranean oregano has anti-inflammatory, antiviral, antibacterial, antiparasitic, and antifungal effects. It has been shown to be more effective against the parasitic amoeba giardia than the drug tinidazole[20] and more effective against yeast infections than the commonly prescribed antifungal drug Diflucan.[21]

- **Olive leaf (*Olea europaea*).** Olive leaf extract has been shown to be effective in animal and in vitro studies against numerous microorganisms, including viruses such as upper-respiratory infections, Coxsackie viruses, and influenza; fungi, including *Candida albicans*; and bacteria, including *E. coli, C. jejuni, H. pylori, S. aureus,* and Methicillin-resistant *Staphylococcus aureus* (MRSA).[22]

- **Wormwood (*Artemisia absinthium L.*).** Wormwood, one of the most bitter of all plants, has antiparasitic properties and is frequently used in conjunction with clove and black walnut extract to eliminate intestinal worms, especially pinworms and roundworms. Wormwood also has antimalarial, antibacterial, and antifungal properties. Studies show that wormwood may be as good as or better than prescription medications at treating SIBO.[23]

- **Berberine.** Berberine, a yellow compound found in several plants including goldenseal (*Hydrastis canadensis*), Oregon grape root (*Berberis aquifolium*), barberry (*Berberis vulgaris*), and Chinese goldthread (*Coptis chinensis*), is antibacterial, antiviral, antiparasitic, and antifungal. It is often used to treat infections in the gastrointestinal tract such as bacteria, viruses, parasites, and yeasts like *Candida albicans*. Berberine has exhibited antiviral effects on the influenza virus in the lab and in humans.[24]

- **Silver.** Hippocrates first described its antimicrobial properties for wound healing in 400 BC. Today silver is used to safely treat infections on its own; or, if antibiotics are used, silver can enhance the effect of antibiotics against gram-negative (often antibiotic-resistant) bacteria called *super bugs.*[25] There are many different types of silver, and according to Raphael d'Angelo, MD, a retired holistic medical doctor who specializes in the diagnosis and treatment of parasites, top types for clearing parasites, yeast, viruses, bacteria, and spirochetes are Silver 500, which is available online from www.HealthMasters.com, and Results RNA's ACS 200 Extra Strength (ES), a strong colloidal silver, available on Amazon, purported to "achieve 99.9999% (complete) kill against *Borrelia burgdorferi, Bartonella henselae* and coinfection microorganisms Powassan virus, MRSA and more without harming healthy flora or damaging human tissue."

Extra Step: Explore "Big Guns" to Clear Stubborn Infections

If you have already dialed in your diet, healed your gut, and addressed infections with the help of an experienced practitioner, and you are *still* not making progress, you may want to consider these adjunctive therapies. Do make sure to discuss these treatments with your practitioner and/or qualified subject matter experts before pursuing them.

- **Explore Helminth Therapy.** If you suffer from asthma, autoimmune liver disease, celiac, Crohn's, MS, type 1 diabetes (T1D) or ulcerative colitis (UC), you may want to explore helminth therapy, a promising treatment that helps to reconstitute a depleted microbiome with a controlled number of benign intestinal worms (helminths) or worm eggs (ova). As unappealing as it sounds to ingest helminths or their ova, people are having remarkable results using helminth therapy.

  Since 2000, small studies have demonstrated success treating autoimmune conditions with helminths, including achieving remission in MS and reversing symptoms of Crohn's disease, ulcerative colitis (UC), and celiac disease.[26] It's still early days, but emerging science and anecdotal evidence for helminth therapy is compelling, if limited. Citizen scientists have been experimenting with helminth therapy for more than a decade and sharing their journeys on a number of websites and forums including:

  helminthictherapywiki.org/wiki/index.php/Helminthic_
    Therapy_Wiki
  www.helminthictherapy.com

- **Address Oral Infections.** David Minkoff, MD and Lyme expert, considers oral health a top priority because if the immune system is dealing with issues in the mouth, like gum disease, root canal teeth, or cavitations (a hole or cavity in the jawbones that may be infected), it can't fight other infections appropriately. He and many other holistic doctors assert that people don't heal unless they clear oral infections, even if the infections are asymptomatic.

Find a biological (also called holistic) dentist by zip code at the International Academy of Biological Dentistry and Medicine (IABDM), iabdm.org/, and inquire about getting a cone beam CT (CBCT) scan of your mouth. The cone beam provides a detailed 3-D image, allowing qualified dental experts to clearly see inflammation, infections, abscess, bone loss, decay, or dead teeth.

- **Consider Hyperbaric Oxygen Therapy (HBOT) for Chronic Lyme Disease.** HBOT is a medical treatment that uses 100 percent oxygen at controlled pressure, as in sixty feet below sea level, for a prescribed amount of time—usually sixty to ninety minutes. The Food and Drug Administration (FDA) has approved HBOT for specific medical uses, including decompression sickness, aka "the bends" suffered by divers, persistent wounds, and burn injuries. Yet there are many other conditions not yet officially approved that may benefit from HBOT as an adjunctive healing therapy, including persistent Lyme. The Lyme bacteria, *Borrelia burgdorferi*, is an anaerobe, meaning it thrives *without* oxygen and, conversely, it cannot survive in an oxygen-rich environment. Additionally, Lyme spirochetes often hide in biofilms, making the infection particularly resistant to antibiotic and herbal remedies. HBOT can penetrate biofilms, especially in combination with a biofilm-busting drug like Alinia (nitazoxanide), which is often prescribed for protozoal (single-celled organism) infections. One study demonstrated compelling findings: eighty-five percent of sixty-six patients with persistent Lyme either experienced partial or complete elimination of Lyme symptoms after undergoing a series of about twenty-two hour-long HBOT sessions.[27]

As you improve your metabolism and adopt healthy lifestyle habits, you'll be shifting your terrain for the better, and your immune system can often eliminate—or at least reduce the magnitude of—persistent infections on its own. By proactively working to clear infections, you are taking a critical step in reversing and preventing autoimmune conditions.

Summary: Top 5 Actions to Address Infections

1. **Stop eating sugar and processed carbs** and unburden your immune system.
2. **Take at least three grams of vitamin C (as ascorbic acid) per day** in divided doses to strengthen your immune system.
3. **Get your vitamin D levels to between 70 and 100 ng/ml,** ideally with sun exposure, but also with supplemental D3 and K2 when you don't get enough sun. Don't forget to check your D levels a few times per year.
4. **Work with an integrative practitioner and get the data** on possible infections.
5. **Consider herbal antimicrobial therapy** instead of gut-harming antibiotic therapy.

CHAPTER 4

Minimize Toxins

Chronic illness is basically a failure of containing the toxic soup in us.

—DIETRICH KLINGHARDT, MD, Ph.D.

Our health is the sum of our relationship with the environment—what we eat, drink, absorb, think, breathe, put on our skin, and how and where we live—and how well our body's natural detoxification system works. Unfortunately, the environment is becoming ever more toxic, we are becoming more and more saturated with toxins each passing year, and we're getting sicker than ever, earlier than ever. As we'll learn in the coming pages, evidence is mounting that our environment's increasing toxic load is having a huge negative impact on our health. Furthermore, our increasing exposure to environmental toxins appears to be fueling the explosive growth of autoimmune conditions.

This toxic assault has greatly intensified over the last century. In 1930, there was virtually no large-scale manufacturing, and thus, there were almost no man-made chemicals in the environment. Experts estimate that there are now more than one hundred thousand synthetic chemicals in commerce in the United States and maybe a million in the environment.[1]

It may surprise you to learn that *fewer than 5 percent of the chemicals used in everyday consumer products in the United States are tested for safety in humans before they are released into commerce.* By contrast, Europe generally follows the "precautionary principle," requiring testing chemicals *before* releasing them for commercial use. Unlike the United States, the European Union (EU) also limits the production, import, and domestic sale of most genetically modified (GM) crops and bans the import of beef and dairy produced from hormone-treated cattle.

No one knows the full picture about how this loosely regulated environment is impacting our health, but we have strong indicators that our collective well-being is taking a dive. Some estimate the average American adult is loaded with 700 contaminants[2], and, more startling, researchers at two major laboratories found an average of 200 toxic chemicals in the cord blood of ten newborns, including flame retardants, mercury, and wastes from burning coal, gasoline, and garbage.[3] Talk about an unfair start!

If you're a parent, it won't surprise you to learn that more than half of our kids, aged zero to seventeen, have at least one chronic health condition. The long list of maladies includes allergies, ADD, ADHD, asthma, autism spectrum disorder, autoimmune conditions, learning disabilities, IQ impairment, obesity, and now, diabetes. Ask any grade school teacher to name a class without food sensitivities, learning challenges, or attention issues, and she or he will be hard pressed to answer you.

Let's consider some specific examples: What used to be called *adult onset diabetes* is now just *type 2 diabetes* because kids are developing it. Children as young as five are getting rheumatoid arthritis (RA), and we even have a new name for it: *juvenile rheumatoid arthritis* (JRA), also known as *juvenile idiopathic*—which literally means *don't know the cause*—arthritis.

Equally troubling is the rising incidence of hypothyroidism in girls and adolescents. Pediatric endocrinologist Andrew J. Bauer, MD, medical director of the Pediatric Thyroid Center at Children's Hospital of Philadelphia, has observed this troubling increase: "We used to think that one or two in one hundred kids and teens would develop hypothyroidism, but now it looks like two to three in one hundred." That's a doubling of thyroid disorders within one practitioner's career.

Autism spectrum disorder (ASD) presents even more shocking statistics. In the 1980s, about one in two thousand children was diagnosed. By 2000, that number jumped to one in one hundred and fifty. By 2008, the number doubled, with one in eighty-eight reported; and today the number has doubled again to about one in forty-five.[4] At a projected annual growth rate of 13 percent, by 2033, one in four children may be afflicted with ASD. Massachusetts Institute of Technology (MIT) senior research scientist

Stephanie Seneff, Ph.D., thinks that's a low estimate. She believes one in two children will have ASD by 2025, thanks mainly to the ubiquitous use of the herbicide (weed killer) glyphosate, the most heavily used agricultural chemical in the history of the world.[5, 6]

What the [Bleep] is Going On?!

These numbers are alarming, and it's understandable if you're feeling shocked. But rather than panicking, we need to ask some tough questions. After all, the better we understand our predicament, the easier it is to make any necessary changes. Sticking our heads in the proverbial sand certainly won't solve any problems. So, let's start with the biggies: *Why is this happening?* And *what can we do about it?*

The best answer we have for the former question is that we are living in a toxic soup that our bodies have never before faced. This unappetizing stew is an accumulation of all the things we are exposed to on a daily basis over our lifetimes: air pollution, chemicals in or added to our water and food, our constant use of plastic, and our frequent use of chemical-laden home and body care products. Each of these is a straw that eventually can break the camel's back. And as we'll see, some are way more than straws.

Our bodies are built to withstand some toxic insults—like the natural phytochemicals in vegetables or small doses of stress—but our natural detoxification systems are becoming overwhelmed by things they have never seen before. These toxins are a top trigger for autoimmune disorders, and given the massive and growing number of chemicals we are exposed to each day, they may well top the list. If you have an autoimmune condition or a genetic predisposition to get one, or if you have a genetically weak detoxification pathway, like nearly half the population, then you may be at greater risk of harm from toxins.

Before you throw up your hands in despair, know that you are *far* more in control of your environment than you ever thought possible. Even if you're already dealing with a crushing body burden, you *can* recover your health. Many people with autoimmune conditions have healed by cleaning up their personal environment. You can, too! It starts with awareness and then some simple shopping changes.

The bottom line: to heal from or prevent disease, you must minimize your exposure to toxins, reduce your toxic load, and optimize your body's

---

Defining Toxins

Toxin: Often used as a catchall for all harmful or poisonous substances. Technically, it refers to any harmful protein produced naturally by living organisms, like snake venom, bacterial waste, and other internally produced chemicals.

Toxicant: Any harmful or poisonous, man-made or naturally occurring substance, like chemicals, metals, mold, or radiation.

Toxic: Capable of producing harmful or poisonous effects.

Neoantigen: New compound, often a combination of a toxicant that binds to human tissue (e.g., BPA binds to human protein), which the immune system views as dangerous and attacks in an autoimmune response.

Exposome: The full range of environmental exposures that influence our health.

---

natural detoxification systems. I'll help you become aware of what toxins you may be exposed to—inside and out—so you can limit your exposure, reduce your likely already-overloaded body burden, increase your body's detoxification ability, strengthen body systems adversely affected, and assist your body in becoming more tolerant.

Expanding Our Understanding of Toxins

When you think of a "toxicant," what leaps to mind? Perhaps a poisonous chemical like rat poison or a smokestack billowing out industrial pollution. I'll bet you never imagined your lipstick or favorite cologne or that paper cup holding your morning coffee contains toxicants, but think again.

Did you know that many lipsticks contain lead? Or that most fragrances contain phthalates (pronounced THALL-ates)—chemicals used in making plastic? Or that disposable paper cups are often lined with polyethylene, a type of plastic? While one tube of lipstick, a few spritzes of cologne, or several paper cups of coffee are not going to trigger an autoimmune condition, the steady exposure to these kinds of low-level toxicants that seep into your skin, get inhaled up your nose, or flow into your gut can, over time, bind to human tissue, result in inflammation and a leaky gut, spark an outsized immune system reaction, and spiral into an autoimmune cascade.

When defining toxins, we must include any substance that is poisonous or toxic—that is, any substance that can harm living organisms and which is capable of inducing antibody formation, meaning it can cause our immune system to mount a defensive reaction. We tend to think of toxins as harmful elements somewhere out there in the environment, but under this broader definition, we must consider any substance that has potential to harm us, including what's produced within our bodies. Toxins known to trigger autoimmune conditions are both "out there" and "in here." Let's zoom in to get a closer look:

Exotoxins (outside toxicants) include chemicals found in air, water, and food:

- **Chemicals** used in industrial production and farming, water treatment, dry cleaning, home cleaning, and body care products.
- **Metals**, including mercury, lead, aluminum, arsenic, and cadmium, which are found in water, fish, soil and the air we breathe.
- **Medications**, including many prescription drugs, antibiotics, and vaccines.
- Many **food additives**, preservatives, and sweeteners, like monosodium glutamate (MSG) and artificial sweeteners.
- Many **genetically modified organisms (GMO)** contain built-in pesticides or herbicides.
- Many **allergenic foods**, including gluten, dairy, soy, etc., can be especially toxic to people prone to autoimmune issues.
- **Air pollution**, including secondhand cigarette smoke and vehicle exhaust.
- **Mold**, which produces poisonous mycotoxins (e.g., aflatoxin and Ochratoxin A [OTA]).
- **Heterocyclic amines (HCAs) and polycyclic aromatic hydrocarbons (PAHs)**, chemicals formed when you use high-heat cooking or char-grill meat, poultry, or fish.
- Chronic or heavy exposure to **electromagnetic frequencies (EMF) and "dirty electricity"**—high-frequency voltage variations/spikes on electrical wiring—may be associated with many chronic health disorders, including autism, infertility, heart disease, and brain cancer.[7]

Endotoxins (inside toxins), also known as biotoxins, are byproducts made by your own body and/or by critters that live inside you:

- **Bacteria, fungus, and yeast** in high proportions and/or harmful species in your gut can be toxic.

- **Yeast and *Candida*** produce a toxic chemical related to formaldehyde (used in embalming fluid) called *acetaldehyde*.

- **Lipopolysaccharides (LPS)**, bacterial toxins, can leak into your bloodstream and even cross the blood-brain barrier, causing an outsized immune system reaction in your body and brain. LPS has been detected in higher levels in the brain of people with late-onset Alzheimer's disease, compared with controls.[8]

- **Poorly detoxified hormones, like estrogen or xenoestrogens** (toxic chemicals that compete with estrogen) may recirculate and bind to estrogen receptor sites, blocking normal hormone function.

- **Chronic stress and negative thinking** can disrupt your neuroendocrine system and the balance of your microbiome, edging out beneficial bacteria and setting the stage for harmful bacteria to take over.

- **Lasting, unresolved, or unexpressed negative emotions** like anger, grief, or resentment can get stored in our nervous systems. Maybe you've heard the phrase, "the issue is in the tissue." Many integrative cancer experts can attest that unresolved emotional pain contributes significantly to the development of cancer.

What's in Your Personal Exposome?

Ever heard of the exposome? It's the word scientists are using to describe the full range of environmental exposures that influence our health. Each one of us has our own exposome that varies in size depending upon the number of chemicals we encounter on a daily basis. How many chemicals do you think you've encountered today? Hundreds, maybe thousands? They're in the air, the water, in our personal care products, our food, our clothes, our furniture, our buildings, our vehicles, our smart phones and computers. Some are simply unavoidable, and many are a choice you can make once you have the information.

While the government does not require advance testing and only loosely regulates many toxins, the Environmental Working Group (EWG) fills an important gap. EWG.org is a nonprofit, nonpartisan organization dedicated to educating and empowering people about the hidden toxins in our environment. A 2004 EWG study found that the average woman uses twelve personal care products per day, containing 168 different synthetic chemicals. While most men use fewer products, they're still exposed to about eighty-five different man-made chemicals daily—and that's just in personal care products like toothpaste, shampoo, shaving cream, deodorant, cologne, and hair products.[9] There's also the water you shower in, which, if unfiltered, likely contains chlorine, chloramine, and/or fluoride, two known cancer-causing compounds.[10] And we haven't even left the bathroom!

If you decide to have fruit-flavored yogurt, it may contain twenty grams of sugar (a toxicant, according to our definition), which contributes to obesity, diabetes, and immune dysfunction. Or if sugar-free, it contains artificial sweetener, which is a neurotoxin (toxic to the brain), along with multiple artificial flavors, preservatives, gums and colors—each of which are known autoimmune triggers. That plain, unsweetened, organic yogurt—ideally coconut and stored in a glass jar—is sounding better all the time!

KEY CONCEPT: *Practice the precautionary principle and consider toxicants guilty until proven innocent.*

Perhaps you have a new car? That "new car smell" is actually a chemical cocktail of more than two hundred compounds that have not yet off-gassed or dissipated into the surrounding environment. If you commute, you'll likely encounter other cars and trucks that emit hazardous exhaust, the worst of which is diesel. If you decide to have *farmed* salmon for dinner, you may encounter PCBs—chemicals known as *persistent organic pollutants*, linked to cancer and autoimmune disease; and if you grill it, you will encounter cancer-causing heterocyclic amines (HCAs) and polycyclic aromatic hydrocarbons (PAHs)—chemicals formed when muscle meat is cooked using high-temperature methods.

I can hear you sighing. You might even be tempted to throw this book across the room, thinking, why even bother? We're doomed anyway! Please bear with me; I know it can be a lot to take in. Rather than being resigned, use this information to empower yourself so you can take actions to protect yourself and your family.

We'll get to the Detoxification Toolkit shortly, but first, let's examine what we're up against. We'll look at the ways a heavy toxic load can impact our health, including two short stories that illustrate how heavy toxic loads led to autoimmune conditions. Then we'll get three experts' insights into toxicants as primary drivers of chronic disease and look at a snapshot of the top toxicants linked to autoimmune conditions. And finally, we'll meet a woman who was brought down by a crushing body burden and who healed by embracing a detox lifestyle.

Our Buckets Runneth Over

Under normal circumstances, our bodies are designed to detoxify themselves, primarily through the liver. When not overburdened, your liver can transform potentially harmful toxins into harmless biological products that are escorted out of the body via your colon and kidneys into the toilet. But when the toxic load becomes overwhelming, your liver can't keep up. To add insult to injury, many individuals have a genetic glitch that hampers their ability to detoxify, which amplifies inflammation and increases the risk of disease. Unprocessed toxins accumulate in the body, getting stored in fat cells and other tissues, setting the stage for inflammation and disease.

Scientists use the phrases *total toxic load* or *total body burden* to refer to the total amount of external and internal stressors on your system at any one time. If our cumulative exposure to toxins is high and our detoxification system is compromised—due to environmental factors, genetic predisposition, or both—then our total body burden will be high.

Think back to that bucket I had you imagine when I shared my story in chapter one. Over the years, toxins, infections, emotional traumas, and other stressors of modern life fill your bucket, until one day the bucket overflows. The overflowing bucket is a metaphor for an overloaded detoxification system. Once the liver, a primary organ for detoxification, can't keep pace with the toxicants coming in, symptoms begin to arise. As your bucket teeters on the brink, there are many ways your body responds. Different toxins can have different effects, depending on the amount, timing, duration, and pattern of exposure.

Naturally, the greater your total toxic load, the greater the risk of harm to your body. As the toxic burden increases, your body may become overwhelmed; your immune system may become more impaired and less able to produce protective antibodies and to generate the master antioxidant, glutathione. The less glutathione you have available, the more vulnerable you are to the harmful effects of toxins, and in a vicious cycle, the less able you will be to get them out of your system.

When the toxic load overwhelms the detox organs, which include the skin, lungs, liver, kidneys, and colon, a cascade of health problems may ensue, including chronic inflammation, leaky gut, DNA damage, autoimmune reactivity, full-blown autoimmune disease, and even cancer and Alzheimer's.

Chemicals can have toxic effects through a variety of mechanisms and even at very low doses. They can:

- Harm the gut—disrupt microbiome balance and cause a leaky gut
- Impair the immune system
- Damage mitochondria, our cells' internal energy source
- Damage cellular DNA and cell membranes, changes that can even get passed to the next generation
- Disrupt hormone balance, blocking thyroid function or estrogen levels
- Cause oxidative stress, which means your body breaks down faster than it can repair
- Block insulin receptor sites, promoting obesity, diabetes, and cancer
- Hamper detoxification via poisoned enzyme systems
- Hamper the body's ability to make and recycle glutathione, the master antioxidant, which your body needs for detoxification
- Bind to your tissues and form a new, foreign molecule called a *neoantigen*, which the immune system views as dangerous and attacks in an autoimmune response

With enough time and buildup, any one of these issues will cause symptoms. When the last drop finally causes the bucket to overflow, the first major signs of ill health often appear.

Even worse, some people with genetically weaker detoxification pathways, like me, may have *smaller buckets*. That means it doesn't take as much or as long to fill the bucket, which may explain why the MS emerged when I was nineteen. My personal body burden included a hefty dose of chronic stress, probably beginning in utero (my birth mother was only fifteen and likely very overwhelmed); extra vaccines for international travel; multiple mercury fillings, thanks to my big sweet tooth; and sensitivities to gluten and casein.

How Toxicants Trigger Autoimmune Conditions: Two Short Stories

We now understand how our bodies' natural detoxification systems can get overwhelmed and stop functioning properly. And we know the various ways toxicants can harm us. The following real-life stories vividly illustrate how chronic exposure to toxins can eventually lead to autoimmune and other inflammatory disorders.

Terry Wahls, MD, is well known for healing her progressive form of MS with food, as documented in her book *The Wahls Protocol: A Radical New Way to Treat All Chronic Autoimmune Conditions Using Paleo Principles*. What may not be so well known is that she suspects that toxic chemicals were the biggest culprits in the development of her MS.

Terry grew up on a family farm in Iowa. In order to meet growing production demand, Terry's father began using pesticides and herbicides like atrazine, the second most widely used herbicide in the United States, to control weeds. Atrazine is a potent endocrine (hormone) disruptor and has been shown to chemically castrate male frogs at low doses.[11] After she left the farm, she experienced further chemical exposure: in medical school, Terry came in frequent contact with high levels of formaldehyde. By her second year, she began to experience strange symptoms, including hearing problems, trouble with her balance, and increasing facial pain. Looking back, Terry has no doubt that long-term exposure to toxic chemicals in childhood and young adulthood created a heavy body burden that greatly contributed to the development of her MS.

Sometimes the sheer load of long-term exposure to toxicants can fill a normal-sized bucket, and sometimes the bucket itself is smaller or more sensitive to the harmful effects of toxicants, and it may take fewer insults for troubling symptoms to surface.

Functional Medicine pioneer Mark Hyman, MD, developed debilitating chronic fatigue syndrome (CFS) as a result

Signs of a Heavy Total Body Burden

The signs and symptoms of a heavy body burden are identical to symptoms reported by people suffering from autoimmune disorders; you may not be aware that these are also telltale signs of toxin overload:

- Energy problems: profound fatigue, lethargy
- Sleep troubles
- Digestive problems: bloating, constipation, diarrhea, foul-smelling stools, gas, heartburn
- Aches and pains: headaches, muscle aches, joint pain
- Sinus problems: chronic post-nasal drip, congestion
- Mental issues: depression, brain fog, trouble concentrating
- Neurological problems: dizziness, tremors
- Weight problems: unexplained weight gain or weight-loss resistance
- Skin problems: rashes, eczema, psoriasis, acne
- Hormonal issues
- High or low blood pressure

of low-level mercury poisoning that may have built up in his body for more than twenty years. As a child, Mark ate "endless" tuna fish sandwiches (tuna is the most common and biggest source of mercury in the diet), and he had a mouthful of silver fillings. In his thirties, Mark spent a year in China to develop a medical center in Beijing, where homes were heated by coal, and black skies on summer days were common. While he was in China breathing polluted air and eating lots of sushi, he was unaware that mercury was slowly but surely accumulating in his system. At the time, Mark also had no idea that he is among nearly half the population missing a key gene—GSTM1 (glutathione S-transferase M1)—that controls production of enzymes necessary for detoxifying mercury and many other toxins.

When he returned to the United States, Mark started having a number of perplexing and seemingly unrelated symptoms. He felt weak, exhausted, and had trouble thinking. He developed muscle pain and twitches, insomnia, digestive problems, food allergies, anxiety, and depression. For a previously bright, energetic, and confident doctor, this was an especially frustrating and confusing time. Unable to find a doctor who could properly diagnose and treat him, Mark began to do his own research, searching for clues to his collection of symptoms, which he finally determined was CFS. A colleague told him that many people with CFS have a big burden of heavy metals, so Mark took a urine test and was shocked by the results. Normal levels of mercury are less than three micrograms per liter (mcg/L), and anything over 50 mcg/L is considered mercury poisoning. Mark's level was nearly 200 mcg/L!

Mark consulted with many experts and then underwent a careful, deliberate detoxification process that included healing his gut, adding detoxifying foods, supplements, intravenous glutathione, and vitamin C, oral chelators (compounds that bond to metals to help escort them out of the body), and saunas. While he began to feel better within weeks, it would take over a year for Mark to rid his body of mercury, heal his damaged mitochondria, and return to his normal high energy levels.

The Toxin-Disease Connection

The list of diseases linked to toxin overload is long—arthritis, CFS, digestive disorders, fibromyalgia syndrome, heart disease, menstrual problems, Parkinson's, and type 2 diabetes, among many others—but let's look at some specific examples that disclose an explicit relationship between toxins and chronic illness.

Doctors Joseph Pizzorno, Walter Crinnion, and Aristo Vojdani have each witnessed the epidemic growth of chronic disease for more than forty years. Today, they all make compelling connections between toxicants and our ill health.

Joseph Pizzorno, ND, is a unique voice in the toxin discussion because over the half century during which he's been practicing medicine, he's witnessed massive changes in the drivers of disease. In 1975, when he first started seeing patients, people got sick primarily due to nutritional deficiencies or poor lifestyle habits. In his first year as a doctor, he had only one diabetic patient, and that pretty much correlated with the national average.

Sixty years ago, only about 1 percent of the U.S. population had type 2 diabetes. Today, that number has grown to approximately 10 percent. Some projections say more than a third of the population will have diabetes by 2050—and that's only people who are diagnosed. If you include undiagnosed diabetics and the insulin resistant or prediabetic, the majority of the population may be afflicted by 2050!

Concerned about the diabetes explosion, Dr. Pizzorno dug into the research. The more he studied, the more he discovered that most chronic disease, including diabetes, is due to environmental toxins. To test his hypothesis, he compared people with the highest levels of specific toxins to those with the lowest levels and discovered strong correlations. For example, people with the highest level of organochlorine pesticides, which are commonly sprayed on conventionally grown fruits and vegetables— especially kale—had *twelve times the incidence of diabetes* compared to people with none of these chemicals in their bodies.[12] As he dug deeper, he found that toxic chemicals—like pesticides, arsenic, and plastics— bind to insulin receptor sites, preventing insulin from entering the cells, and harm the gut microbiome and metabolism. Dr. Pizzorno now believes toxins are mostly to blame for the increasing incidence of diabetes over the past fifty years.

Another doctor with a front-row seat to the impact of toxins on health is Walter Crinnion, M.D., author, toxin expert, and a practitioner of environmental medicine since the early 1980s. When he started his practice, many of his patients were young women who wanted to have a baby but couldn't conceive. Back then Dr. Crinnion just cleaned up their diet and put them on a multiple vitamin. He had a success rate of 90 percent where his patients were finally able to get pregnant within six to twelve months. Today, he claims, you can't do that because of the big and worsening load of environmental toxins. Now, Dr. Crinnion reports seeing men in their twenties and thirties with the testosterone level of sixty-year-olds—young men with clinical hypogonadism, simply because they're breathing air!

Research indicates that the incidence of male infertility has been steadily increasing in industrial countries from 7 percent to 8 percent in 1960 to 20 percent to 35 percent today[13]; and a 2017 meta-analysis confirms that air pollutants indeed lower reproductive capacities of both animals and humans.[14]

Exposure to Toxicants Triggers Multiple Chemical Sensitivities (MCS): Aristo Vojdani's Story

Autoimmunologist Aristo Vojdani, Ph.D., has been both personally affected by and professionally interested in the effects of environmental toxins on the immune system. In the early 1980s, as a postdoc at UCLA, Dr. Vojdani was studying the effect of toxic chemicals on mice. By injecting a tiny amount of chemicals into three different strains of mice—one sensitive to chemicals, one resistant to their effects, and one in the middle—he observed that the sensitive mice developed a large tumor, the middle ones developed a small tumor, and the resistant ones did not develop cancer at all. Dr. Vojdani says human beings, like mice, have different vulnerabilities. He goes on to say that twenty percent of the population, when exposed to chemicals, will develop multiple chemical sensitivities (MCS), maybe 20 percent will be resistant, and 60 percent are somewhere in the middle.

Dr. Vojdani personally identifies with the sensitive mice. After working in the lab for about five years, he began to develop severe headaches and fibromyalgia-like pain all over his body. Doctors told him he was stressed out and just needed to take a vacation; so he took two weeks off and felt much better—not, he says, because he was more relaxed, but because he got a break from the chemicals in the lab! Finally, he saw Gunnar Heuser, MD, a neurotoxicologist who diagnosed him with MCS and told him that if he really wanted to help people, he should start a lab to do testing for people like himself. And that's how Dr. Vojdani got started developing chemical antibody testing, which eventually evolved into Immunosciences Laboratories and Cyrex Laboratories, two companies focused on detecting problematic environmental factors often implicated in autoimmune disorders—like chemicals, viruses, Lyme infections, food and dietary components.

Dr. Vojdani told me in an interview how chemicals are changing our bodies' tissues and triggering the autoimmune response:

"Chemicals get into our body, bind to our tissue, and change the very structure of our body parts, whether it be our thyroid, adrenal gland, or myelin sheath, etc., into a structure that our immune system doesn't recognize. This new structure becomes a neoantigen—a new foreign substance or enemy bound to human tissue for the immune system to attack. Just doing its job, the immune system then produces "autoantibodies" ("soldiers" that destroy our own cells) to attack the new antigen—that is, our own new, foreign-looking tissue."

Dr. Vojdani and his colleague Datis Kharrazian, DHSc, DC, MS—aka Dr. K.—explain the reason why some people develop autoimmune conditions and others do not. The difference comes down to a concept called *immune tolerance*, and that's related directly to the immune system, which decides which elements to tolerate and which to attack. Dr. K. says that by urinary measurements, *everyone* is exposed to high levels of chemicals from plastic and mercury, but that doesn't tell you whether someone will develop an autoimmune condition or whether the plastic or metals are the reason behind someone's existing autoimmune condition. The key issue, Dr. K. emphasizes, is whether they've lost immune tolerance to the chemical; once immune tolerance is lost, the immune system starts producing antibodies to the toxicant.

So, levels of any particular toxicant in a person's system may not be as significant a factor in the disease equation as the levels of antibodies to the toxicant. It follows that the higher the level of antibodies roaming in the bloodstream, the greater the possible damage from the autoimmune attack. And conversely, the lower the levels, the less damage expected from an autoimmune assault. Good news, then, that testing is now available to measure antibody levels to common chemicals and metals (see pages 154–59). As for restoring immune tolerance? That's a natural byproduct of addressing all of F.I.G.H.T.S.. We lower levels of inflammation as we remove the bad stuff, and we increase our resilience to a broad array of stressors as we embrace nourishing habits.

Toxicants and Autoimmune Conditions: The Science

While there are many more environmental toxins that have been implicated in or proven to trigger autoimmune conditions, including asbestos, dioxin, lead, trichloroethylene (TCE), and silicone breast implants, for practical purposes, I'm highlighting some of the most common toxicants scientifically linked to autoimmune disorders:

Pesticides: DDT, Atrazine
Main sources of exposure: water and conventionally raised (nonorganic) foods
Conditions they're linked to: ADHD, Alzheimer's, type 2 diabetes, early menopause, Parkinson's, RA, lupus, and cancers

Many different kinds of synthetic (human-made) pesticides are used to kill insects in agriculture or in products used in homes, schools, parks, and gardens. Organophosphate pesticides, originally developed in the 1940s as highly toxic biological warfare agents, are the top insecticide used in the United States. The Environmental Working Group offers an annual "Dirty Dozen" list of the produce with the most pesticide residue. Some fruits, like conventionally grown strawberries and grapes, may have residue from up to fifteen pesticides!

DDT, an organochloride pesticide, was banned in the United States in the 1970s, as it was linked to cancer and reproductive harm, but DDT is a persistent organic pollutant, or POP for short, meaning it's extremely difficult to remove it from the environment and our bodies. The half-life (the time it takes to degrade half of the chemical) of DDT in the human body is ten years. Dr. Pizzorno suspects that nearly 45 percent of Alzheimer's cases are linked to DDT alone.

In a study of three hundred thousand death certificates in twenty-six states over a fourteen-year period, researchers examined links between occupation and death from autoimmune disease. They found that farm workers who worked in fields where pesticides were used were more likely to die from an autoimmune disease, including RA, lupus, and systemic sclerosis. But it's not just farm workers who are affected. A long-term study of seventy-seven thousand post-menopausal women showed that women who used or were exposed to pesticides at home or in the workplace were at greater risk for developing lupus, RA, and other autoimmune conditions.[15]

Bisphenol A (BPA)
Main sources of exposure: plastic beverage bottles, canned foods, sales receipts

Conditions it is linked to: multiple autoimmune conditions, cardio-vascular disease, type 2 diabetes, and neurodegenerative diseases

BPA is an endocrine-disrupting chemical used to harden plastic. It's ubiquitous in consumer products, and the long list includes plastic water bottles, food containers, and canned foods—especially canned soup, cooking utensils, and toys. And it's also in *us*. In one study, more than 90 percent of Americans were found to have detectable levels of BPA in their urine. BPA can leach into liquids and food—especially when containers are heated. Studies show it causes many immune reactions involved in the expression and progression of autoimmune disease.[16] Don't be fooled by "BPA-free" labeling. Something could be BPA-free but contain newer versions like BPAF, BPB, BPF, and BPS, which may be as or *more* harmful than BPA.[17] Certainly makes you want to make your own soup!

Mercury

Main sources of exposure: seafood (especially large, predatory fish like shark, marlin, swordfish, king mackerel, tilefish, and tuna), dental amalgam fillings, coal dust in air

Conditions it is linked to: CFS, headaches, depression, autism, cardiovascular disease, Alzheimer's disease, ALS, MS, Parkinson's disease, cancer

Mercury is a naturally occurring element and ubiquitous environmental contaminant released from the combustion of coal and fossil fuels, and from mining and industrial chemical production that contaminates lakes, rivers, and the ocean, bioaccumulating in bigger fish that are high on the food chain. Scientific literature published within the past fifty years continues to implicate mercury exposure from fish and dental amalgams, as well as from any other chronic low-grade mercury exposure, as a contributing factor in the development of MS.[18] Patrick Kingsley, MD, a leading MS expert, reported that of the nearly four thousand patients he had seen with MS, *only five didn't suffer from mercury poisoning.*[19]

PCBs (polychlorinated biphenyls): used in electrical equipment like transistors and capacitors

Main source of exposure: farmed (e.g., Atlantic or Scottish) salmon

Conditions they are linked to: autoimmune conditions, especially thyroid and RA, type 2 diabetes, chronic infections, cancers, lowered IQ

PCBs are POPs that are no longer produced in the United States because they are linked to cancer in humans; yet they are still found in the environment because the half-life of PCBs is up to twenty-five years. PCBs bioaccumulate (increase in concentration) as they move up the food chain to levels millions of times higher in fish and animals than levels found in water or soil. Studies confirm that PCBs harm tight junctions, creating a leaky gut and contributing to the advent and progression of many diseases, including diabetes, allergies, asthma, and autoimmune disorders.[20, 21]

Medications: many over-the-counter and prescription drugs
Main sources of exposure: antibiotics, antifungals, antihypertensives, anti-inflammatories, cholesterol-lowering meds, synthetic estrogens, oral contraceptives, biologics like TNF blockers, and chemotherapy
Conditions they are linked to: leaky gut, autoimmune conditions like lupus, Parkinson's, RA, and cancer

We know medications often come with side effects, and sometimes those effects can be especially unwanted, like an autoimmune condition—especially when you are taking a medication to treat an existing autoimmune condition or cancer! Some common over-the-counter medications, like non-steroidal anti-inflammatories (NSAIDs), create a leaky gut, which opens the gate to the autoimmune cascade. More than ninety medications, including drugs to treat heart disease, thyroid disease, hypertension, and neuropsychiatric disorders, have been implicated in causing drug-induced lupus erythematosus (DILE). Statins used for lowering cholesterol can trigger autoimmune myopathy (muscle disease), and oral contraceptives may precipitate RA.[22, 23, 24, 25]

Aluminum
Main sources of exposure: antiperspirants, aluminum-based household products, and vaccines
Conditions it is linked to: dementia, Alzheimer's, autism, Parkinson's disease, autoimmune syndrome induced by adjuvants (ASIA) spectrum, multiple autoimmune conditions

Aluminum salts, the most widely used vaccine additive, can trigger a post-vaccine syndrome called autoimmune syndrome induced by adjuvants (ASIA) spectrum, or Shoenfeld's syndrome, for the autoimmunologist who discovered it. Initial symptoms may include chronic fatigue, pain, weakness, and cognitive impairment; and it may eventually lead to any number of autoimmune diseases, including MS, systemic lupus erythematosus, and RA.

Phthalates

Main sources of exposure: flexible plastic (like shower curtains), food packaging, and storage—especially food microwaved in plastic, and personal care products, including lotions, nail polish, hair gel, deodorant, cosmetics, and fragrances
Conditions they are linked to: Obesity, infertility, birth defects in baby boys, asthma, endometriosis, fibroids, type 2 diabetes, lupus, cancer—notably of reproductive organs: prostate, uterus, ovary, and breast

Phthalates are chemicals used to make plastic flexible and to maintain color and scent in home and personal care products, cosmetics, and fragrances. They harm human physiology by disrupting hormones and blocking insulin and thyroid receptors. One study of phthalates in young men found that just two weeks' use of chemical-containing personal care products including lotion, cologne, deodorant, and mouthwash raised the body burden of phthalates *three hundred times,* not merely 300 percent.[26]

Food additives: added glucose (sugar), sodium (salt), emulsifiers (chemicals that make products creamier or more stable), gluten, transglutaminase (an enzyme that serves as food protein "glue"), nanoparticles, artificial sweeteners, monosodium glutamate (MSG), and soy extracts
Main sources of exposure: processed, packaged and fast foods and beverages
Conditions they are linked to: Leaky gut, autoimmune conditions, metabolic syndrome (obesity, insulin resistance, elevated cholesterol, heart disease risk, etc.), and cancer

A recent study of industrial food additives aimed at enhancing qualities like taste, smell, texture, and shelf life found a significant connection between the increased use of processed foods, the advent of leaky gut, and an increase in the incidence of autoimmune diseases. Some food additives, like MSG and aspartame (artificial sweetener), are excitotoxins, excitatory neurotoxins that overstimulate neuron receptors and may trigger autoimmune disease.[27, 28]

Arsenic

Main sources of exposure: water, chicken, brown rice, mining, wood preservative, pesticides

Conditions they are linked to: autoimmune conditions, diabetes, cardiovascular disease, gout, and lung, prostate, and liver cancer

Arsenic is a natural component of the earth's crust and is widely distributed throughout the environment in the air, water, and land. It is highly toxic in its inorganic form—the type that is naturally found in soil and groundwater as a result of minerals dissolving from weathered rocks. (Note: here, *organic* and *inorganic* are chemistry terms and should not be confused with food sold as organic.) People are exposed to elevated levels of inorganic arsenic through drinking contaminated water (especially well water); using contaminated water in food preparation and irrigation of food crops; eating contaminated food—especially conventionally raised chicken and brown rice, which has higher levels of arsenic than white rice; and smoking tobacco. Although national standards for drinking water exist, in 2015, thirty-two states were found to have arsenic levels above the legal limit.[29]

Mold and mycotoxins: *Cladosporium*, *Penicillium*, *Alternaria*, *Aspergillus*, and *Stachybotrys chartarum* (sometimes referred to as "toxic black mold")

Main sources of exposure: water-damaged buildings

Conditions they are linked to: allergies, asthma, mold illness, now commonly called chronic inflammatory response syndrome (CIRS), autoimmune conditions

When we think of air pollution, we typically think of outside air, like smog, smoke, and vehicle exhaust, but experts say indoor air quality may be an even bigger health risk. It's estimated that indoor air pollutants, including mold and mycotoxins, may be contributing to more than 50 percent of illnesses. A large investigation of patients with multiple health complaints attributable to confirmed exposure to mixed-molds infestation confirms that exposure to molds and their associated mycotoxins in water-damaged buildings can lead to multiple health problems involving the central nervous system and the immune system, including increased risk for autoimmunity. [30, 31]

Factors That Increase Your Risk of Harm

Many factors can make you more susceptible to the harmful effects of toxicants. You may want to consider this list as a way to gauge whether or not you're more or less susceptible:

- Increased or ongoing exposure
- Nutrient deficiencies (B vitamins, antioxidants, magnesium, selenium, etc.)
- High-carbohydrate, low-protein diet
- Heavy metals
- Chronic stress and emotional trauma
- Intestinal dysbiosis
- Single nucleotide polymorphisms (SNPs) (pronounced SNIPS)— common genetic variants in detoxification gene enzymes that indicate impaired detoxification capacity

What can you do when faced with the seemingly insurmountable barrage of toxicants and other factors that make you more susceptible to harm? Practice the precautionary principle and take proactive action to safeguard your health. While you may feel saturated with information right now, I want you to feel empowered that you can gain new levels of freedom by following what others have successfully done. The following story offers hope for anyone concerned about the status of his or her own bulging toxin bucket.

Detoxifying to Heal: Amie Valpone's Story

Amie Valpone, Functional Medicine nutrition and wellness expert and author of the best-selling cookbook *Eating Clean, The 21-Day Plan to Detox, Fight Inflammation and Reset Your Body,* has been there and back. Amie was terribly sick for ten years, until she discovered that she has a genetic weakness that about a third of us share—a defect in the swear word–sounding MTHFR (methylenetetrahydrofolate reductase) gene that makes you more susceptible to environmental toxins—and did what she could to correct for it. Amie's story is a testament to the power of daily detoxification to empty the bucket and recover vibrant health.

For ten years, Amie suffered from multiple chronic illnesses and a heavy toxin burden, including Lyme disease, systemic *Candida*, polycystic ovarian syndrome (PCOS), hypothyroidism, chronic fatigue syndrome, and small intestinal bacterial overgrowth (SIBO), a load of heavy metals, parasites, and mold toxicity. As she explained in an interview, what made this so baffling to her was that she was a "good girl who lived a pretty clean life." She avoided obvious toxins like drugs, alcohol, processed foods, and fast foods, and other than being lactose intolerant, she was unaware of any sensitivities.

The first sign that anything was wrong showed up in her early twenties when her legs swelled with forty pounds of water weight that left her "unable to wear anything but spandex." First, she was misdiagnosed with leukemia, and then she contracted a deadly infection (*Clostridium difficile* or *C. diff*) and was given twenty-four hours to live. She survived, but barely. She went on disability for a year, saw doctors all over the country, including at the Mayo Clinic, and accumulated nearly half a million dollars in out-of-pocket medical expenses, all in a quest to figure out why she was sick in the first place. It wasn't until she came upon integrative and Functional Medicine that Amie discovered the glitch in her detox genetics; she had the swearword-sounding MTHFR (methylenetetrahydrofolate reductase) gene mutation.

Amie explains that carriers of this genetic mutation are unable to detoxify efficiently and, as a result, toxins can accumulate and lead to a host of autoimmune conditions and even cancer. Studies estimate that 40 percent of the population may have the MTHFR mutation, meaning they are more susceptible to harm from environmental toxins like herbicides, pesticides, antibiotics, and heavy metals. An MTHFR mutation hampers methylation, a complex process that's involved with detoxification, DNA repair, and regulating inflammation. Simply put, you need to be able to methylate to stay healthy, and Amie was not methylating.

To give herself a fighting chance, Amie educated herself and embarked on a whole-life detox. She examined everything in her life and made intentional choices about everything she put on and into her body. She started with food, removing gluten, dairy, soy, refined sugar, corn, eggs, processed food, and food additives, and she healed her gut. She removed all chemical-laden home and body care products and only used nontoxic alternatives. She stopped drinking tap water and started filtering her drinking water and shower water.

In short, Amie got back to basics, eating real food and drinking real water—without added chemicals. To help remove the metals, Amie worked with a detox expert and underwent careful IV chelation treatments over two years. She also had her mercury fillings safely removed by a biological dentist who made sure Amie did not inhale any harmful mercury vapors during the procedure.

As she slowly detoxed, she started feeling better, her blood work improved, and within four years, Amie felt well enough to go back to school to officially study nutrition. In 2009, Amie quit corporate America to launch The Healthy Apple, LLC, where she now cooks for clients and helps them recover from seemingly insurmountable health conditions, like she did.

Amie is proof that living a detox lifestyle can help us transcend symptoms and diagnoses. The bonus is you don't need to spend ten years and half a million dollars to get well. It can be far simpler. Keep the bad stuff out and let the good stuff in, just as much as you can.

Detoxification Toolkit

You can't turn back the clock or avoid toxicants altogether, but you can learn more about your personal exposures, make lifestyle changes to minimize further exposure, and strengthen your body's defenses. There is enormous hope that you can regain your health, even after dealing with the negative consequences of a huge body burden.

Experts agree that the best approach to removing toxins is proactive, gentle, and continuous detoxification rather than a few harsh and quick cleanses per year. True, cellular detoxification takes time. You don't accumulate a heavy body burden overnight, nor should you expect to unload the burden all at once. Detoxification experts Dan Pompa, PScD, Chris Shade, Ph.D., and Wendy Myers, FDN-P, NC, CHHC, are careful to set expectations with their clients that it may take up to a few years to significantly lighten heavy loads of molds, metals, and chemicals. Even though detoxification may take time, the process is pretty straightforward and, as Amie Valpone, Dr. Hyman, and many others can attest, the effort is well worth it.

There is much you can do on your own to reduce your body burden, while other areas require expert guidance. Dr. Crinnion says that about 80 percent of the chemical toxicants in our blood are nonpersistent and can be reduced by 84 percent in three weeks, just by cleaning up our homes and our diet.[32]

To minimize harm from toxicants and regain or protect your health, follow these five steps. And, a strong word of caution: If you are dealing with a big toxin burden like the trifecta of metals, mold, and Lyme disease and coinfections, please work with a qualified practitioner to investigate toxic exposures, nutrient deficiencies, and genetic detoxification status. The risk of dislodging metals into your bloodstream before your gut and detoxification organs are prepared can lead to disastrous consequences, like mercury getting deposited in your brain.

Step 1: Take a body-burden self-assessment.
Step 2: Get the data.
Step 3: Turn off the tap.
Step 4: Optimize your organs of elimination.
Step 5: Reduce your body burden.
Extra Step: Consider "Big Guns" in detoxification.

Step 1: Take a Body-Burden Self-Assessment

Consider the following statements. If you don't know an answer, just skip it. Rate your responses as 0 or 1, where 0 means "no" or "never" and 1 means "yes" or at least "sometimes":

0 1 I have an autoimmune condition, type 2 diabetes, or metabolic syndrome.

0 1 I have a family history of Alzheimer's, ALS (amyotrophic lateral sclerosis), Parkinson's, or MS.

0 1 I have one or more of the following symptoms: profound fatigue, muscle aches, headaches, focus or memory problems.

0 1 I have mercury amalgam fillings.

0 1 I am bothered by chemical smells like gasoline, perfumes, cleaning products, etc.

0 1 I drink unfiltered tap water.

0 1 I use plastic water bottles and/or canned foods (e.g., soups, vegetables, fruits from a can).

0 1 I eat conventionally grown produce and animal products most of the time.

0 1 I eat large or farmed (e.g., Atlantic or Scottish salmon) fish once a week or more often.

0 1 I eat rice.

0 1 I store food in plastic containers, and/or microwave food or drinks in plastic containers.

0 1 I live in a house or building that was built before 1978.

0 1 I live within five miles of farms or orchards, or in an agricultural farming area.

0 1 I live in an urban or industrial area.

0 1 I live in a house or work in a building that has known mold or prior water damage.

0 1 I use or am exposed to chemical-based household cleaning products or lawn garden chemicals.

0 1 I have my clothes dry-cleaned.

0 1 I smoke or am regularly exposed to secondhand smoke.

0 1 I often take medications like NSAIDs, acid blockers, synthetic hormone replacement (e.g., the Pill, estrogen, prostate meds), or steroids.

0 1 I'm under chronic stress or have experienced traumatic stress which is not yet resolved.

0 1 I'm overweight.

0 1 I find it hard to break a sweat.

0 1 I know I have weaknesses in my detox genetics (e.g., MTHFR, GSTM1, COMT).

Anything else you'd like to add?

1 _____

1 _____

Total _____

TOXIN ASSESSMENT KEY:

0–1 Outstanding! You're a role model for living a detox lifestyle. Keep up the great work!

2–5 Not bad! Looks like you're living a pretty clean lifestyle and may only be dealing with a relatively small load of toxins. You will benefit from practicing the precautionary principle, continuing to minimize your exposures, and reducing the load you may already have acquired to prevent future health issues.

6–9 Detoxification is a priority for you. You may already have autoimmune symptoms or may be at greater risk of developing them given your exposure to toxicants. Now's a great time to get ahead of further health issues by minimizing your exposures and reducing your body burden. Consider working with a qualified practitioner to assist you.

10+ Detoxification is very much a priority for you. Take heart in knowing you're not alone. Many people have healed in part or fully from many chronic illnesses by prioritizing detoxification and keeping at it for the long haul. Please work with a qualified practitioner to collaborate in the process, be committed to the process, and have patience.

Step 2: Get the Data

Unfortunately, there is not a single lab test (at this writing) that can assess your overall body burden of metals, chemicals, molds, and endotoxins. There are, however, a number of tests that can give you a pretty good picture of your load of each of those individual toxicants. Keep in mind that while testing can offer a snapshot of your exposure and even your immune system's reaction to that exposure, it won't indicate what the effects of any burden will be. Again, this is why working with an expert can be extremely helpful.

- **Detoxification Genetics**

  Common genetic mutations, called SNPs (pronounced SNIPS), associated with increased risk of impaired detoxification capacity include: CYP (drug metabolism), MTHFR (methylation), GSTM1 (glutathione), COMT (neurotransmitter processing), SOD (oxidative protection), and VDR (vitamin D receptor). To see whether you have detoxification SNPs, consider the following tests; but keep in mind, your genes are not your destiny. They are controlled epigenetically by your nutrition and lifestyle choices.

  - **Genetic test by www.23andMe.com** (saliva) provides raw genetic data. You must upload your raw data to apps that interpret SNPs. There are numerous apps that offer interpretation, and to date, I have found NutraHacker to be the most helpful, as it offers useful tips on what to encourage and what to avoid.

  - **DetoxiGenomic Profile by Genova Diagnostics** (saliva) offers your genetic detoxification profile directly without requiring 23andMe raw data.

  - **PCR by LabCorp** (blood) can provide your HLA-DR (human leukocyte antigen—antigen D-related) status, markers that reveal whether you are genetically more susceptible to mold, Lyme, and/or multiple biotoxins.

- **Chemicals**

  - **Cyrex Array 11 Chemical Immune Reactivity Screen** (blood) tests for increased antibodies to mold, chemicals, and heavy metals, providing insight into which may be challenging your immune system and promoting autoimmune processes.

  - **Great Plains Laboratory's GPL-TOX** (urine) screens for the presence of 172 different toxic chemicals.

- **Metals**

  - **Doctor's Data toxic metals panel** ("provocation-based" urine test) uses an oral chelator to pull metals out of tissues for collection in urine over a twenty-four-hour period.

  - **Quicksilver Scientific (QS) Mercury Tri-Test** (blood, hair, and urine) measures excretion abilities and exposure to inorganic and methyl mercury. The **QS Blood Metals Panel** (blood) screens for a broad range of potentially toxic and nutrient metals to show elevated exposure to toxic metals and nutrient elements.

- **Mold**
  - ○ **Visual contrast sensitivity (VCS)** online eye test is a biotoxin screening tool that can be performed for a ten dollar donation to www.vcstest.com
  - ○ **Great Plains Laboratory MycoTOX Profile** (urine) detects seven different mycotoxins from four mold species.
  - ○ **Realtime Laboratories** (urine) detects fifteen different mycotoxins from four mold species. Realtime Labs provides direct-to-consumer testing in many states.

Step 3: Turn Off the Tap

You can make big progress in lightening your toxic load by minimizing your toxicant exposures. Rather than feeling like you have to do everything at once, just start where you can and use the following as a guide to help you minimize the most common or problematic ones. As you begin to swap your usual products and choices for safer alternatives, you'll find that the process gets easier over time. You may even notice you have more energy and fewer symptoms, and that can be just the motivation needed to keep going.

Food

Dr. Pizzorno says that *70 percent of your toxin load comes from food*—specifically SAD foods and food additives, as well as how we cook, store, and reheat food. Studies show that switching from conventional to organic fruits and vegetables, even for just a few days, reduces pesticide levels in children's bodies up to 50 percent.[33, 34]

✔ **Eat organic food.** The most important step you can take in reducing your body burden is to eat organic food. And the most important food to buy organic is meat—that means 100 percent grass-fed and grass-*finished*. According to Lee Cowden, MD, board-certified cardiologist and integrative medicine expert, there are five to twenty times more pesticides in conventionally raised meats than there are in conventionally grown fruits and vegetables.

If you can't afford to go all organic, at least buy 100% grass-fed meat, 100% pastured chicken and eggs, and organic versions of what EWG calls the "Dirty Dozen" fruits and vegetables: strawberries, spinach, nectarines, apples, peaches, celery, grapes, pears, cherries, tomatoes, sweet bell peppers, and potatoes.

✓ **Filter your water.** Tap water contains toxicants and contaminants including fluoride, chlorine, aluminum, arsenic, herbicides, and even prescription medications. Consider a solid carbon block filter as a countertop device or a whole-house water filter if possible. And get a reasonably priced shower filter like AquaBliss, Homspal, or Starbung. Head's up that not every water filter or pitcher removes fluoride, a pernicious toxin, so read labels carefully before buying.

✓ **Cook with lower heat.** High-heat cooking or barbequing damages oils and proteins, which can lead to advanced glycation end products, appropriately known as *AGEs* because they age you prematurely. Bake, simmer, gently sauté, or steam your food, and add oils *after* you've plated your food.

✓ **Use stainless steel, cast iron, or ceramic cookware.** Nonstick pans like Teflon contain PFOA, a chemical shown to harm the immune system, liver, and thyroid.[35]

✓ **Use glass food storage containers.** Plastic leaches chemicals into your food, especially when heated.

Body

✓ **Use chemical-free body care products and cosmetics.** A good rule of thumb: don't use it if you don't recognize the ingredients. A step further: don't put it on your body if you wouldn't eat it. For example, coconut oil is a great moisturizer! Refer to EWG's Skin Deep database for information on more than seventy thousand personal care products. And download Think Dirty, a free mobile device app that scans barcodes of your personal and skincare products to get the product's potential harm rating on a scale of one to ten.

✓ **Work up a sweat.** A review of fifty studies found that sweating in a sauna and/or from exercise can help cleanse the body of toxicants, including lead, cadmium, arsenic, mercury, and BPA.[36] Far or near infrared saunas support detoxification safely without the high heat of a regular sauna. Low-EMF saunas include the Relax

Sauna, Clearlight, and Sunlighten; and SaunaSpace offers a no-EMF option.

✔ **Minimize medications.** Work with your doctor to gradually reduce your dosages and quantities of medications as you experience the beneficial effects of healthful lifestyle changes.

✔ **Consider having your mercury amalgam fillings removed** and replaced with nontoxic composites. Experts agree, before addressing mercury toxicity, you must remove sources of exposure, including silver amalgam fillings and fish. Find a dentist trained in proper removal procedures at iabdm.org/location/.

Home

According to the EPA, indoor air pollutants may be present at levels two to five times higher—and occasionally more than *100 times higher*—than outdoor air pollutants. Given that the average person spends nearly 90 percent of his or her time indoors, indoor air pollution is a major source of environmental chemicals exposure. Sources of indoor air pollution include: poor ventilation, chemical-based cleaning products, foam in couches and under carpets, air fresheners, scented candles, radon, and volatile organic compounds (VOCs) like mold.

✔ **Vacuum your floors.** One of the best things you can do to reduce your body burden is to keep your floors free of dust, dirt, and mold spores. Environmental consultant John Banta advises clients to get and use a high-quality HEPA (high efficiency particulate air) vacuum, and to "ban the broom" to avoid redistributing particles into the air. Don't forget to empty the vacuum canister outside.

✔ **Clean up your indoor air.** Another tool to help reduce your body burden is to use HEPA air filters for rooms you use most often like your bedroom, kitchen, and office. HEPA air filters are capable of removing ultrafine particles (<0.1 microns)—which represent 90 percent of all airborne pollution that you breathe, including mold, dust, formaldehyde, pet dander, volatile organic components (VOCs), and even viruses from the air. Consider Intellipure, Air Oasis, IQAir, Austin Air, or Blueair air filters.

✔ **Use nontoxic cleaning products.** EWG tested 2,500 products and found that more than two-thirds fell short, receiving a D or F for both human and environmental toxicity. Consider making your own inexpensive and effective all-purpose home cleanser: to four parts pure water, add one part white vinegar and ten to twenty drops essential oils like lavender, cinnamon, or lemon. Store in a glass bottle so oil does not degrade plastic.

- ✔ **Check for and eliminate sources of mold.** If you live or work in a building that has had water intrusion, a damp basement, or musty smells, it's highly likely you have mold and VOCs (volatile organic compounds) produced by mycotoxins. Jill Carnahan, Functional Medicine MD and autoimmune expert, has personally recovered from CIRS (chronic inflammatory response syndrome) due to mold exposure and recommends getting the EPA-approved ERMI(SM) (environmental relative moldiness index) test done through myco-metrics.com because it measures more species of mold. Safe removal of mold, called *remediation*, can be daunting and pricy but imperative to assist in health recovery. As harsh as it may sound, you may not heal unless you remove the mold or relocate.

- ✔ **Remove shoes at the door.** It's not just a Zen concept, but a very practical way to keep your home free of weed killers, fertilizers, coal tar dust, and harmful bacteria and parasites from dog waste, etc.

- ✔ **Minimize your electromagnetic field (EMF) exposure.** Science has linked exposure from artificial or non-native EMF from cell-phones and Wi-Fi networks with chronic diseases including heart disease, obesity, and inflammatory bowel disease.[37] While our homes are getting smarter with Wi-Fi–enabled appliances, convenience may come at a growing risk to our health. Put your electronics on airplane mode when not in use, consider turning off your Wi-Fi router at night, use a wired headset with your cell phone, and keep your phone far from your body.

Step 4: Optimize Your Organs of Elimination

Prime your body's inherent ability to detoxify by supporting the main organs of elimination:

- ✔ **Liver/gallbladder:** Your liver is your body's chemical processing factory, responsible for changing most of the food you eat into components that your body can use, and for getting rid of the things that are of no use or are toxic. The gallbladder stores and regulates bile flow to help you digest fat. To assist both, start each day with warm water and lemon, minimize alcohol and caffeine, and increase hydration with pure water and a splash of organic, sugar-free cranberry juice. Eat organic, nutrient-dense foods like leafy and bitter greens (e.g., arugula, chard, and collard greens), cruciferous vegetables (e.g., kale, broccoli, cauliflower, and cabbage), sulfur-containing foods (e.g., garlic, onions, and eggs), and amino acid-rich foods that support phase two (bind and excrete) liver detoxification (e.g., bone broth, gelatin or collagen, meat, poultry, fish, spinach, and pumpkin seeds).

- **Kidneys:** Your kidneys are in charge of filtering things in your blood to be excreted in your urine. To assist your kidneys, minimize alcohol, caffeine, and excess protein consumption. Adequate hydration is key for optimizing excretion through the kidneys. Nourishing foods for the kidneys include those that are very dark in color, like dark berries—especially 100 percent unsweetened cranberry juice (add stevia for sweetness), beets, seaweed, black sesame seeds, and black walnuts.

- **Colon:** Your colon, or large intestine, is responsible for absorbing water to make waste more solid, and then excreting that waste through bowel movements, ideally one to three times per day. The main idea is to keep things moving daily. Three keys to supporting colon health include increasing hydration, eating more fiber, and moving your body throughout the day.

- **Skin:** The skin is your largest organ of elimination, which is why it's sometimes referred to as the "third kidney." Do what you can to work up a sweat daily and use a sauna a few times per week, if possible, to promote sweating. Keep well-hydrated and rinse off immediately after with cool or cold water to prevent toxins from reabsorbing.

- **Lungs:** Indoor air pollution may be worse than outdoor air pollution, so if you can, use a HEPA air filter like Intellipure, Air Oasis, IQAir, Austin Air, or Blueair in the room(s) where you spend the most time. Practice breath-holding: take ten conscious breaths with a 1-4-2 ratio. For example, inhale for four seconds, hold for sixteen seconds, and exhale for eight seconds. Get regular, moderately intense exercise and use herbs and oils that relieve congestion and improve circulation to the lungs, like ginger, oregano, and eucalyptus.

✔ **Lymph/glymph systems:** The lymphatic or lymph system is your body's inner drainage system, a network of lymph nodes, glands, organs, and blood vessels that transport waste away from tissues into the bloodstream and then to the spleen for purification. Your brain has its own lymphatic system that removes waste called the glymphatic or glymph system. The best ways to support your lymph system is to eat an anti-inflammatory, Paleo-template diet, increase hydration, exercise daily—any way you can and *will*—dry brush your skin toward your heart, and soak in Epsom salts baths. The best way to support your brain's glymph system is to get plenty of restorative sleep since that's when it takes out the trash.

In addition to the food, herbs, and lifestyle recommendations above, consider adding one or more homeopathic and herbal drainage remedies to your detoxification toolkit. I recommend the following brands and personally rotate these tinctures: BIORAY NDF and Liver Life; and Energetix homeopathic formulas Drainage-Tone and Lymph-Tone III. Some formulas are only available through practitioners: Apex Energetics ANTITOX drainage formulas for liver, kidney and lymph; PEKANA homeopathic Big 3 Detox and Drainage Kit; and Beyond Balance, Inc. TOX-EASE GL.

Step 5: Reduce Your Body Burden

There are many simple habits you can adopt on your own to reduce the majority of circulating nonpersistent toxins, like phthalates, BPA, and other chemicals.

SUPPLEMENT STRATEGICALLY TO ASSIST DETOXIFICATION

Dr. Pizzorno has been quoted as saying that if we're alive today and merely breathing, chances are near certain that we have toxins in our bodies, even if, like Amie Valpone, we are doing everything "right." This is why integrating proactive detox strategies into your daily health routine is so important. By supporting your bodies' natural detox pathways and incorporating detox "binders"—elements that bind to toxins to help excrete them without being reabsorbed—you help unburden your body from ongoing exposure to chemicals, molds and metals.

Gently Push Out Toxins

In addition to eating detoxifying foods, upping hydration, and supporting your organs of elimination, certain nutrients can assist your body in successfully *pushing out* toxins:

- ✓ **Glutathione (GSH)**, the body's most important antioxidant, helps to strengthen liver and immune function, neutralize free radicals, and bind to and excrete toxins. If you're in pretty good health, a good option to boost your glutathione stores is taking the glutathione precursor N-acetylcysteine (NAC). If you're dealing with health challenges, premature aging, or chronic stress, you may be deficient in glutathione and might benefit more by taking liposomal glutathione, a more bioavailable form than oral glutathione capsules. I take both NAC and liposomal glutathione when I feel like my liver needs extra loving care.

  NAC dose: 200 to 600 mg twice a day on an empty stomach.

  Liposomal glutathione dose: 100 mg reduced glutathione as two pumps or one teaspoon twice per day on an empty stomach. Hold in the mouth for thirty seconds to initiate absorption in the capillaries under the tongue. Look for high-quality brands in glass bottles like Quicksilver Scientific or Designs for Health.

  Note: Keep liposomal glutathione refrigerated and take along with vitamin C and E (if the formula does not contain both) to keep glutathione at optimal levels.

- ✓ **Omega-3 essential fatty acids** (EPA + DHA) found in fish oil are required in all functions of the liver, including detox, supporting cellular membranes, and nerve and brain tissue repairs. Take supplemental omega-3 EFAs and eat more omega-3–rich fish like wild salmon and sardines.

  Dose: 2,000 to 4,000 mg of EPA and DHA in divided doses daily with food and vitamin E. Look for a high-quality, refrigerated oil from wild salmon or krill that has been tested for and is free of metals, like OmegaBrite, Nordic Naturals, Green Pasture and Dr. Mercola.

  Note: All oils are at risk for rancidity (spoilage) due to oxidization. Purchase high-quality supplements and minimize their exposure to air, heat, and light. Keep refrigerated, ideally in glass containers, and toss if cod liver oil or fish oils smell or taste fishy.

Caution: Omega-3 fatty acids may increase the effects of blood-thinning medications.

✔ **Magnesium** promotes healthy bowel movements in a gentle, non-addictive way.

Dose: Start with about 100 mg magnesium (one capsule) with or without food, ideally at bedtime, and increase one capsule each day up to 2,000 mg in divided doses throughout the day. Preferred types include malate, glycinate, ascorbate, and threonate. Natural Calm is a widely available magnesium citrate powder that contains organic stevia.

Note: If you take too much, or if your body saturates with magnesium, you may experience stool loosening or diarrhea. Just back off a little but don't stop completely.

Cautions: The most common side effects include temporary GI symptoms including diarrhea, abdominal cramps, and bloating. Magnesium citrate may also decrease absorption of some antibiotics and will decrease thyroid hormone if taken at the same time.

Pull Toxins Out Gently

Binders are an important component of effective detoxification protocols. When the liver processes toxins, they get excreted through bile and into the small intestine. If the toxins are not bound to anything, they can get reabsorbed into circulation, where they may wreak more havoc. The role of binders is to grab and safely escort toxins out of the body, avoiding harmful retoxification.

✔ **Eat more fiber.** One of the most important ways to assist your body in clearing toxins is to increase your fiber intake. Not only does fiber feed your beneficial gut bacteria as we learned in the Gut chapter, but it also binds waste products and helps escort them out of our colon and into the toilet. Good sources of fiber include larch arabinogalactan powder, organic psyllium seed husk, organic and freshly ground chia or flax seeds, and organic fruits and vegetables like avocados, artichokes, coconut, and raspberries. Aim for forty to fifty grams of fiber per day if your system can handle it. And, remember to ramp up slowly.

✔ **Use a gentle "cocktail" of binders.** Detoxification experts recommend taking a cocktail of safe and gentle binders to address multiple toxins in the GI tract. Ideally, you'll want to use a combination of activated charcoal, chlorella, cilantro, and a food-grade clay to cover all the bases: metals, mold, chemicals, volatile organic compounds (VOCs), and other biotoxins. Just make sure to take supplements and medications at least two hours before or after taking binders to ensure they don't get bound up and excreted too!

Consider taking the following binder cocktail at least once a day thirty minutes before eating: Put a teaspoon of the powders and several drops of cilantro tincture into a small glass jar (with lid), add about four ounces of pure water and a few drops of stevia, as desired. Seal, shake thoroughly for about thirty seconds, and drink immediately. Wait thirty minutes before eating. There is no rule on how long to take binders, so listen to your body and consult with your health practitioner for additional guidance.

○ **Activated charcoal** from coconuts or hardwood is a carbon-rich, broad-spectrum binder that binds endotoxins (bacterial waste), mycotoxins (except aflatoxin), BPA, and pesticides. Charcoal will also bind to vitamins and minerals, so take at least two hours away from supplements. I like Takesumi Supreme, Viva Doria, and Zen Charcoal powder forms.

Dose: 600 mg one to three times per day on an empty stomach, thirty minutes before meals.

Note: Charcoal can be constipating and may stain your poop black. Drink extra water and take extra magnesium (away from binders).

○ **Chlorella**, chlorophyll-rich green algae, is an effective chelator (pronounced KEY-lay-ter) for heavy metals, VOCs, pesticides, herbicides, and mycotoxins. Consider these powdered forms, which mix nicely in the binder cocktail: Micro Ingredients Pure Organic Chlorella Powder, Sun Potion Transformational Foods, and Organic Clean Chlorella SL powder.

Dose: 500 mg broken cell wall (for best absorption) organic chlorella powder one to three times daily thirty minutes before meals.

○ **Cilantro** is the Spanish word for coriander leaves, the fragrant herb that looks like parsley. It helps detoxify the body by binding with heavy metals such as mercury, lead, and aluminum and aiding in their elimination. Three high-quality organic tinctures include Bioray's NDF Gentle Heavy Metal Detox Tonic, BioPure cilantro, and Planetary Herbals' Cilantro Heavy Metal Detox.

Dose: Start with a few drops, monitor your response, and ramp up slowly to the recommended dose.

○ **Clay** (food grade bentonite, zeolite, or pyrophyllite) binds mold toxins—specifically aflatoxin—and other biotoxins. I rotate BioPure's ZeoBind, which is broad-spectrum, and Living Clay's Detox Clay, which is a finer powder that dissolves better than most clays.

Dose: one teaspoon pure food-grade clay in two ounces of water—shaken and drunk immediately.

General caution on binders: Drink extra water with binders and consider taking extra magnesium and vitamin C to avoid constipation. Make sure to take thirty minutes before eating; and take medications or other supplements at least two hours before or after taking binders.

Extra Step: Consider "Big Guns" for Detoxification

If you have already followed the above steps and believe you are still dealing with a stubborn toxin burden, you may greatly benefit from working with an integrative practitioner skilled in the fine art of detoxification.

Heavy duty "push" strategies:

✔ Nutritional IVs are often used by integrative and naturopathic physicians because they can "push" much-needed vitamins, amino

Lose Belly Fat to Detoxify

In a brilliant strategy to keep your vital organs safe, your body sequesters fat-soluble toxicants like pesticides, heavy metals, and plastics in your fat cells. Many toxicants are aptly called *obesogens* because they create fat cells, promoting obesity—especially in your abdomen. Losing weight, especially belly fat, helps to reduce your toxic load. The problem is, belly fat (and the toxins stored within) is particularly stubborn to reduce without a detox strategy that focuses on increasing lipolysis (pronounced lie-POL-i-sis)—the breakdown of fat cells, and autophagy (ah-TA-fa-gee)—a healthy cellular cleanup process that clears dysfunctional cells and makes way for new cells. What can you do to engage lipolysis and autophagy and lose stubborn belly fat and the toxins stored within? The short answer is to break your addiction to carbohydrates and become an efficient body fat burner.

To increase lipolysis and autophagy and reduce your toxic load, follow three strategies:

1. **Go keto periodically**—either a few days per week or a few weeks per year, and reduce your net carbs (carbohydrates minus fiber) to twenty to fifty grams per day (see Consider Ketosis sidebar on p. 70).

acids, minerals, and other nutrients directly into the bloodstream, bypassing digestion, which is often impaired in people with autoimmune conditions. Favorite push IVs to support detoxification include glutathione, phosphatidylcholine (PC), vitamin C, and the Myers cocktail (vitamin C, magnesium, minerals, and B vitamins).

Heavy duty "pull" strategies:

✔ For some people, the gentle binder cocktail isn't enough. Detox experts may suggest a moderate pull strategy like oral chelation (pronounced key-LAY-shun) or an extra-strength pull strategy like IV chelation. In either case, before embarking on *any* chelation protocol, it is critical to prepare detoxification pathways, making sure they are open and able to excrete metals properly. This is why it is imperative to work with a well-trained detoxification expert.

2. **Practice intermittent fasting** and eat only during a six- to eight-hour window, like from eleven a.m. to seven p.m. Periodically, extend the fast to seventeen, twenty, or twenty-four hours, or even five days for additional health benefits like lowered insulin levels and increased lipolysis and autophagy.

3. **Do high intensity interval training** (HIIT) if you are able, or high intensity interval *resistance* training (HIIRT) two or three days per week.

To enhance these strategies, drink green tea, which increases lipolysis and autophagy, reduces inflammation, and shrinks adipose fat mass; take omega-3 fatty acids to reduce fat mass and increase lean body mass; and consider taking the amino acid L-carnitine to shuttle fatty acids into your cells' mitochondria, where fat can be used for fuel.

Finally, to assist your body in clearing out toxins and cellular debris, make sure you drink half your body weight in ounces of pure water each day and enjoy a binder cocktail (page 174) at least once a day to grab and escort released toxins out of the body as you slim down.

Chelation involves ingesting capsules (oral) or having an injection (IV) of a strong binding agent like EDTA (ethylenediaminetetraacetic acid), DMSA (dimercaptosuccinic acid) or DMPS (2,3-Dimercapto-1-propanesulfonic acid) into the body so it can grab all metals, including aluminum, lead, and mercury, from tissues and help escort and excrete them out of the body via urine and stool. Different chelating agents have varying success in removing metals. For example, DMPS was shown to remove 86 percent of mercury in rabbit kidney tissue, DMSA removed 60 percent, and EDTA removed just 26 percent.[38]

Recent research suggests that EDTA chelation may be a well-tolerated and effective treatment method for multiple diseases associated with toxic metals, including Alzheimer's, cardiovascular disease, diabetes, and MS. In fact, in one study of mice with an experimental model of MS, EDTA was shown to reduce demyelination plaques, slow disease progression, and significantly reduce disease severity.[39, 40]

I know this has been a particularly daunting topic, and I want to congratulate you for making it this far! If you're still feeling overwhelmed or resistant to do anything else, consider getting started with just one of the top five actions below. And keep in mind the words of wisdom from Sherry Rogers, MD, who wrote in *Detoxify or Die*:

"Every night you can go to bed knowing you have made your cumulative load better, same or worse. The choices you make every day add to that total package. You are truly captain of your own ship."

Summary: Top Five Detoxification Actions

1. **Eat organic food**—especially animal products—to minimize your exposure to pesticides, antibiotics and growth hormones.
2. **Eat more fiber** to both bind and remove toxicants from your body. Don't forget to drink more water when you increase fiber to keep things moving!
3. **Use filtered wat**er for drinking and showering to avoid fluoride, chlorine, and other chemicals.
4. **Use a HEPA (high efficiency particulate air) vacuum** to remove ultrafine toxic particles from carpets and floors.
5. **Use chemical-free home and body care products** to avoid plasticizers and other hormone disruptors.

CHAPTER 5

Address Stress

When you can maintain a level of inner tranquility no matter what is happening around you, you can avoid the damage that stress causes to your health.

—GERALD S. COHEN, DHom, DC, FIHI,
founder of the Center for the Healing Process

When people with autoimmune disorders recall what was happening in their lives before the onset of their condition, they almost always have a story of unusual emotional stress or a shocking event. For Jacob Teitelbaum, a family meltdown and drop-dead flu in quick succession triggered his chronic fatigue and fibromyalgia. For Toréa Rodriguez, the triple whammy of a traumatic experience while piloting her plane, losing her mother, and a bad bicycle accident—all within one year—preceded her Hashimoto's diagnosis. Donna Eden, energy medicine pioneer, was a vivacious teenager who suffered an excruciating emotional shock after a seemingly inconceivable betrayal. She experienced the first symptoms of MS within months. While all of these experiences are unique, stress is not.

No one escapes stressful events. We share common human burdens of illness, life disruptions, or loss of loved ones. Thankfully, our bodies are built to weather those storms, and most of the time, we emerge whole. Whatever form stress takes—physical, mental, emotional, and/or traumatic—we are designed to withstand it and even thrive or *grow* from it in small doses.

Unfortunately, it's all too common for many of us to experience longer-lasting and more damaging effects of stress. Whether it's a traumatic or shocking event, like a natural disaster or sexual assault; repeated bouts of acute stress, like arguments with a spouse; or the unrelenting type, qualified as chronic stress, like ongoing abuse, financial pressures, or social isolation, toxic stress alters body chemistry in ways that can harm your immunity, contribute to inflammation, early aging and chronic illness, and even cause premature death.[1, 2]

"Seriously?" you may be asking. You just finished reading the Toxins and Infections chapters, which, by the way, were pretty stressful, and now it's time for *more* stress? In a word, yes. Here's the deal: Most doctors, functional and conventional alike, avoid or only minimally address the topic of stress be-cause it's usually easier and less murky to address straightforward topics like food or toxins. But not fully addressing stress does a disservice to anyone who is eager to heal; and as I have personally experienced and learned from studies and my own clients, plus experts who work with thousands of clients with autoimmune conditions, ignoring stress or emotional pain is a setup for health problems to emerge downstream. Try as you might to suppress or bury negative emotions, your body can't lie, and just like trying to submerge a cork in water, when you remove your hand, the cork bobs back to the top.

Maybe you intuitively know what I mean? Maybe you have your own experience doing anything you can to avoid facing emotional pain. Perhaps you've developed some unhealthy coping strategies, like eating too much sugar or drinking too much alcohol; or maybe you've repressed your anger and become a people-pleaser, because short-term relief and conflict avoid-ance is much easier than dealing with the realities of an unhappy marriage, an unfulfilling job, or traumatic memories from childhood. And maybe those strategies work for a while—until they don't.

Here's the startling truth: science shows that three types of stress—whether ongoing daily stressors of modern life, a major stressful event, or emotional trauma from childhood—are deeply connected to the advent and perpetuation of autoimmune disorders, even *decades* later. Your doctor may not have inquired about stress in your life or educated you about the strong connections between stress and autoimmune issues, and that's a gap-ing hole in modern medicine. As much as we may want to ignore it, there is ample evidence that the mind and body are inextricably linked. To bor-row from the title of Donna Jackson Nakazawa's powerful book *Childhood Disrupted*: your biography truly becomes your biology.

So, now I invite you to get cozy with a cup of tea, take a few slow, deep belly breaths, and walk with me through the science and stories of how stress can lead to and worsen autoimmune conditions. I promise to provide hope and resources on the other side, so that you have a soft landing into the realm of relaxation, which is where healing happens.

What Is Stress?

Let's start with the basics, like *what is stress*? We each know it when we feel it, but nailing down a consensus definition of stress is tough. For help, I turned to Heidi Hanna, Ph.D., author of *Stressaholic: 5 Steps to Transform Your Relationship with Stress* and executive director of the American Institute of Stress, the organization founded by the "father of stress research" and the man who coined the term *stress* in 1936, Hans Selye. Selye was an Austro-Hungarian medical researcher who led many experiments on rats, testing various hormones and placebos. What he discovered was that rats not only responded to his tests, but also to the stress of the experiments. It was stress, Selye observed, that caused the rats to become ill and die. His 1936 paper introduced the concept of general adaptation syndrome, three phases for how organisms respond to stress: phase one is the alarm stage, where the body prepares to fight, flee, or freeze; phase two is the resistance stage, where the organism makes efforts to cope, slowly depleting its reserves; and phase three is the exhaustion stage, which occurs if the organism is unable to muster the resources to overcome the threat.

When we spoke, Hanna summed it up for me this way: "Stress is what happens when perceived demands on you exceed your capacity."

Stress is not something that happens *to* you, but rather how you respond, or put more accurately, how you *react* to a stressor—that is, a situation or event you *perceive* as threatening. Your reaction sets off a process that changes the physical chemistry of your body, the type and duration of which determines whether and how stress helps or harms you.

Tame stress, also known as *good stress* or *eustress*, is a normal, essential, and ultimately *positive* response to stress. It's that nervous tension or excitement you may feel when rising to the occasion, like taking an exam, giving a presentation, or finally mustering up the courage to ask for something outside your comfort zone. Your heart rate goes up, your stress hormones get a little elevated, your immune system gets a boost; but the event passes and you're none the worse for wear. In fact, you may feel empowered by the situation. This is where personal growth happens.

Tolerable stress is less comfortable, but you still muster the resources to bounce back. Examples might include the stress one feels as a result of divorce, the death of a loved one, or a frightening diagnosis. In this case, the body's alert systems are triggered to a greater degree, but provided the event is time-limited *and* you have sufficient emotional support, you get through and the body recovers. You may even learn some important life lessons.

KEY CONCEPT: *It's not the size of the stress that matters so much, it's whether we adapt to it or not.*

Toxic stress is just what it sounds like: unhealthy and very harmful. It's what happens when the body's stress response gets stuck in the on position for too long—becoming chronic—and stressful events far outweigh a person's ability to cope. Examples include ongoing physical or emotional abuse, childhood trauma, or enduring financial hardship. When

Common Stress Terms

Stressor: The thing or event that's stressing you out. It can be real, perceived, or imagined.

Acute stress: A feeling of emotional distress, pressure, and sometimes excitement that lasts up to a month and usually does not cause lasting damage—unless it is frequently repeated. Could be the pressure of a big deadline, a public speaking event, an unresolved argument with a loved one, or getting an audit letter from the IRS.

Allostasis: The adaptation process to physical, psychosocial, and environmental challenges or stress. Your *allostatic load* refers to level of wear and tear chronic stress wreaks on your body. *Allostatic overload* is harmful and can lead to disease processes. Examples include excess belly fat, immune system suppression, or acceleration of heart disease.

Chronic stress: The grinding kind of stress that lasts longer than a month can lead to mental, emotional, and physical breakdown, and a person is stuck in a toxic stress response for too long, the consequences include prolonged activation of the fight-flight mechanisms, impaired immune function, and a greater likelihood of developing depression, heart disease, autoimmune disorders, and even early death.

We Are Getting More Stressed and Sicker Than Ever

Collectively, our toxic stress response is making us sicker than ever. It's estimated that between 75 percent and 90 percent of all doctor visits are due to stress-related symptoms, and research suggests that about half of all sick days are due to stress.[3] What's behind all this stress? To get a sense of the root causes—that is, the demands on us that outweigh our resources—I looked to the American Psychological Association (APA). Over the past decade, the APA has commissioned an annual survey to examine the state of stress across the country and its resulting health impact. The Stress in America survey reports the top six stressors to be:

chronic disease. Chronic stress may come from unrelenting daily demands, having a chronic illness or caring for someone who does, persistent feelings of hopelessness or helplessness, sleep deprivation, and/or unresolved traumatic experiences from childhood.

Coping: The many strategies people use to manage, deal with, or minimize the effects of stressful events. These may be healthy, effective, unhealthy, or ineffective ways of dealing with stress.

Homeostasis: The ability of the body to seek and maintain equilibrium or balance when dealing with external changes. One example of homeostasis is the body's ability to maintain an internal temperature around 98.6 degrees Fahrenheit, regardless of the outside temperature.

Resilience: Successful allostasis or the ability to adapt, cope, and even grow and thrive despite adverse experiences.

1. Money
2. Work
3. Family responsibilities
4. Personal health concerns
5. Health problems affecting family members
6. The economy

Hanna adds that the perception of not having enough time may, in fact, be the number one stressor today.

Recent survey results also shine a light on the growing connection between stress and worsening health of Americans:

- In 2017, 80 percent of Americans reported experiencing at least one symptom of stress in the prior month, up from 71 percent in 2016.
- That year, 67 percent reported having at least one diagnosed chronic illness, compared to 60 percent in 2014.
- And 23 percent reported that their health was just "fair" or "poor," up from 19 percent in 2012.[4]

These findings were corroborated by Vivek Murthy, MD, the former surgeon general of the United States under President Obama. Dr. Murthy started his time in office with an unusual strategy: He went on a "listening tour" of the country to learn how he could help. Across generations, geographies, and income levels, he heard a common refrain: Americans were feeling high levels of emotional pain. The causes for the pain varied depending upon the specific situation, but broadly, they included illness, economic uncertainty, addiction, or isolation. Regardless of the source of stress, the resulting feeling of great emotional pain was the same. Dr. Murthy describes a single event, which he said was representative of what he saw "everywhere." At the University of Texas, Dr. Murthy addressed five hundred students in an auditorium. He asked how many in the past month had experienced "unbearable stress." About 95 percent of the students raised their hands. He followed up by asking how many of those who had raised their hands felt that they had the tools for dealing with that stress in a healthy way. Only 5 percent answered affirmatively.

Dr. Murthy warns that if we don't proactively address stress and emotional well-being, then we risk missing a major contributor to not just our personal health and well-being, but also to the health of our country.[5]

How Does Stress Lead
to Disease in the Body?

To appreciate what all this stress is doing to us, it helps to understand how stress works in the body. Gabor Maté, MD, author of *When the Body Says No: Exploring the Stress-Disease Connection,* in a video with the same title on Youtube, describes the stress experience as having three components. First is the triggering event, the physical or emotional stressor that we interpret as threatening. Second is how our brain processes and interprets the meaning of the stressor. Third is the stress response, both our physiological and behavioral adjustments made in reaction to the perceived threat. How or whether we recover depends upon our ability to shift back into a resting state. Here's how I visualize it:

Healthy stress response:
Stressor → Meaning → Stress response → Resolution →
Relaxation response → Rest, digest, and heal

Unhealthy stress response:
Stressor → Meaning → Stress reaction → NO resolution →
Stuck in fight-flight mode → Increased risk of autoimmune
disease, and/or unhealthy coping behaviors, which add
to the risk of disease

Physiologically, our bodies react to a stressor with the "fight, flight, or freeze" response, a series of chemical reactions involving a cascade of hormonal changes. The adrenal gland releases stress hormones cortisol, epinephrine—also known as adrenaline—and norepinephrine into your bloodstream, preparing your body to fight or run. Your sympathetic nervous system activates, causing your heart rate and blood pressure to go up, your muscles to tighten, and digestion to stop—all in an attempt to increase your chances of survival. If the event is short-lived and you outran the bear or avoided an accident or learned that the strange noise in your house was your cat and not a burglar, your stress response subsides and, ideally, you return to the relaxation response, your body's "rest and digest" mode under the control of the parasympathetic nervous system.

But what happens if you don't go back to a relaxation response? What if your stress reaction gets stuck in the always-on position?

Stress without relief leads to *distress*, and prolonged distress leads to physiological breakdown. Studies have shown that chronic stress—that long-term toxic stress response—can have negative impacts on just about every system and organ in the body. It disrupts gut function and detoxification, raises blood pressure, elevates cholesterol, changes brain chemistry, upsets hormone and blood sugar balance, disrupts deep sleep, and harms immune function. When your immune system is suppressed, you become more susceptible to infections, and wounds take longer to heal. With prolonged stress, the body's tissues—including immune cells—can become less sensitive to the regulatory effects of cortisol, reducing cortisol's ability to manage the inflammatory response. This can lead to uncontrolled inflammation, which is associated with the onset and progression of autoimmune disorders.[6]

> **KEY CONCEPT:** *Chronic stress → systemic inflammation → autoimmune conditions*

Without addressing it, ongoing stress can lead to just about any disease under the sun, from the merely annoying to the life-threatening, including:

- Acne
- Alzheimer's
- Autoimmune conditions
- Cancer
- Dementia
- Depression
- Headaches and migraines
- Heart disease or sudden heart attack (stress cardiomyopathy)
- Obesity
- Parkinson's
- Stroke
- Weight gain or loss
- Weight loss resistance

The Stress-Autoimmune Connection

The evidence is in that stress plays a starring role in the development and perpetuation of autoimmune conditions. Studies show that 80 percent of people report uncommon emotional stress before autoimmune disease onset; and not only does stress *cause* disease, but the disease itself also causes significant *stress*, creating a vicious cycle.[7]

Here is a snapshot of the science linking stress with the onset and amplification of autoimmune disorders:

- A longitudinal study of fifty-four thousand women over twenty-four years showed that those who had been exposed to any kind of trauma—from car crashes to sexual assaults—were three times more likely to develop lupus compared with women who had experienced no trauma.[8]
- A study of 2,490 Vietnam veterans found that those with chronic PTSD (post-traumatic stress disorder) had a 174 percent increased risk for autoimmune diseases, including rheumatoid arthritis (RA), psoriasis, type 1 diabetes, and autoimmune thyroid disease, compared to those without PTSD.[9]
- People who experienced more negative life events in the past year were 6.3 times more likely than controls to develop Graves' disease.[10]
- People with RA frequently note the occurrence of stressful or traumatic life events prior to the onset of their illness and/or disease flares.[11]
- The incidence of emotional disorders is higher in people with Crohn's disease and ulcerative colitis compared to the general population. Moreover, depression and anxiety influence the course and the severity of the underlying intestinal disease.[12]
- Family conflict and job-related problems are strongly correlated with the development of new brain lesions in MS patients eight weeks later.[13]

When it comes to autoimmune conditions, three types of stress come up again and again in the literature. These include:

1. **Chronic stress**, the unrelenting type that lasts longer than a month and wears you down, like ongoing relationship or work troubles, financial pressures, or burdensome family responsibilities like caregiving for a loved one with a serious illness.
2. **Major stress or shock**, a one-time event from which you have trouble recovering, as in an accident, the death of a loved one, a natural disaster, or loss of an important job or relationship.

And last but far from least is …

3. **Childhood trauma**, perhaps the most treacherous type of stress because it occurs during formative years when children don't have the resources to effectively cope. Whether or not the traumatic events in childhood are remembered, their impact has been shown to have devastating consequences, including altered brain development and lifelong effects on health and behavior—unless and until interventions are made to resolve emotional pain. While it may seem hard to believe that something that happened decades ago might impact your physical health today, it's important to understand this relationship in order to improve your well-being. Still skeptical? Let's take a closer look.

Adverse Childhood Experiences (ACEs) and Autoimmune Conditions

Maybe you haven't made the connection between what happened in your childhood and your present-day health, but research reveals powerful linkages that can't be ignored. In the mid-1990s, the CDC and the Kaiser-Permanente Health Maintenance Organization of San Diego set out to examine potential links between physical, emotional, and mental trauma experienced in childhood and later development of chronic disease. More than seventeen thousand men and women, mostly white, educated, and middle- or upper-middle class, participated in a study that ran for two years, with fifteen years of follow-up. Participants were asked about ten types of childhood trauma, including:

- Physical, emotional, and sexual abuse
- Physical and emotional neglect
- A family member who is depressed or diagnosed with other mental illness; addicted to alcohol or another substance; in prison
- Witnessing a mother or stepmother being treated violently
- Parental separation or divorce

When the results started coming in, study cofounder and medical epidemiologist at the CDC Robert Anda, MD, was shocked to see how much people had suffered. What Dr. Anda learned was that 64 percent of adults had experienced at least one adverse childhood experience (ACE), and of those, 87 percent had experienced two or more ACEs. That meant, for example, that a child who witnessed her mother being verbally or physically abused was also very likely to have personally experienced abuse of one type or another. And if the father was an alcoholic who abused both the mother and the child, that counted as three ACEs. Each type of adverse childhood experience counted as one point. If a participant had no adverse childhood events, the score was zero.

The greater the point score, the greater the risk for health and behavioral problems down the road. The higher the ACE score, the greater the risk of autoimmune conditions, cancer, Alzheimer's, and even early death, regardless of a person's behavior. In other words, having a high ACE score is a big risk factor for developing lung cancer *whether or not the person smoked*:

- 2+ ACEs → 70 percent increased risk of MS, type 1 diabetes, Hashimoto's
- 2+ ACEs → 80 percent greater risk of lupus, eczema, IBS, asthma
- 2+ ACEs → 100 percent greater risk of rheumatic diseases
- 4+ ACEs → 2.5 times more likely to develop cancer
- 4+ ACEs → 4.22 times more likely to develop Alzheimer's
- 6 ACEs → reduced lifespan by twenty years
- 7 ACEs → 360 percent increased risk for heart disease
- 8 ACEs → triple the risk for lung cancer[14]

The ACEs study also provided insight into the coping methods people use to escape emotional pain. Those who reported four or more ACEs, compared to those who had experienced none, had a four- to twelvefold increased health risk for alcoholism, drug abuse, depression, and attempted suicide; a two- to fourfold increase in smoking, self-assessing as being in "poor health," and reporting fifty or more sexual partners; and a 1.4- to 1.6-fold increase in physical inactivity and severe obesity. Self-medicating with substances and potentially unhealthy habits, it seems, is a normal human response to serious childhood trauma.[15]

The data imply that ACEs can consciously or unconsciously drive subsequent behaviors, determine health outcomes, and even shape your personality.

I know it's a lot to take in, especially if you think you have a high ACE score (see Appendix C for the ACE questionnaire). Take heart: we'll soon see that no matter your score, there are things you can do both on your own and with an expert that are proven to help shrink your perception of the trauma(s) and expand your capacity to cope. First, let's explore the autoimmune personalities that many adopt in childhood as a means to control their environment. Then we'll see how two women transcended childhood traumas and decades of chronic stress as a big part of their autoimmune healing journeys.

The "Autoimmune Personality"

Dr. Gabor Maté, CM, Hungarian-born Canadian physician and author, has spent more than two decades serving thousands of patients in both family practice and palliative care. He claims to know, "with near 100 percent certainty," which patients will go on to develop chronic disease and even early death. Maté observes four significant risk factors in his patients who develop autoimmune disorders that he says "are quite capable of killing you." These include:

1. Automatic concern for the needs of others, often ignoring your own
2. Impulsive and rigid identification with duty, role, and responsibility, rather than being your authentic self
3. Suppression or repression of so-called "negative" emotions (in quotes because the expression of anger, for example, in the present moment can be a valid emotion)
4. Taking responsibility for how other people feel, never wanting to disappoint them, feeling that you can never say no

People who can't say no, who put everyone else first, or who suppress who they are to please others, Dr. Maté says, have not developed healthy boundaries. In other words, they become "too permeable," allowing everything in, often overriding their own desires. Remind you of anything from the Gut chapter? An intact gut barrier is capable of determining which nutrients pass through and which do not. A gut barrier that becomes too permeable or permissive loses its ability to regulate what should or should not enter the bloodstream, like large protein molecules and bacterial waste.

Healing happens when we reestablish and maintain healthy boundaries, selectively choosing what to let in and what to keep out. As we learned from Jacob Teitelbaum's story, pleasing his mother and suppressing his authentic self was a setup for developing chronic fatigue and fibromyalgia. It wasn't until he removed himself from his family environment and took a step back and time off that Jacob learned to listen to and follow his inner guide, which led to his healing and full recovery.

Dr. Maté emphasizes that there is no blame or shame here. These are not deliberately chosen patterns; these are adaptations that children make unwittingly to survive great stress. However, he warns, if the adaptations become lasting personality traits, children may be at greater risk for pathologies later on. The personality types often associated with autoimmune conditions include the following:

> **KEY CONCEPT:** *Leaky barriers, both physically* and *emotionally, pave the way for autoimmune expression.*

- **Perfectionist.** There are *positive* qualities associated with perfectionism, including being driven, being responsible, and having high standards. The traits of perfectionism that are more likely to be associated with the development of autoimmune conditions include having a merciless inner critic, being judgmental of others, and being prone to anxiety and depression.
- **Workaholic.** Workaholics are compulsively work-obsessed and can become addicted to power and control in order to gain approval and public recognition.
- **Overachiever.** Traits of this personality can be similar to those of perfectionists and include being motivated by a fear of being judged inadequate, incompetent, or unworthy.
- **Chronic overgiver.** These individuals typically put the needs of others ahead of their own needs. Overgivers often have great difficulty receiving and may give out of a desire to feel loved, admired, or appreciated. An overgiver regularly sacrifices his or her own needs for the sake of others, which can lead to exhaustion, a sense of unworthiness, depression, resentment, and conflict in important relationships.

- **Substance abuser.** Childhood trauma is linked to personality traits including anxiety, compulsive behavior, frequent negative emotions, and impulsiveness.

Letting Go of the Need to Be Perfect: Susan Blum's Story

What follows is a story of an accomplished Functional Medicine doctor who, as a child in a stressful family environment, adopted the classic autoimmune personality of perfectionist to avoid emotional pain. While it seemingly served her well for many years, allowing her to achieve great things, the burden of being the "perfect one" finally took its toll. We can learn from Susan Blum, MD, MPH, that doing "everything right" may come at great cost, and that healing requires both the courage to examine our lives and a willingness to let go of the need to be perfect.

Raised in a stable family with two sisters and a brother, Susan was an easygoing, optimistic, and self-sufficient child. She avoided conflict, and instead, attempted to smooth things over on behalf of her siblings or parents if tensions flared, as they often did, especially when her father was involved. His quick, powerful response to anger left young Susan feeling nervous and insecure. "I definitely was afraid of him when I was younger," she recalls.

"There was a lot of stress in the house. My father was a good guy, but he would just blow, and we would all scoot out of his way. Though he never touched me, he took a strap to my elder sister on occasion, and there was definitely some sort of emotional stress from observing that physical abuse. The way I dealt with everything was to run and hide. I made sure I was an A-plus student so that my parents would not find any problems with me. I became the 'perfect one' in the family. That was my way of dealing with stress at home."

Driven and competitive, Susan excelled in science and math and decided early on that she wanted to be a doctor, a goal she pursued passionately all the way through medical school. But during her two-year residency, she quickly became disillusioned with what she saw as an "impersonal, cookie-cutter approach" in the conventional medical field. The feeling nagged at her, but life was too busy for much introspection.

By her early thirties, Susan had two sons, one of whom had significant ADHD. Susan spent her thirties feeling overwhelmed as she raised two active boys and worked part time at New York's Mount Sinai Hospital in the Department of Preventive Medicine, all while traveling frequently with her family for her husband's business. "There was a lot of stress in the family during those years, and I really had to look at my whole perfectionist thing; I had this kid, he's not perfect. Our family was not perfect. I was not perfect. The situation revealed a lot of things that I really needed to look at."

At thirty-eight, after her third son was born, Susan buckled under the weight of so much stress and decided to stop working. She was desperate for a new perspective and wanted to explore all the factors contributing to the mounting stress in her life.

"Finding and cultivating ways to prevent stress from coming into the body and making us sick is our job. That's the task that we're presented with to stay healthy and resilient throughout our entire lives. I started working on addressing the stress thing."

In 1998, she found and participated in a professional training program at The Center for Mind-Body Medicine (www.CMBM.org) in Washington, D.C. Through the training, she discovered that some aspects of her personality were no longer serving her. Among those was the compulsion to be the "perfect one" in her family. She embarked on a mission to tell her family, "I'm not going to be perfect anymore" and to change her role in family dynamics. But even after the training, Susan was still out of balance.

While she was fitter than ever, Susan was plagued with persistent fatigue and a pesky extra ten pounds. Her mental fortitude allowed to her to push through her exhaustion, when one day, a friend noticed that Susan's hands were yellow. A thyroid test revealed that Susan had an autoimmune hypothyroid condition: Hashimoto's thyroiditis. Her underactive thyroid didn't allow her to fully clear beta-carotene, an antioxidant present in yellow and orange produce. After she went on Armour Thyroid, a natural hormone derived from pigs, subsequent tests showed

even worse results. Troubled, Susan embarked on a quest to figure out why she had developed an autoimmune condition in
the first place. She couldn't simply turn off her perfectionist
personality and expect everything to change; she knew she
needed to dig deeper to uncover her physical limitations and
the ways in which she'd allowed stress to overload her life. She
reflects on the time of her diagnosis: "I thought I was doing
everything right, eating a lot of fish, exercising and sleeping
pretty well. It turned out, kind of like an iceberg, I had all this
stuff under the surface that I didn't know about, so I set about
trying to figure it out."

Susan's journey led her to study at the Institute for Functional Medicine (IFM). Focused on addressing the root causes
of chronic disease, the coursework provided Susan with the perfect opportunity to explore her own autoimmune triggers. She
determined that her autoimmune setup was a combination of
toxin overload and chronic stress. The toxin overload was due
to high levels of accumulated mercury in her body, thanks to a
lifetime of eating big fish, coupled with a genetic variant that
causes her to be a super-slow detoxifier. The chronic stress? That
was an accumulation of challenging events in childhood that
shaped her perfectionist personality, combined with a demanding family life and a dispiriting job in reactive medicine. The
chronic stress led to dysbiosis and a leaky gut, which has been
shown to lead to Hashimoto's thyroiditis.[16]

"My biggest autoimmune triggers were probably a combination of stress, gluten, soy, mercury, genetic detox challenges, and
gut issues. Food, stress, gut, and liver issues are the four big
pieces that everyone has to work their way through to repair the
foundations of their immune system. It took me two years to
fully address each area, but the work paid off. I felt better, I slept
better, my energy improved, my digestion resolved, and I even
lost those ten stubborn pounds."

Eighteen months after she was diagnosed, the antibodies to
her thyroid were back in the normal range and her Hashimoto's
condition was reversed. She is so passionate about minimizing
the harmful effects of stress, today she is on the faculty of The
Center for Mind-Body Medicine (CMBM) where she teaches

people worldwide how to become more resilient in the face of big or small stressors.

To maintain her health, Susan employs multiple stress-reducing strategies: She receives acupuncture every week, meditates each morning, follows a low-grain, plant-focused diet, drinks green tea daily, and has cut back on her work hours. She walks or runs in nature with her dog every day without her cell phone and enjoys reading and relaxing with her husband in their screened-in porch on weekends. Her commitment to maintaining this routine 90 percent of the time has allowed her to be very productive, healthy, and happy.

"The silver lining for me is that an autoimmune diagnosis just wakes you up to realizing the importance of putting yourself first. And it wakes you up to what's important in life. Living in balance, and the importance of reducing your stressors and managing what you can't let go of. Even when you have addressed toxins, the gut, and other triggers, too much stress can derail things."

Sometimes the pain of accumulated childhood stress can give rise to a profound sense of unworthiness, and that deep-seated belief can lead to unhealthy coping behaviors, which further add to the risk for developing chronic disease. For Michelle Corey, functional mind-body medicine practitioner and autoimmune recovery expert, having experienced more than two ACEs in childhood increased her risk for developing lupus and Hashimoto's thyroiditis by more than 70 percent. It also explains why she adopted personality traits like "workaholic" and "people-pleaser" and developed unhealthy coping strategies. In other words, Michelle's story illustrates how the effects of childhood trauma reach into adulthood. It also speaks to the powerful possibility for healing when emotional pain is met with a devotion to self-love, compassion, empathy, and forgiveness—key elements of emotional well-being.

Childhood Trauma Leads to Unhealthy Coping Behaviors and Autoimmunity: Michelle Corey's Story

Michelle was born to a single, teenage mother. Her mother later married a man who emotionally, physically, and sexually abused

Michelle, her siblings, and her mother for years. As an adult, Michelle was debilitated by feelings of self-loathing and shame, and believed herself unworthy of love. To cope, she drank too much wine and coffee, and, true to her driven personality, she worked way too many hours at her own advertising consulting firm. She followed a strict, low-calorie, vegetarian diet and was a yo-yo dieter. In spite of her diet, daily hot yoga, and regular runs on the beach, she was overweight and stressed out. In addition to her draining daily habits, Michelle also entered into an unhappy, codependent relationship. Michelle recalls, "I was totally stressed out most of the time. I was addicted to stress and unhappiness. I didn't know any other way of being in the world."

In her midthirties, Michelle's eyebrows and hair began to fall out. She developed rashes on the palms of her hands and soles of her feet, drenching night sweats, transient fevers, and aching joints. She saw several doctors who ran the classic TSH (thyroid stimulating hormone) test, which really only shows late-stage thyroid damage, and told her she was fine.

"I was treated like it was all in my head. That's a very real thing in medicine; when an otherwise healthy woman comes in with a set of aggravating symptoms that can't really be pinpointed to any one thing, she's lumped into this 'crazy woman' category. 'She's just self-indulgent, that's why she has all these problems, so we'll just give her Ativan or something for her anxiety or depression.'"

As Michelle approached her thirty-sixth birthday, her unhappiness grew and so did her symptoms. Instead of putting her needs first or following her intuition, she ignored her symptoms and stayed in her dysfunctional marriage, until a doctor's appointment for her husband led her to confront some tough questions of her own.

At the appointment, her husband's doctor noticed Michelle's puffy face and freckled melasma mustache, so he recommended an ANA test, a full thyroid panel, and a *Candida* test. The results revealed that Michelle had both a systemic *Candida* infection as well as Hashimoto's thyroiditis, plus markers for early-stage lupus, an autoimmune condition that presents with a multitude of symptoms, including profound fatigue, joint pain, hair loss, rashes, fevers, swelling, and sensitivity to the sun.

Then the doctor presented her with the compelling question, "Why do you think you got this disease?" First, Michelle felt victimized, and then she was filled with rage. *How* dare *he insinuate that* I *caused this!* But, his question resonated and wouldn't fade. She didn't know it at the time, but that irksome question put Michelle on the path to healing.

"I thought, 'There's something to be explored here.' I realized there wasn't anyone outside of myself who could figure this out. He was asking me the question because I'm the only person who could answer it. I went inward, and I journaled. It seemed like every part of my life was the reason I was sick. On every level, it was a mess. 'Everything's wrong in my life, and I'm living a lie. No wonder I'm sick!' "

Michelle realized that in order to heal, she would have to change her life, so change she did—massively. She sold her business, and when therapy didn't work, she left her unhappy marriage. Then she delved into mind-body-spirit healing.

Michelle's first introduction to mind-body medicine was Network Chiropractic, a gentle, holistic technique that taps into the body's ability to heal itself. Her chiropractor introduced her to somatic breathing exercises that helped ground her in her body and enabled Michelle to release long-stored emotions.

"It was very dramatic for me. I hadn't been connected to what was going on with me physically. I wasn't 'in my body,' which is a common experience for many survivors of sexual trauma. I find this with a lot of my female clients, people who have said, 'I just got a hysterectomy. I just wanted to get rid of it. If it's going on down below the waist, I don't want to know about it.' That's how I was. I was afraid of what my body might tell me."

As she freed herself from the shackles of childhood wounds, Michelle began to seek and create a nourishing lifestyle. She moved to the mountains of New Mexico with the intention to heal her life. She gave up alcohol and coffee for two and a half years. Instead of burning the midnight oil, she went to bed by ten thirty p.m.; and she replaced her intensive cardio workouts with Pilates, gentle weight training, and long walks in nature. She cut out all news and media consumption, and instead played uplifting, healing music that promoted joy. She listened to inspirational CDs from spiritual teachers, attended healing workshops and lectures, and devoured books by scientists, researchers, and doctors like Candace Pert, Ph.D., who taught that we have the ability to consciously choose our responses to life situations, rather than living in unconscious, reactive states. As her heart opened, she experienced "spontaneous forgiveness" of others, and finally, she forgave herself.

"I view my journey as a gift. I have learned that in order to heal, we must focus on the positive aspects of our lives, forgive ourselves (and others), and learn to love ourselves enough to make our own needs a priority.

"There is one thing I know for sure: no matter how sick you are or how bad your life situation may seem, things can get better. Every day presents you with the amazing response-ability to make new choices. Illness is the body's way of communicating to you that something—perhaps many things—in your life need to change. Take the opportunity to listen. Take the opportunity to heal."

Whether you have experienced a lifetime of stress like Susan and Michelle, or whether you're just dealing with the pressures of a busy modern life, it is never too late to address stress in all its forms.

Bottom line: If you want to heal from or prevent the advent or progression of autoimmune conditions, *you must tend to your emotional well-being.*

Emotional Well-Being Toolkit

If stress is what happens when perceived demands on you exceed your capacity, then the way to minimize the negative effects of stress is either to reduce the (perceived) demands on you or increase your capacity—or *both*. While you may not always be able to control the demands in your life, it makes sense to do what you can proactively to reduce your stress *and* increase your capacity to cope with stress, ideally before, but especially after, symptoms arise. In the coming pages, you'll learn practical, proven strategies you can use to address both sides of the equation: A. better managing (perceived) demands, plus B. strengthening your resilience.

While most of the strategies I include are simple do-it-yourself techniques, they only work if you *do them consistently*. Tony Robbins, human behavior expert and performance coach, says the secret to success is to start with little rituals you do each day, like a ten-minute morning practice. As momentum builds, the little rituals are more likely to become daily habits that you can't imagine not doing, the same way you can't wake up or go to bed without brushing your teeth.

We all have ten minutes a day that we can give to ourselves. But deciding to prioritize that time and actually *doing it* requires commitment to your well-being above everything else. Consider the wise words of airline personnel: *put your own oxygen mask on first!* Many people, especially women with the classic autoimmune personality traits, resist taking care of themselves first because they think it's selfish. But it's actually the opposite: prioritizing your emotional well-being gives you *more* energy for your daily roles and responsibilities. Beyond increasing your energy capacity, studies show that the strategies we'll explore lower inflammation, strengthen your immune system, increase happiness, and build a better brain.

While the number of stress-reducing and relaxation-promoting techniques seems practically endless, I include only those that are both scientifically proven to reduce stress and relatively simple to adopt. A study at Harvard-affiliated Massachusetts General Hospital confirms that relaxation-response techniques, like meditation, yoga, and prayer, could reduce the need for health care services by 43 percent.[17] Imagine how simple relaxation practices might reduce your need for medication or help you avoid the doctor altogether!

The Emotional Well-Being Toolkit is meant to provide you with a variety of options that you can adopt and practice over time. Some of these suggestions are easier to embrace than others, which is why I recommend that everyone begin by gaining awareness of their emotional stress levels and establishing a solid resilience-building foundation. If that's all you can do right now, that's okay! For those eager to progress further, steps 3 and 4 will help you more deeply engage your mind and heart to enhance your emotional well-being.

Explore the four steps below and consider the extra step if you require extra-strength help.

Step 1. Take a stress self-assessment.
Step 2. Get a solid foundation in place.

Step 3. Harness the power of your mind.

Step 4. Increase positive emotions.

Extra Step: Consider "prescription-strength" emotional support.

Step 1: Take a Stress Self-Assessment

You probably already know whether you feel a little or a lot of stress in your life. There's also a pretty good chance that you've gotten used to feeling the way you do and may even consider it normal. Or, maybe you're resigned that there's nothing you can do about it. The following self-assessment will help you gain greater awareness about the specific sources of stress in your life. I hope it will motivate you to prioritize stress reduction; plus, by recording the date you take the assessment, you'll be able to measure how your stress levels shift over time.

Consider the following statements. If you don't know an answer, just skip it. Rate your responses as 0 or 1, where 0 means "no" or "never" and 1 means "yes" or "sometimes":

0 1   I go to bed after ten p.m. most days.

0 1   I often get less than eight hours sleep.

0 1   I often feel wired and tired.

0 1   I often wake up tired or feel sluggish during the day.

0 1   I don't get much or any exercise.

0 1   I lack time or energy for personal hobbies and activities.

0 1   I often feel muscle tension in my neck or back.

0 1   I sit for long periods during the day (more than four hours).

0 1   I am a mouth breather, and/or my breathing is mostly shallow, from my chest.

0 1   I feel like I lack control over my schedule or daily priorities.

0 1   I work more than eight hours a day.

0 1   I rarely take vacations or long weekends.

0 1   I often feel anxious.

0 1   I worry a lot.

0 1   I often feel depressed.

0 1   I often feel guilt or shame.

0 1   I consider myself a perfectionist or frequently expect things to be perfect.

0 1   I frequently feel impatient or irritable.

0 1   I am a Type A overachiever.

0 1   I experienced one or more ACEs in childhood (see ACE assessment in Appendix C).

0 1   I currently have PTSD or believe I have unresolved trauma.

0 1   I have recently lost a partner, spouse, pet, or loved one.

0 1   I carry resentment(s), regret, or unresolved grief.

0 1   I find it hard to say no.

0 1   I rarely make time to play or be in community.

0 1   I don't make time to relax or have a daily relaxation practice.

0 1   My life has little meaning or purpose.

0 1   I don't feel loved.

0 1   I feel lonely, isolated, or unsupported much of the time.

0 1   I often feel hopeless or helpless.

List any other relevant stressor(s):

1   _____

1   _____

Total _____

STRESS ASSESSMENT KEY:

0   Incredible! You may be among the very few living virtually stress-free. Keep up the great work and positive attitude.

1–5   Congratulations! You may feel some stress or emotional pain, but you seem to have a pretty good handle on it. Now's a great time to get ahead of health issues by prioritizing your emotional well-being.

6–15   Make your emotional well-being a priority. Take heart in knowing you're not alone. Many people have healed in part or fully from chronic illnesses by prioritizing their emotional well-being.

16+   It's time to take make your emotional well-being your highest priority. Many people find themselves dealing with an overload of stress and emotional pain, which can understandably feel overwhelming. You may be one of those individuals who would benefit from taking the Extra Step on page 214. No matter what, please treat yourself with compassion as you embark on this journey, and have patience with the process. Remember, there are many who have experienced years of stress and unimaginable trauma and yet have *still* succeeded in achieving a state of emotional well-being and full healing.

Step 2: Get a Solid Foundation in Place

A foundation is the base on which everything else stands. It's the ground-level support onto which you can add other layers. Carrying the architectural metaphor forward, if you were going to build a house, you wouldn't start with the roof; you would start with a sturdy foundation. Your emotional well-being foundation includes lifestyle elements that will help you swap habitual fight-flight-freeze mode for rest-and-digest relaxation mode, where repair and restoration happen. Once you're able to regularly get better sleep, breathe more deeply, and move your body—ideally in nature—you will likely feel the energy and motivation necessary to move onto steps 3 and 4.

✔ **Prioritize sleep.** Chronic sleep deficiency can lead to a slew of negative health outcomes, including cardiovascular disease, diabetes, obesity, cancer, and potentially a shortened lifespan. Even a few hours of lost sleep in *a single night* causes inflammation and insulin resistance, and harms your immune system.[18] On the other hand, a good night's sleep is imperative for helping our bodies and brains repair, reorganize, reset, restore, and regenerate. According to American Academy of Sleep Medicine (AASM) past president Safwan Badr, MD, eight to nine hours is critical, not indulgent, *especially* if you have an autoimmune condition.

Give it a try: As the Paleo Mom Sarah Ballantyne, Ph.D., scientist and author, advises, *having a bedtime is not just for kids!* Make a habit of going to bed before ten p.m. (if you can) to get the most restorative sleep. Create a sleep sanctuary by putting your phone in airplane mode (some experts recommend shutting off your Wi-Fi router), unplugging other electronics, and using ear plugs and eyeshades or blackout curtains for total darkness and quiet. Consider getting some early morning sun without sunglasses to support a healthy circadian rhythm, increase HGH (human growth hormone), strengthen your eyes, and boost your immune system.

My successful sleep ritual includes getting into bed by nine p.m., winding down with a good book, wearing silicone ear plugs and a comfortable eye mask, and taking magnesium before bed along with 125 mg of progesterone to both balance my hormones and help me sleep. Most mornings I go for a walk or at least stretch on the deck to get some morning sun in my eyes to help with serotonin and melatonin production.

✔ **Breathe consciously and slowly.** One of the fastest paths to stress relief is right under your nose. It's something you do every minute of every day; it's automatic and free, and yet sadly, breathing is overlooked. Slow, controlled breathing calms the brain's arousal center, activates the calming rest-and-digest parasympathetic nervous system, and sends the message to your mind and body that all is well.

Give it a try: Practice conscious breathing by breathing in through your nose, feeling your in-breath filling your lower abdomen like a balloon, and then slowly exhaling through your nose, deflating your abdomen. Try "5 x 5" breathing right now: Slow your breathing down by slowly counting to five on the inhale and the exhale. Repeat six times to complete one minute. The 5 x 5 breathing technique was proven to significantly increase feelings of relaxation compared with baseline breathing, as well as increase heartrate variability (HRV), an important indicator of health, resilience, and youthfulness.[19] The hardest part of conscious breathing is remembering to do it. I find it works best by having a few cues that automatically remind me—for example, when I'm stopped at traffic lights, in line at the market, or even while I'm walking. Any way you choose to breathe consciously and slowly is a natural tranquilizer for the nervous system.

✔ **Move more.** Science shows that prolonged sitting, defined as more than four hours per day, and lack of movement are associated with greater incidence of poor health outcomes, including cardiovascular disease, diabetes, cancer, and early death.[20] On the other hand, consistent, moderate exercise like thirty minutes or more of daily walking, cycling, swimming, or strength training is anti-inflammatory, immune system–enhancing, and a powerful buffer against stress. Moderate exercise also helps to significantly reduce fatigue, prevent or improve autoimmune conditions, depression, and dementia, and trigger the growth of new brain cells.[21]

Give it a try: Start wherever you are and build from there. If you're bed- or wheelchair-bound, or too ill to even contemplate thirty minutes of exercise, experiment with micromovements or chair/bed yoga and gradually increase the duration and number of times you move per day. If you're physically able and have energy for more activity, pick and schedule exercise you enjoy and will do consistently. Make it easy to add movement throughout your day, like taking the stairs, walking with a friend, or working out at home. Set a reminder on your electronic devices to take hourly stretch or jumping jacks breaks. Get some free weights and an exercise or yoga mat, and find online videos for your fitness level. For variety and proven stress-relief, consider yoga, qigong, or tai chi classes, in person or online. I enjoy working out at home and frequently use free, online options like FitnessBlender.com or GymRa.com, which offer videos with a variety of skill, duration, and intensity levels, including high intensity interval training (HIIT), an efficient way to gain exercise benefits in a shorter time.

✔ **Spend time in nature.** Most people spend about 90 percent (twenty-two hours) of each day indoors; and a growing body of research shows that the air within homes and office buildings may be more seriously polluted than outdoor air, leading to or worsening health problems, especially for the young, elderly, and chronically ill. Research also confirms that spending time in nature has a long list of health benefits, including lowered cortisol, reduced inflammation, improved immune function, decreased feelings of depression and anxiety, and even improved memory.[22] The Japanese practice of "forest bathing"—basically, opening up all your senses in the presence of trees—has been proven to lower blood pressure, glucose levels, and cortisol levels, strengthen the immune system, reduce stress and anxiety, and improve overall feelings of well-being.[23]

Give it a try: Wherever you live, make it a priority to get outside and spend time in nature. Allow yourself to relax into the scenery, taking in the fresh air and scents, ideally without being tethered to an electronic device. Enjoy the calming, restorative effects. Even a one-day trip to a suburban park boosts natural killer (NK) cells and anticancer proteins for seven days afterward![24]

And whenever you can, get a little sun to increase your vitamin
D levels, improve your mood, and improve your sleep, which is
the first of the foundational elements to dial in.[25]

Step 3: Harness the Power of Your Mind

Once you've built up your foundation, it's time to delve deeper and lift
off those extra sticky layers of stress patterns. The greatest source of stress
is arguably our own minds, specifically our imagination, which tends to
create all kinds of negative stories and worst-case scenarios. But conversely,
the fastest path to peace is also our imagination—if we can learn how to
use it in our favor. Harnessing the power of your mind requires awareness,
intention, and some reflection on what's most important to you. Once you
get clear about what you value most, you'll be more aligned with the positive future you envision, and it may be easier to let go of things that are not
aligned with that possibility. Maybe you'll be able to start saying no to ex-
traneous things and free up more time for yourself. Imagine that!

> ✔ **Know your *why*.** In the wise words of nineteenth-century German
> philosopher Friedrich Nietzsche, "He who has a why can withstand
> any how." When it comes to beating the odds of a chronic disease
> like autoimmune conditions or cancer, researcher and author Kelly
> Turner, Ph.D., found that one common trait among survivors and
> thrivers was having strong reasons for living. Your reasons for liv-
> ing inspire and keep you motivated, even when you feel low.
> *Give it a try:* Contemplate the questions:
>
> - What or who do you live for?
> - When you think about the future, what do you look for-
>   ward to?
> - What's on your bucket list—experiences or achievements
>   that you hope to have or accomplish during your lifetime?
>
> There is no shame in not having immediate answers, and there
> is no one right answer. Some of us have spent so much time taking
> care of other people that it seems impossible to even consider our
> own needs. Heed the sage advice of Jacob Teitelbaum, MD, who
> offers: "Do more of what appeals to you and less of what doesn't."

In time, you may notice yourself discovering new passions, which may fuel your own reasons for living. If you can't identify your *why*, ask a close friend or therapist to help.

It took me ages to find my path and purpose. While I spent many years working successfully in jobs I enjoyed, it wasn't until I took a sabbatical and started filling myself up with things I love, like spending more time in nature, learning how to paint, and exploring more healing modalities, that it dawned on me that maybe I could help people become empowered to take greater control of their health outcomes.

For some, children and grandchildren may be the strongest reasons for living. Many people may have causes they care deeply about and even live for. And for others, simply being the best person/partner/friend they can be is enough.

✔ **Surrender your stressors.** You can't rid your life of all stressors, and you wouldn't want to. Increasingly, researchers are identifying the upsides to stress, demonstrating the truth of that old adage, "What doesn't kill you makes you stronger." Moderate amounts of acute or short-term stress—bursts of energy produced by stress hormones—have been found to strengthen the immune system, increase mental performance, protect against some diseases, like Alzheimer's (by keeping brain cells working optimally), and prevent breast cancer (by suppressing the production of estrogen).

Give it a try: Get out a blank sheet of paper and on the left-hand side, list all the things that are stressing you out. Categories might include money, work, family responsibilities, personal health concerns, health problems affecting family members, world events, the news in general, and social media. Don't forget to include any experiences from your childhood that are still causing you emotional pain.

Consider each element on your list and write down on the right-hand side how you plan to handle each. Are there items you can eliminate, minimize, outsource, or just need to accept? Do you need help with anything? For the things you can't control, consider surrendering them to a higher power or the universe. Are there items that require your action, like researching a holistic doctor, finding more fulfilling work, or limiting your exposure to news or social media? Are there places where you're stuck and might benefit from talking with a trusted friend or therapist? Maybe the action required is a shift in perspective, viewing your stressors as strength-promoting challenges or learning opportunities rather than feeling disempowered by circumstances.

Here's a sample from my own stress surrender sheet, which I created during a particularly difficult time, when I was managing a sales team while simultaneously caring for my ill parents and experiencing MS symptoms:

Thing that is stressing me out / What I will do about it

- My mom needs more help with bathing, dressing, and moving around the house. / I will hire an eldercare expert to help me evaluate Mom's needs.
- I am feeling so sad about my mom's declining health. / I will find a local grief counselor.
- I am hypervigilant in the middle of the night in case the phone rings. / I will give this one to God and gently remind myself there's no value in me catastrophizing and losing sleep.
- Frank on my sales team requires so much of my time. / I will make a plan with our HR VP to let him go by the end of next week.
- I am concerned about a new MS symptom of heavy legs on waking. / Whenever I feel the heaviness, I will thank the symptom as a messenger that is reminding me to breathe more, stress less.

An increasing number of studies show that just the act of writing about emotional experiences is healing, and that's certainly been true for me. By deciding proactively what to do with each stressor, I feel less like a victim of circumstance and more in control of my emotional well-being.

✔ **Tap away stress.** Tapping, also called *Emotional Freedom Techniques* or just *EFT*, is a relatively new technique that marries principles of ancient Traditional Chinese Medicine with modern belief-shifting and positive affirmations. By tapping on specific acupuncture meridian points while evoking an anxiety-producing thought and positive affirmation at the same time, signals are sent to the brain to shift out of the stress response. Numerous studies have demonstrated the efficacy of tapping for relief from anxiety, PTSD, phobias, pain/physical symptoms, and depression.[26] Harvard Medical School psychiatrist Rick Leskowitz, Ph.D. calls tapping "the most impressive intervention I've encountered in twenty-five years of work."

Give it a try: The best way to learn tapping is to follow a skilled practitioner. Watch intros with Brad Yates www.youtube.com/watch?v=JiD72cZ5mcU or Julie Schiffman www.youtube.com/watch?v=C7fXY5CPmFw to learn how to tap out stress, anxiety, or fear in less than ten minutes. May sound too good to be true, but you'll never know unless you try it! For me, tapping is one of the easiest and fastest stress-relieving tools in my toolkit. It even helped me to deliver the eulogy for my mom with more grace and peace and fewer tears.

✔ **Meditate—even a little.** Mind chatter, commonly called *monkey mind*, is the default mode network (DMN) of our brains. For some lucky people, the default mode is creative, while in others the pervasive thoughts are a steady, ruminative loop of worries, anxieties, and fears. The science is definitely in on meditation as a means to tame mind chatter by engaging the relaxation response, the parasympathetic counterbalance to the fight-or-flight stress response. Meditation has been shown in numerous studies to decrease stress, anxiety, and depression, increase resilience and empathy, increase the size of your brain, and produce beneficial and immediate changes in the expression of genes involved in immune function.[27] For people who have experienced ACEs, studies have demonstrated that practicing mindfulness reduces depression, anxiety, and trauma-related symptoms; enhances coping and mood; and improves quality of life as well as mental, behavioral, and physical outcomes in children, youths, and adults.[28] Explore and find which type of meditation practice works best for you: following your breath, using a mantra—a sound, word, or phrase you repeat—or mindfulness meditation, a nonjudgmental moment-by-moment awareness.

Give it a try: You may appreciate that meditating would be beneficial, and yet you don't get around to doing it, maybe because you think you don't have time, or because you feel like it would be too hard. But a recent study shows that just ten minutes of daily mindfulness meditation can help prevent your mind from wandering and is particularly effective if you tend to have repetitive, anxious thoughts.[29]

For ten minutes, ideally when you wake up, simply sit in a relaxed position in a quiet place, if possible. Close your eyes. Focus on your breath as you breathe into your belly, consciously and slowly. Repeat a word or sound, like *peace* or *om*. When your mind wanders, gently bring it back to the word or sound. If you want to use a timer, consider a lovely bell, bowl, or chime sounds from apps like Zen or Insight Timer.

Don't think you have ten minutes? Start with five. If that still sounds daunting, start with one minute. Any time you dedicate to stillness and self-compassion, ideally before you check your e-mails or turn on the news, is a gift to savor. For additional guidance and online meditation resources, please refer to resources in Appendix F.

✔ **Use guided imagery.** Your imagination can be your biggest source of stress or your greatest ally in finding emotional freedom. Guided imagery, sometimes called *guided hypnosis* or *guided visualization*, is a gentle mind-body practice that helps to direct your mind to a relaxed, focused state, which is optimal for healing. More than two hundred studies in the past thirty years have shown that guided imagery can dramatically help people who experience fear, anxiety, panic, loss of control, helplessness, and uncertainty. So, it's not surprising that more and more health institutions are embracing guided imagery as a complementary therapy for their cancer, pain, and surgery patients.

Give it a try: Martin Rossman, MD and acupuncturist, is an expert in helping people harness their minds to transform from constant states of worry and anxiety into more consistently calm, healthy, and happy states using guided imagery and creative visualization. He has a deep, soothing voice, perfect for gently guiding people into relaxed and positive states. He has a few free videos online, including this fifteen-minute evocative guided imagery demonstration that he gave at UCSF: www.youtube.com/watch?v=dL96FeiL1Xs. At thehealingmind.org, you'll find numerous CDs to address anxiety and stress, pain relief, sleep, and health and wellness. Another source of numerous guided imagery CDs is www.healthjourneys.com. To find a trained professional near you, look into the Academy for Guided Imagery (acadgi.com/).

Step 4: Increase Positive Emotions

Science confirms that our brains are hardwired to recall and dwell on negative experiences over positive ones as a survival mechanism.[30] To counterbalance the natural tendency toward the negative, we need to proactively work on increasing positive emotions.

> ✔ **Cultivate social connections.** Recent research indicates that actual or perceived loneliness or social isolation are both associated with increased risk for early mortality and are perhaps deadlier than obesity.[31] John Cacioppo, Ph.D., social neuroscientist and author of *Loneliness: Human Nature and the Need for Social Connection,* says loneliness affects one in four people. He warns, "The mortality rate for air pollution is 5 percent. For loneliness, it's 25 percent."
>
> Fortunately, we can change our situation and our perceptions. Strong social connections have been shown to strengthen the immune system, help people recover from disease faster, and help to lower levels of anxiety and depression, and can lead to a 50 percent greater chance of longevity.[32]
>
> *Give it a try:* If you feel isolated, muster the courage to reach out and connect with others. Or, you may need to examine why you feel lonely despite having sufficient social connections. Here are some ideas to help you find greater connection:
>
> - Consider a class at a local community center: yoga, qigong, meditation, art, etc. Talk to the teacher and other students before or after class to get acquainted.
> - Find a local recreational group: walking, hiking, dancing, bridge, mah-jongg, etc. Using the social media site Meetup.com is a good way to find a group based on area of interest. Again, when it comes to gathering with like-minded strangers, you'll gain more from the experience if you introduce yourself and get acquainted with others.

- Join or create a book club.
- Volunteer at a soup kitchen, food pantry, hospice, or a local school. Introduce yourself to other volunteers and the volunteer coordinator and/or staff.
- Explore a faith community that resonates with you. There are many spiritual and nonreligious organizations that meet weekly. When you attend, introduce yourself to someone, or stay for the social program following the structured service.
- Reconnect with old friends.
- If you're home-bound, ask friends and neighbors to visit; and if you're part of a faith-based community, inquire about community outreach programs.

Once you've dipped your toe in, be open to connecting further with the people you meet. Find more opportunities to bond over shared experiences. We are, after all, social creatures, and for most of us life is more deeply satisfying—and healthy—when it's a shared journey.

✔ **Start a gratitude journal.** When you're feeling low, chances are the last thing you're thinking about is what to be thankful for. Science suggests, however, that people who practice gratitude consistently report numerous benefits, such as stronger immune systems, lowered blood pressure, reduced aches and pains, higher levels of positive emotions, reduced anxiety and depression, and better sleep. While it may feel contrived at first, cultivating an attitude of gratitude grows stronger with use and practice.

Give it a try: Keep a gratitude journal to help establish the habit of greater appreciation for people and experiences in your life. There's no one best practice for how often or when to write in your journal, except to really feel the depth of your gratitude while adding to your list. And if writing things down doesn't appeal to you, just make an extra effort to pause, mentally note, and deeply feel what you appreciate. When Mary Ruddick, certified nutrition consultant and ancestral lifestyle expert, was bedridden and attempting to heal from twelve painful disorders, including postural orthostatic tachycardia syndrome (POTS), Ehlers-Danlos syndrome (EDS), polycystic ovary syndrome (PCOS), Hashimoto's thyroiditis, Graves' disease, and fibromyalgia, she kept a gratitude journal and faithfully wrote in it every night, even when she was feeling down. Her entries included the smallest milestones and events, such as riding the stationary bike for ninety *seconds* or appreciating that her sister called. By spending a little time focusing on and appreciating what you have instead of what you lack, as Mary did, you'll increase your own health and happiness.

✓ **Laugh more.** Studies show that laughing releases feel-good endorphins, relieves pain, decreases stress hormones, improves immune function, and may help you live longer. No wonder more health providers are recommending laughter therapy as a complementary intervention for cancer and other disorders. Norman Cousins wrote a book called *Anatomy of an Illness as Perceived by the Patient: Reflections on Healing and Regeneration* about proactively using laughter (and high-dose vitamin C) to help him heal from his "incurable" and painful autoimmune condition, ankylosing spondylitis (AS). He found that ten minutes of laughter would give him two hours of pain relief. During the weeks of my initial MS diagnosis, my parents and I adopted Cousins' laughter strategy and spent evenings watching sitcoms like *I Love Lucy* and *Cheers*, all in an effort to reduce fear and uncertainty. It helped! Even today, free of all MS symptoms, I still make it a priority to find silly things to laugh about every day.

Give it a try: Humor is very individual, so find what works for you and do more of it. It might be connecting more often with a good friend who makes you laugh, cozying up with a David Sedaris or Bill Bryson book, or watching silly cat videos, sitcoms, funny movies, stand-up comedy specials, or my favorite belly laugh–producing TV show, *America's Funniest Home Videos*. And don't worry if laughter turns into crying. Crying can help you release pent-up trauma!

✓ **Get more hugs.** In some of the saddest research findings, studies show that infants deprived of human touch grow more slowly, fail to thrive, and are more likely to die. On the other hand, recent research demonstrates that premature infants who were massaged for fifteen minutes three times a day gained weight 47 percent faster than those who were left alone in their incubators, with no difference in diet. The massaged infants were released earlier from the hospital, and eight months later, maintained their weight advantage, plus greater mental and motor function. Science confirms that nonsexual touch like hugs or massage supports the immune system, decreases stress, and improves heart health. A simple touch releases oxytocin, known as the bonding or cuddle hormone and dubbed the "elixir of health" by Dr. Kelly Turner, Ph.D. and author of *Radical Remission*. David Hamilton, a former medical researcher and author of *Why Kindness Is Good for You*, studied the healing effects of increased oxytocin levels and found evidence that the hormone lowers inflammation, strengthens the immune system, aids digestion, lowers blood pressure, heals wounds faster, and even repairs damage to the heart after a heart attack.[33]

Give it a try: One ten-second hug can significantly improve your health by reducing stress, easing depression and fatigue, strengthening your immune system, and helping you fight infection.[34] Make a concerted effort to hug people close to you. Animals count, too, since just a few minutes of petting your cat or dog can release oxytocin. Research shows that just staring into your dog's eyes is therapeutic for both the canine and their human companions, raising oxytocin 130 percent in the dog and 300 percent in the human![35]

If you're not in a situation where hugs are readily available, you may want to consider getting massages more often. In addition to daily hugs, I make it a priority to get massaged a few times a month at an inexpensive, yet thoroughly relaxing, local Chinese foot massage place.

✔ **Forgive everyone.** Did you know that unforgiveness is classified in medical books as a *disease*? According to Steven Standiford, MD, chief of surgery at the Cancer Treatment Centers of America, refusing to forgive makes people sick and keeps them that way. According to research by Dr. Michael Barry, a pastor and the author of the book *The Forgiveness Project*, 61 percent of cancer patients have unforgiveness issues. While harboring emotions like anger, resentment, or regret is harmful or even deadly, forgiveness can lead to huge health rewards: lowering the risk of heart attack, improving cholesterol levels and sleep, and reducing pain and bouts of anxiety, depression, and stress.[36]

Give it a try: Good news: forgiveness can be learned. Fred Luskin, Ph.D., director of the Stanford University forgiveness project, has successfully explored forgiveness therapy with people who suffered from unimaginable violence in Northern Ireland, Sierra Leone, and in the 9/11 attacks on the World Trade Center. Dr. Luskin explains that forgiveness does not necessarily mean reconciliation with the person who hurt you or condoning their action. The key, he emphasizes, is to find peace.

Forgiveness can be defined as a conscious, deliberate decision to release feelings of resentment or vengeance toward a person or group who has harmed you, regardless of whether they actually deserve your forgiveness. It does not mean you must forget, deny, or excuse the behavior; it just means that you free yourself of deeply held negative feelings.

If people personally affected by abusive acts or violent events can forgive, like Michelle Corey and those in Dr. Luskin's studies, then there is hope that we, too, can forgive.

One of the most effective forgiveness practices I know is a short but powerful ancient Hawaiian prayer called Ho'oponopono: *I'm sorry. Please forgive me. Thank you. I love you.* Just saying those four lines—in any order—when thinking about people who have harmed you, is heart-opening. If it feels good, put one hand on your heart and the other on your belly while feeling the healing emotion of forgiveness permeate your body and soul. Be sure to say the prayer for yourself! Self-forgiveness may be even more powerful, reducing the risk of clinical depression and improving health by lowering markers of inflammation.[37]

Extra Step: Consider "Prescription-Strength" Tools

✔ **Explore EMDR (eye movement desensitization and reprocessing).** EMDR is a therapy that allows people to reprocess and transform the meaning of traumatic events so they are no longer psychologically disruptive. In an EMDR session, the client is asked to conjure up part of a painful memory or thought while intently tracking the therapist's hand moving back and forth in front of the client's field of vision. In a successful EMDR session, for example, a woman who previously felt victimized and shameful about a sexual assault may feel self-compassion, empowerment, and safety.

Some studies show that up to 90 percent of single-trauma victims no longer have PTSD after only three ninety-minute sessions. Another study, funded by the HMO Kaiser Permanente, found that 100 percent of the single-trauma victims and 77 percent of multiple-trauma victims no longer were diagnosed with PTSD after only six fifty-minute sessions.

There has been so much research on EMDR therapy that it is now recognized as an effective form of treatment for trauma, PTSD, and other disturbing experiences by organizations such as the American Psychiatric Association, the World Health Organization, and the U.S. Department of Defense.

To learn more and find an EMDR-trained therapist, check out Trauma Recovery EMDR Humanitarian Assistance Programs (Trauma Recovery/HAP) at www.emdrhap.org/content/what-is-emdr.

✔ **Explore neurofeedback.** Neurofeedback, biofeedback for the brain, is deeply healing to the central nervous system (CNS). It has been shown to effectively treat severe developmental traumas, including childhood abuse, neglect, or abandonment—or anyone with a fear-driven brain. A growing body of research attests to the effectiveness of neurofeedback for ADHD (attention-deficit hyperactivity disorder), PTSD (post-traumatic stress disorder), ASD (autism spectrum disorder), chronic pain, brain injuries, and epilepsy.[38]

Unlike talk therapy, a person receiving neurofeedback therapy has the experience of playing a video game with their brain. With repeated sessions, users can learn to regulate their brain waves, enabling them to feel calmer, more centered, and less reactive, and even sleep better. Over time, neurofeedback can even grow neural connectivity.

Find an experienced neurofeedback provider at EEG Education and Research Inc.: www.esiaffiliatesforum.com/providers or EEG info: directory.eeginfo.com.

✔ **Explore DNRS (Dynamic Neural Retraining System).** DNRS takes a different approach to healing, asserting that trauma to the limbic system, the brain's emotional center, leads to a stuck brain pattern of fight-flight, which can promote chronic and mysterious illnesses like MCS, CFS, IBS, and Lyme disease. DNRS is a neuroscience-based therapy, focused on rewiring the brain to restore limbic system functionality to improve cognitive function, sensory perception (sensitivities to smell, taste, sound, light), emotional regulation, detoxification, absorption of nutrients, and cellular communication.

There are two ways to experience DNRS: 1. an on-site, five-day immersive, interactive DNRS Neuroplasticity Bootcamp, which includes all training, meals, and lodging (available locations and dates listed on website); or 2. a home-based, fourteen-hour DVD series. Expect the investment of time following the five days or fourteen-hour DVD series to be a minimum of one hour a day for six months. From my investigation and discussion with people who have done both the in-person training and the videos, the in-person, shared experience is worth the extra money. Check out the success stories and see if this is a fit for you at retrainingthebrain.com.

My hope is that these resources will help you not only to cope but also to *thrive*, no matter what's happening around you. Imagine yourself in the eye of a hurricane, where you are able to exist peacefully at the still, calm center. Maybe you've been able to reframe your stress levels and what you once perceived as a Category 5 hurricane is now merely a 1 or 2. Regardless of the force of the storm swirling around you, your commitment to foundational self-care and emotional well-being will enable you to fill your sails with the winds rather than be tossed around by them.

Summary: Top Five Emotional Well-Being Strategies

1. Get eight or more hours of sleep.
2. Move throughout the day, ideally in nature.
3. Meditate—even a little bit—every day.
4. Cultivate meaningful connections.
5. Forgive everyone, including yourself.

CHAPTER 6

Balance Your Hormones

It's easier to fix your hormones than to live with the misery of imbalance.
—Sara Gottfried, MD, hormone expert, and author of
The Hormone Cure: Reclaim Balance, Sleep, Sex Drive and Vitality Naturally with the Gottfried Protocol

Like a symphony where all instruments play in harmony, when your hormones are balanced, everything's in tune. You feel good, look good, sleep well, wake up refreshed, you're energetic, and your clothes fit pretty well. Your immune system is strong, your metabolism is optimal, and your nervous system and mood are steady, too. That's because everything is connected and working together, a feel-good equilibrium called *hormonal homeostasis*.

But when things are out of whack for women, the sound becomes dissonant, and if it gets worse, a cacophony. You have trouble sleeping, wake up tired, need a cup of coffee to get moving in the morning and a glass of wine or two in the evening to relax. Your pants seem to have shrunk, you're anxious all the time, and you'd kill for a nap, if only you could find the time to lie down while trying to tackle your mounting to-do list. If you're dealing with an autoimmune condition on top of a busy life, chances are you're feeling pretty stressed about that, too.

When things are out of balance for men, the tune also changes, albeit more subtly. You don't have the energy you used to, exercise feels harder, and you notice your muscle mass has declined. A spare tire has inflated around your middle, and—*good grief!*—are your breasts growing? You may feel depressed and experience memory problems, too. Thanks to declining testosterone, a result of aging and rising levels of estrogen (due mostly to a diet high in conventionally raised red meat, alcohol, and environmental toxins), your risk for autoimmune conditions goes up.

If you resonate with these scenarios, you're not alone. In fact, this is how many Americans feel, because we're living out of harmony with our natural biological rhythms. While it's true that hormones naturally decline with age, our modern lifestyle has sped up the decline. We stay up too late, live under artificial light, sit too much, rely too heavily on caffeine, and eat too much sugar. We're dealing with more stress than ever before and are confronted every day with an onslaught of environmental toxins. It's a perfect storm for hormonal havoc, leaving us tired, miserable, fatter than ever, and more susceptible to autoimmune disorders.

And women are most vulnerable. If you're female, the odds of developing an autoimmune condition are about three times greater than if you're male. The jury's not completely in on *why*, but it's pointing to women's stronger immune systems, naturally higher levels of estrogen, increased sensitivity to inflammation, and greater exposure to endocrine (hormonal) disrupters called *xenoestrogens* (pronounced ZEE-no-estrogens)—toxic chemicals found in pesticides, plastics, body care products, and makeup—that mimic the molecular structure of estrogen and bind to and hijack estrogen receptors in our bodies.

Hormones may be tiny molecules, but their impact is huge. They're involved in almost every function of our body, including regulating appetite, cravings, digestion, sleep, resilience to stress, immune function, tissue repair, reproduction, stamina, moods, cognitive function (clear vs. foggy thinking), and whether or not we develop autoimmunity.

If you're feeling bad, naturally you go to the doctor. Maybe he runs a standard TSH (thyroid stimulating hormone) test to check your thyroid, which unfortunately is not a complete picture of thyroid function. If your TSH is five or less, he assures you, "Everything's in the normal range. You're fine." Or, he may suggest some combination of the following:

- Just eat less and exercise more.
- Depressed? Here's an antidepressant.
- Anxious? Here's antianxiety medicine.

- Not sleeping? Here's a pill.
- Rashes? Try some cortisone.
- Blood sugar's up? There's a pill for that, too.
- Blood pressure's up? Here's another pill.
- Cholesterol's high? Let's put you on a statin. (Yikes—if you knew that your hormones are made from cholesterol and your doctor wants to *lower* your cholesterol, you might think twice before taking something that both interferes with your hormone production and puts you at risk of some serious downstream complications, like heart disease, diabetes and cancer.)[1]

Or, he may just assure you, "What you're feeling is normal; you're just getting older."

While it's true that most hormones decline with age and lowered hormones accelerate aging, it's *not* normal or inevitable that we develop blood sugar problems, diabetes, sleep problems, or autoimmune disorders.

I suffered from hormonal imbalances from adolescence to perimenopause and followed my doctors' orders, taking birth control pills for decades to smooth out irregular cycles, calm awful PMS, clear up acne, and prevent pregnancy. I had no idea that the synthetic hormones were basically tricking my body into believing it was pregnant for thirty years (anything natural about that?), while increasing my risk of heart disease, cancer, osteoporosis, and autoimmunity.

If I had known then what I know now, I would have tried to balance my hormones naturally with the right lifestyle approaches and would have strongly considered natural birth control methods. When I learned about the risks, I beat myself up for harming my body, but that only created more stress. So, I stopped blaming myself, apologized to my body (especially my poor liver, which had to process all that synthetic estrogen), and channeled my frustration into this book with the hopes that you (and your daughters) will be aware of underlying root causes and adopt natural approaches earlier.

Here's the very good news: hormones are *downstream* from everything else we've covered so far, which is why they're the focus of the last F.I.G.H.T.S. chapter. If you've read the prior chapters, most of what follows will likely be a new spin on familiar topics. In any event, I hope this chapter will serve as additional motivation for you to carefully address each of the F.I.G.H.T.S. root causes.

In the Hormone Balance Toolkit, you'll find proven strategies for balancing hormones naturally, starting with a review of beneficial lifestyle elements that we've already covered. For example, F.I.G.H.T.S. hormone-balancing strategies include eating your optimal foods, shoring up nutrient deficiencies, reducing stress, getting restorative sleep, moving more, removing toxins, and supporting the health of your gut and liver. If you've already started implementing strategies from previous toolkits, congratulations! You've already begun promoting hormone balance, so additional efforts may be minimal. If you haven't gotten started yet, no worries—hormonal balance will naturally follow beneficial lifestyle changes, once you're ready for action.

To be clear, the topic of hormones is vast and complicated, and I am not attempting to cover everything. This chapter focuses on the main hormone imbalances implicated in autoimmune conditions, most of which occur for women in particular, especially during the reproductive years. For more comprehensive resources on hormones, please refer to Appendix F for recommended books and videos.

Putting the H in F.I.G.H.T.S.

The fastest path out of hormonal hell and back to hormonal homeostasis is to address each of the F.I.G.H.T.S. categories head-on. In fact, many integrative hormone practitioners believe added hormones, like bioidentical ones, are the icing on the cake, not the cake itself, and won't take on clients who refuse to change their diet and lifestyle. (I know, bad metaphor, since cake is not on the menu—unless, of course, it's a gluten-free, organic Paleo cake sweetened with stevia or birch wood–derived xylitol).

All of the components of F.I.G.H.T.S. can contribute to hormonal imbalance and immune dysfunction and can set the stage for autoimmunity. Let's examine how:

Food: You've probably heard of insulin and know that it's connected to diabetes, but did you know it's a *hormone*? The Western diet, high in sugar, low in fiber and micronutrients, promotes high levels of insulin and is the main reason half of Americans today have prediabetes or diabetes—and may not even know it.

Infections: This one is a double-edged sword. Hormone imbalances can lower our normal protection against infections, and infections themselves can create hormonal imbalances. For example, excess estrogen can promote the unregulated growth of *Candida*; and *Candida* overgrowth encourages estrogen dominance (a state of high estrogen relative to progesterone).

Gut: When you think about your gut, chances are you're not thinking about your hormones. But the microbiome itself has been recently deemed an endocrine (hormonal) organ because gut flora is intimately connected with hormone production and function, including thyroid, estrogen, cortisol, and insulin, to name a few. An imbalanced gut microbiome can create imbalances in your hormones, including low thyroid, estrogen dominance, lowered serotonin (the "happy" neurotransmitter), appetite regulation problems, and insulin resistance.

Hormones: When even a single hormone is out of balance, others are impacted, creating a downward domino effect. For example, increases in the stress hormone cortisol can lower sex hormone production, raise blood sugar, increase both inflammation and insulin resistance, and make you gain belly fat, which, in a vicious cycle, produces *more* estrogen, leading to higher insulin and greater risk for all kinds of chronic disease.

Toxins: Toxicants are huge drivers of insulin resistance, elevated estrogen, obesity, and autoimmune conditions. The ubiquitous presence of endocrine disruptors in our environment—like pesticides, plastic, and BPA—are causing girls to go through puberty earlier, driving the increased incidence of diabetes and doubling the risk of MS in adolescent girls.[2]

Stress. Perhaps the biggest villain of all, chronic stress in all its forms disrupts hormonal balance across the board. Ongoing daily stress, unresolved emotional pain, poor sleep, minimal movement, and other physical, chemical, and emotional stressors lead to high and then low cortisol, insulin resistance, disrupted sex hormones, a leaky gut, and runaway inflammation, which is the perfect setup for obesity, diabetes, autoimmune conditions, and Alzheimer's disease.

As you proactively address each F.I.G.H.T.S. category, you will be moving toward hormonal balance, which is the optimal state for healing and preventing chronic illness.

- By removing gluten, sugar, and dairy and by minimizing carbohydrates, you improve insulin sensitivity.
- By healing your gut, you improve function of numerous hormones.
- By clearing gut infections, you help resolve imbalanced gut flora and inflammation and move toward hormone balance.
- By minimizing exposure to toxins, you decrease estrogen dominance and improve insulin sensitivity.
- By addressing your stress, you move *all* of your hormones toward balance.
- By balancing estrogen, you improve your resistance to infections.

In other words, by attending to each category, you reduce your risk for all chronic disease and move closer to vibrant health. Whew! Ready?

The Main Hormones
Implicated in Autoimmunity

Hormones are chemical messengers of the endocrine system, which is made up of a dozen glands, including the hypothalamus, pituitary, adrenals, pancreas, thyroid, and gonads (ovaries in women and testicles in men). Hormones are your body's way of communicating to distant sites, instructing cells to, among many other things, develop at puberty, repair damaged tissue, regulate your blood sugar, fire up your libido, handle emergencies, and stabilize your mood. In response to signals from the brain, hormones travel through the bloodstream to bind to receptors on or inside cells in a perfect lock-and-key formation. Hormone imbalance happens if your glands don't produce enough of a hormone (key), or if your receptors (locks) are jammed with synthetic, foreign, or toxic chemicals. All it takes is one hormonal imbalance to negatively impact the rest, and a downward spiral of health problems may ensue.

While we have dozens of hormones, the star players when it comes to autoimmune issues are thyroid, cortisol, insulin, and the sex hormones: progesterone, testosterone, and three primary estrogens (estrone, estradiol, and estriol). Other important players include DHEA and vitamin D, which you may be surprised to learn is a hormone. Let's take a look at each before we dig into the big hormonal imbalances implicated in autoimmunity.

Meet the Key Players

Estrogen—the "pro-fat hormone." Estrogen is actually a trio of hormones under the umbrella called *estrogen*: estrone, estradiol, and estriol. Estrogen is responsible for the development of breasts, hips, and menstrual periods. Both men and women produce estrogen, although women produce much more—at least until menopause, when levels drop dramatically. Estrogen helps keep your heart, bones, skin, and brain healthy and your cortisol and thyroid hormones in check. When estrogen is balanced, it promotes serotonin, the neurotransmitter that helps keep you content and sleeping well.

Progesterone—the "protective hormone." Made by both men and women, progesterone is the calming counterbalance to stimulating estrogen. It has also been called the "protective hormone," because it is essential for creating and maintaining pregnancy, protecting the developing baby from stress, and may also be protective against cancer. High levels of progesterone during pregnancy also puts many autoimmune diseases, like MS, into remission. Progesterone is found in high concentrations in our brains, where it exerts a calming, sedative effect. In optimal levels, it helps with sleep, bone building, and libido, and you feel contentment and a sense of equilibrium.

Testosterone—the "assertive hormone." Testosterone is considered a male hormone, but women make it, too, just in much smaller amounts. Testosterone builds tissue, like muscles, bones, and the heart. It's responsible for your zest for life and sex drive. At optimal levels, testosterone decreases body fat, improves muscle strength, and enhances memory, motivation, and cognitive function. Testosterone naturally declines with age, but insulin resistance, elevated cortisol, and excess estrogen—due to chronic inflammation, belly fat and/or toxic chemicals—hasten testosterone's decline.

Thyroid—the "energy hormone." The thyroid is a butterfly-shaped gland in your neck that has a huge role in your body. It's your master metabolic regulator, responsible for regulating your breathing, body temperature, heart rate, energy level, and weight. Every single cell in your body has thyroid receptors, and if your thyroid is not functioning optimally, *you* won't be functioning optimally. At least, not for long. When your thyroid is working well, your body temperature will feel just right, your metabolism will be revving, your energy levels will be good, and your hair will be growing.

Cortisol—the "stress hormone." Cortisol is known as the "stress hormone" for good reason. It has many functions, but its most important job is to increase blood sugar and blood pressure to get blood to your extremities, so you can fight or flee and survive short-term threats. When balanced and working optimally, cortisol is anti-inflammatory and helps to regulate the immune response. When out of balance due to chronic stress, cortisol has an inflamma-

---

Little-Known Hormone Facts

- Fat cells are the largest endocrine gland in the body.
- Testosterone can be converted into estrogen by a process called *aromatization*.
- "Man boobs" and "beer bellies" are telltale signs that men are aromatizing testosterone into fat-promoting estrogen.
- It's not just sugar that makes you fat. Stress and poor sleep also make you fat.
- All of your sex and adrenal hormones are made from cholesterol.
- When you're chronically stressed, your body preferentially makes the stress hormone cortisol instead of sex hormones. No wonder your libido goes down when you're stressed!

tory and immune-suppressing effect—consider how you're more vulnerable to infections when you're stressed.

Insulin—the "fat fertilizer hormone." While its main function is to enable your body's cells to take up glucose for fuel, too much insulin in the bloodstream—caused by eating too much sugar and carbohydrates that quickly turn into sugar—causes your cells to store fat. Too much insulin—a condition called insulin resistance—is actually a state of prediabetes, which is the path to type 2 diabetes. This unnatural, modern condition is a massive risk factor for all other chronic disease, including Alzheimer's, which is sometimes called type 3 diabetes!

Vitamin D—the "sunshine vitamin." Vitamin D is actually a potent prohormone because it is produced in the skin in response to exposure to sunlight and converted into the hormonally active form by the liver and kidneys. Vitamin D receptors are found in almost every cell because vitamin D plays numerous roles in multiple bodily functions, including insulin regulation, immune function, and inflammation reduction.

Dehydroepiandrosterone (DHEA)—the "foundational hormone." The most abundant steroid hormone in the body, DHEA is the precursor hormone to testosterone and estrogen and is essential for tissue building and repair and supporting healthy immune function. DHEA plays a key role in maintaining hormonal balance and youthful vitality. In normal levels, DHEA supports cognitive function, psychological wellbeing, bone, skin, and heart health, and enhances immunity.

The Six Major Hormonal Imbalances in America

There are six big hormonal imbalances contributing to autoimmune and other chronic diseases today:

1. High insulin
2. High cortisol
3. Estrogen dominance

4. Low thyroid
5. Low vitamin D
6. Low DHEA

And, unfortunately, we frequently have a combination of all six and don't even know it!

But the good news is that these imbalances are mostly within our control.

Let's take a look at the most common hormonal imbalances so we can get our arms around the problem, and then we'll delve into solutions in the Hormone Balance Toolkit. If you've read the prior chapters and/or have been incorporating changes as we go through each chapter, this may be a breeze. As you read about the common imbalances, see if you can spot two primary patterns. *Hint*: both start with the letter *s*.

1. **High insulin—aka insulin resistance.** High insulin is arguably the leading driver of chronic disease in the Western world. High insulin fuels chronic inflammation, promoting obesity, diabetes, heart disease, cancer, autoimmune conditions, and Alzheimer's disease. And the biggest culprit behind insulin resistance is, in a word, sugar.

First, we have to expand the definition of sugar beyond the obvious white table sugar. A recent study showed that nearly 90 percent of the average source of added sugars, in fact, comes from processed (refined carbohydrate) foods, defined as soft drinks, salty snacks, cakes, pizza, and frozen meals.[3] Processed foods often contain high quantities of sugar, fructose, refined flours, man-made fats, excess sodium, and artificial toxic additives.

Here's a very brief history of humanity's sugar consumption: For millions of years, sugar was a rare treat. Our ancestors ate honey from time to time, but normally foods were no sweeter than the occasional carrot. Daniel Lieberman, evolutionary biologist, professor at Harvard University, and author of *The Story of the Human Body: Evolution, Health, and Disease*, explains that farming made starchy foods more abundant, but that it wasn't until very recently that technology made sugar ubiquitous. He cautions that our bodies are not adapted to the amount of sugar that we now consume and that it's making us sick. Obesity and chronic disease were not on our ancestral radar partly because sugar was so scarce and partly because carbs were not constantly available. Fast forward to a hundred years ago, when the average person consumed about five pounds of sugar per year. Twenty years ago, that number leapt to twenty-six pounds of sugar a year; and today, that number has jumped to a staggering sixty-six pounds of added sugar per person, per year.[4]

The American Heart Association (AHA) recommends no more than six teaspoons (twenty-five grams) of added sugar per day for women; nine teaspoons (thirty-eight grams) for men; six teaspoons (twenty-five grams) per day for children aged three to eighteen; and children two and under should not have *any* added sugar. What's actually happening is that the average child in the United States is eating nineteen teaspoons of added sugar *per day*—more than three times the recommended limit. For a little perspective, one can of regular soda has over nine teaspoons (thirty-nine grams) of sugar, and low-fat, flavored yogurts may have up to eleven teaspoons (forty-seven grams) of sugar—each of which by itself is over the daily limit for *anyone*!

KEY CONCEPT: *Key concept: Excess consumption of carbohydrates (carbs) and sugar drives insulin resistance*

When you eat too many refined carbohydrates, your insulin levels surge in an effort to get your cells to take up the sugar. But like in the story of the boy who cried wolf, over time your cells become deaf to the noise. Your pancreas pumps out more and more insulin, in effect screaming at your cells to take up the sugar; but your cells, now insulin resistant, no longer respond, and insulin levels continue to rise in the bloodstream. Because excess sugar can't be stored in the liver or muscles, your body stores the sugar as fat, usually around your abdomen. In a vicious cycle, extra fat raises insulin and estrogen levels, too, increasing the risk for autoimmune conditions and cancer.

Symptoms of insulin resistance include:

- Fatigue after eating
- General fatigue
- Craving sweets, especially after meals
- Weight gain in the abdominal area—an apple shape where waist girth is equal to or greater than hips
- Weight loss resistance

- Frequent urination
- Migrating aches and pains
- Dark patches of skin called *acanthosis nigricans* on the back of the neck, elbows, knees, knuckles, or armpits

If these sound like familiar signs or symptoms, you'll want to get your insulin levels measured, revisit the Food chapter, and examine your daily sugar and total carbohydrate consumption.

Lest you think sugar's the only villain in the high-insulin story, think again. It's not just sugar and belly fat that drive insulin resistance; it's also stress—which is why many thin people are insulin resistant, too, and probably don't know it. Let's take a look at the next extremely common hormonal imbalance: high cortisol.

2. **High cortisol.** High cortisol may be tied for first place with high insulin in the most prevalent hormonal imbalance contest. And the biggest culprit when it comes to high cortisol is also one word: *stress.*

Our adrenal glands produce many hormones, including the stress hormones adrenaline and cortisol. Hormone expert Kathryn Retzler, ND, author of *HormoneSynergy*, uses the metaphor of wind to describe cortisol. In small amounts, cortisol is like the wind that makes it fun to sail; but, in large amounts over time, cortisol can produce destructive hurricane-force winds.

As we examined in the Stress chapter, we are designed to deal with bursts of stress and then recover. But since we're human, we have the capacity for endless fear, anxiety, and worry, which activates and perpetuates the stress response—raising cortisol higher and higher, sometimes for good reason, but usually for no real reason at all. Chronic stress is the cause of the devastating cortisol hurricane Dr. Retzler warns against. The more stress you're under, the more your body is pushed into a catabolic state. This means your body is breaking down faster than it can build up, which leads to faster aging and decline. With ongoing stress, cortisol may first become too high, and then, if stress continues, cortisol resistance can happen, where cells become deaf to increasing levels, and cortisol can drop to below normal levels or flatline. Sometimes cortisol levels can peak and plunge in the same day.

It's not just psychological stress that drives cortisol up. All kinds of stressors increase cortisol, including inflammation, infections, food sensitivities, leaky gut, nutrient deficiencies like magnesium and zinc, overexercising, excess alcohol or caffeine, poor sleep, and toxins.

How do you know if you have cortisol issues? Consider these common symptoms:

- Feeling tired but wired, edgy, or anxious
- Anxiety
- Palpitations
- Trouble sleeping
- Salt cravings
- Dizziness when you stand up
- Low blood pressure
- Sugar cravings, because your body can't regulate your blood sugar properly

If these symptoms seem familiar, you will want to get a salivary cortisol test (learn more in the Hormone Balance Toolkit) and review the Stress chapter for assistance with addressing stress in ways that work for you.

Elevated cortisol has widespread impacts, including throwing your other hormones out of balance. For example, high cortisol from stress can block progesterone receptors, depleting calming progesterone. And what happens when progesterone goes down? Estrogen, by default, goes up, like a seesaw, which you'll see is the next big hormonal imbalance: estrogen dominance.

3. **Estrogen dominance.** Estrogen may endow us with soft, feminine curves, but when she dominates, she can be a powerfully dangerous force. Estrogen dominance, defined as too much estrogen (specifically estradiol) relative to progesterone for women and too much estrogen (estradiol) relative to testosterone for men, is an underdiagnosed, serious health concern, making both women and men more susceptible to disease—especially breast cancer, autoimmune conditions, heart disease, and Alzheimer's.

As a normal part of aging, especially after age thirty-five, progesterone and testosterone levels decline, naturally tilting the balance in the direction of estrogen dominance. Today it is common for women to have too much estrogen (relative to progesterone) before age fifty. Harvard-trained physician and hormone expert Sara Gottfried, MD, says that eighty percent of women over thirty-five are affected by estrogen dominance. The two big reasons? High levels of emotional stress and more exposure to artificial estrogens than ever before.

We've just seen that high levels of stress and, therefore, high cortisol depletes progesterone, making estrogen more dominant. As for the artificial estrogens, we need to shine a bright light on synthetic chemicals in the environment called *xenoestrogens*. What are the biggest culprits in the artificial estrogen pollution arena? You may remember these baddies from the Toxins chapter: Bisphenol A (BPA)—found in food cans and the ink of grocery receipts; phthalates—plasticizers found in everything from plastic wrap to baby toys; and parabens—found mostly in body care products and cosmetics.

One telltale sign that women are being bombarded with additional environmental estrogen is the fact that girls are getting their first periods at younger ages than ever recorded in history. In the nineteenth century, the typical age of menstrual onset for girls was fifteen. Today the average age is twelve, but increasingly, girls are experiencing "precocious puberty," with one in five thousand having her first period before age nine.[5]

Not only does this present potential emotional and behavioral problems, but it also increases the risk for chronic disease. Evidence suggests the longer a woman's exposure to high levels of estrogen in her lifetime, the greater her chance of developing hormone-related disorders in later life, including breast, endometrial, and uterine cancers and some autoimmune conditions like lupus and MS. For example, one large study of 77,300 women showed that the earlier a girl reaches menarche (her first period) and, therefore, the longer her exposure to estrogen, the greater her risk of developing MS becomes; and conversely, the later the menarche, the lower the risk of MS.[6]

What else is causing estrogen dominance? Turns out we're getting more than our fair share of estrogens from a variety of external factors, including birth control pills, synthetic hormone replacement therapy (HRT), and SAD foods—most notably conventional cow dairy, which contains high levels of hormones. Three internal factors also work against us, keeping estrogens high. First, chronic inflammation from any source increases estrogen inside the body by activating an enzyme called aromatase. Second, fat cells produce estrogen, especially after menopause, so the more fat you have, the more estrogen you produce. Third, if your liver is overtaxed, it may have trouble excreting used-up estrogen—if so, the metabolites (estrogen waste products) can recirculate and promote estrogen dominance, thereby increasing your risk for cancer.

Common symptoms of estrogen dominance in women:
- Heavy menstrual bleeding
- Severe menstrual cramps
- Premenstrual breast tenderness
- Premenstrual bloating and puffiness
- Weight gain in hips and butt
- Ovarian cysts
- Endometriosis
- Fibroids
- Migraines
- Miscarriages
- Rosacea
- Insomnia
- Brain fog
- Anxiety, panic attacks, or depression
- Decreased libido
- Gallbladder issues or no gallbladder

Common signs of estrogen dominance in men:
- Fatigue
- Loss of muscle mass
- Urinary tract issues
- Reduced libido
- Erectile dysfunction
- Anxiety
- Depression
- Increased belly fat
- Enlarged breasts (gynecomastia)

If any of these symptoms sound familiar to you, you'll want to explore your sources of added estrogens and review the Toxins chapter in particular to make sure you're avoiding harmful xenoestrogens. You'll also want to consider limiting alcohol and taking estrogen-lowering supplements as outlined in the toolkit.

When estrogen levels are high, the liver produces high levels of thyroid-binding globulin (TBG), a protein which binds to thyroid hormones in the blood, preventing them from getting into cells. Lab tests may not pick up the thyroid hormone deficiency, which is the next biggest hormonal imbalance: low thyroid.

4. **Low thyroid.** Low thyroid function, commonly called *hypothyroidism*, is complex and could fill an entire book, so consider this the highlight reel. Low thyroid function is estimated to affect up to three hundred million people worldwide, with up to sixty million of those in the United States, making it one of the most common modern disorders.[7]

   More than 20 percent of women and 10 percent of men have low thyroid function, yet most remain both unaware of their condition and undiagnosed by medical testing.[8] This is especially concerning as low thyroid function, if unaddressed, is linked with a greater risk for depression, infertility, heart disease, autoimmune conditions, and degenerative brain conditions including Hashimoto's encephalopathy (HE), and Alzheimer's disease.

   Because your thyroid gland is your body's metabolic thermostat, you can think of low thyroid as a s-l-o-w metabolism disorder. Symptoms may come on so gradually that you hardly notice that you're feeling a little more sluggish, tired, and cold than normal. Low thyroid occurs when the thyroid gland does not produce enough of the hormones T4 and T3; and your pituitary—the boss of your thyroid—produces more and more TSH (thyroid stimulating hormone), attempting to stimulate the thyroid into producing more of the needed T4 and T3 hormones.

   It turns out that the vast majority of people with low thyroid function—maybe 90 percent—have an autoimmune condition, known as Hashimoto's thyroiditis, named for the Japanese physician who discovered it in 1912. As with all autoimmune conditions, Hashimoto's is not technically a thyroid problem—it's an *immune system problem* in which your own body attacks your thyroid gland, often due to molecular mimicry. Unfortunately, thyroid tissue is often molecularly similar to an antigen (foreign molecule) being targeted by the immune system.

A primary reason Hashimoto's is underdiagnosed is that conventional doctors typically order only a TSH blood test to evaluate thyroid status, which doesn't catch the problem early enough. Standard reference ranges have considered normal TSH to be between 0.5 and 5.5; forward-thinking doctors now consider TSH over 2.0 to be too high. Which means doctors and endocrinologists have been waiting too long to treat Hashimoto's. And, rather than seek and correct the root causes of the Hashimoto's, the doctor usually just prescribes a synthetic T4 medication. For many people, that may be insufficient because, due to micronutrient deficiencies, stress, toxins, or infections, they are unable to convert the inactive T4 into the necessary active hormone, T3. Functional Medicine practitioner McCall McPherson, PA, says it's like putting crude oil (T4) in your car and expecting it to convert to gasoline (T3). Without the T3 "gas," many people stay stuck in a slow metabolic state, which is why many experts advocate a combination of T4 and T3 thyroid medication, like Armour Thyroid, Nature-Throid, or Westhroid, while patients address their underlying root causes.

What are typical root causes of Hashimoto's? Top triggers include:

- Gluten sensitivity (note that celiac disease is often under-diagnosed)
- Nutritional deficiencies including iodine, zinc, and selenium, which are needed for that T3 conversion
- Environmental toxins including fluoride, bromine, and mercury
- Chronic stress and adrenal dysfunction
- Viral infections including Epstein-Barr virus (EBV) and *Yersinia enterocolitica*

Common signs of low thyroid:

- Weight gain
- Weight loss resistance

- Hair loss, including the outer third of your eyebrows
- Poor concentration
- Brain fog
- Constipation
- Feeling tired on waking
- Cold intolerance or sensitivity to cold
- Depression or anxiety
- Joint aches and pain
- Dry skin, hair, or brittle nails

If these symptoms sound familiar to you, you'll want to have your doctor run a comprehensive thyroid panel including these six markers: TSH, free T3, free T4, reverse T3, and the two thyroid antibodies, TPOab and TGab, which will let you know whether or not you have or are at risk for Hashimoto's. The key to reversing Hashimoto's is to discover your root causes, remove them, and heal your gut. Supplemental thyroid medication—ideally one that combines T4 with the active form, T3—may be necessary to optimize levels and return to normal thyroid function.

Don't forget to get your vitamin D levels tested! In one study, 92 percent of people with Hashimoto's were shown to be vitamin D deficient compared with controls.[9] That's the next big hormonal imbalance we'll explore: low vitamin D.

5. **Low vitamin D.** Vitamin D deficiency may be the biggest undiagnosed health problem in the world. Thankfully, it's the easiest to fix. Worldwide, vitamin D deficiency affects nearly a billion people, and it's been reported that 75 percent of Americans are deficient, including 95 percent of African Americans. People at greatest risk for deficiency include those over age sixty-five, those with darker skin pigmentation, and those who limit sun exposure or those who always wear sun protection. SPF 15 or greater decreases vitamin D production by 99 percent.[10] Additionally, people like me who have mutations in their vitamin D receptor site genes, called *VDRs*, may also be at greater risk for vitamin D deficiency. This genetic glitch means we need even more sun exposure and/or supplementation to ensure sufficient levels.

There is mounting evidence that vitamin D deficiency is linked to increased risk for cardiovascular disease, cancer, dementia, and autoimmune conditions, including rheumatoid arthritis (RA), systemic lupus erythematosus (SLE), inflammatory bowel disease (IBD), MS, and type 1 diabetes (T1D). For example, researchers from the Harvard T.H. Chan School of Public Health who studied health data from more than eight hundred thousand Finnish women found that women with vitamin D deficiency—defined as less than 20 ng/ml (nanograms per milliliter)—were 43 percent more likely to develop MS than their counterparts who had normal levels of the vitamin (more than 20 ng/ml). Of the participants with MS, nearly 60 percent were vitamin D deficient.[11]

Most of the time, vitamin D deficiency is subclinical, meaning it's common to have no obvious symptoms. If you do have any of the following, you may be extremely deficient (< 20 ng/ml):

- Fatigue
- General aches and pains
- Weakness
- Frequent infections
- Osteopenia
- Osteoporosis
- Bone pain
- Bone fractures

The best way to determine your vitamin D levels is with a blood test, technically called a 25(OH)D test or simply a vitamin D test. Optimal levels of vitamin D for preventing and reversing chronic disease appear to be between 70–100 ng/ml. If you get plenty of sun and/or supplement with vitamin D and your levels are below 50 ng/ml, you'll want to check your VDR genetic status. You can do that by getting a genetic test like www.23andme.com and have the raw data interpreted by one of many genetic interpretation sites like NutraHacker.com, StrateGene.com, or LiveWello.com.

Last but not least is one more hormonal deficiency, which, like low vitamin D, is commonly found in people with autoimmune conditions: low DHEA.

6. **Low DHEA.** The foundation hormone known for its immune-protective role and association with longevity, DHEA peaks in young adults around age twenty, and then declines year after year so that by age eighty, levels have dropped to only 5 percent or 10 percent of peak levels.

Two big reasons for the marked decline in DHEA are aging and chronic stress. And the biggest contributing factor to both premature aging and chronic stress appears to be inflammation. As we've seen, when you're under lots of stress for an extended period of time, cortisol goes up and has an inflammatory effect in the body. Your adrenal glands make both cortisol and DHEA, but when demand for cortisol is high, especially over extended periods of high stress, your adrenals get depleted and production of DHEA suffers.

The consequences of elevated cortisol and reduced DHEA levels are devastating: the immune system becomes compromised, aging accelerates, and the risk for numerous health problems goes up. Not surprisingly, low DHEA levels are observed in many degenerative diseases, including chronic fatigue syndrome, diabetes, autoimmune conditions, Alzheimer's disease, cancer, and heart disease. For example, studies show strong correlations between low DHEA and Sjögren's, lupus, MS, and RA.[12, 13, 14]

Common signs of low DHEA:

- Profound fatigue
- Decreased stamina and alertness
- Feeling achy and weak
- Malaise or depression
- Decrease in muscle mass
- Decreased bone density or osteoporosis
- Thinning skin
- Low libido
- Frequent infections
- Dry skin and eyes
- Poor memory
- Difficulty in losing weight

If you believe you may be dealing with low DHEA, you'll want to do a salivary cortisol test that measures both cortisol and DHEA levels.

Multiple Hormonal
Imbalances Driven by Stress

The vast majority of us in this country are dealing with a lot of stress much of the time, so it's not surprising that high cortisol is the biggest hormonal imbalance Sara Gottfried, MD, has seen in her more than twenty-five thousand patients over twenty-five years. Dr. Sara refers to cortisol as the "Dark Lord" because it controls most of the other hormones, including how fast or slow your thyroid works, whether you are more or less insulin resistant, whether your sex hormones are produced or not, whether or not you'll be estrogen dominant, whether or not your vitamin D receptors (VDRs) take up circulating vitamin D, and whether or not you'll produce sufficient DHEA. Given that cortisol is likely ruling the roost most of the time in most of our lives, it's not surprising that many people experience combinations of multiple hormonal imbalances, and sometimes all six, like I did.

Sugar and Stress, A Hormonal Mess: My Story

Until quite recently, I can't remember a time when my hormones were balanced. Most of my life, I didn't have a clue about hormones; I certainly didn't know that my lifestyle could influence my hormones and lead to imbalance or balance. With hindsight, it's easy to see how my always-on stressed state coupled with an addiction to sugar was the perfect setup for the hormonal misery that began in my teens and continued to plague me through perimenopause. File this under: better late than never.

Some of my earliest memories are of my dad yelling at my mom, usually about her weight, and me, child warrior, yelling back at him in an attempt to protect my mom. I became hypervigilant and even endured a long period of insomnia as a child. I am certain that chronic stress was the biggest contributing factor to my developing MS at nineteen. Even today, with a big toolkit of stress-reducing tools, including daily meditation and exercise, lots of hugs, a supportive husband, good friends to laugh with, occasional yoga, and plenty of sleep, wrangling stress remains my top priority.

As for sugar, my mom didn't buy sugary cereals or snacks, so to make the barely sweet whole-grain cereals more palatable, I added sliced banana, sometimes raisins, several heaping teaspoons of sugar or honey, and then drenched it all in nonfat milk. I'd have two big bowls, slurping up the sweetened milk when I finished. The added sugar alone met the AHA's daily recommendation for women of no more than six teaspoons (25 grams). When you add the amount of sugar already in the cereal (18 grams), half a banana (7 grams), 1 ounce raisins (17 grams) plus two cups non-fat milk (24 grams) that's about 91 grams of total sugar—before eight a.m.! Little wonder that my blood sugar was usually over one hundred, in the prediabetic range, and I'm pretty sure my insulin levels were elevated, too, even though I don't think anyone ever checked it in my first three decades.

Puberty hit me like a ton of bricks. When my period finally arrived at age fifteen, I had such excruciating cramps I once passed out in a public restroom. Every so often I'd miss school for a day or two because the pain was so intense, and my mom had to tend to me with heating pads and extra strength ibuprofen. Eventually, my OB/GYN urged me to go on the pill to even out painful, infrequent cycles and worsening acne.

By the time I was in my thirties, my husband and I had decided not to have children, and my OB/GYN said I could just stay on the pill right until menopause. This was the same OB/GYN who wrote "Excellent!" on my lab report next to my total cholesterol of 104. Remember what your hormones are made out of: cholesterol. I was barely producing enough cholesterol to scrape together my sex hormones, let alone repair the damage from all the inflammation that the high cortisol was producing.

It wasn't until 2010, when I discovered I had non-celiac gluten sensitivity, that I began to educate myself deeply about the root causes of MS and other autoimmune conditions. In the process, I learned how sugar, stress, and the pill can wreak havoc on hormonal homeostasis, so I went off the pill, stopped eating sugar, and continued to seek ways to reduce stress and heal any unresolved emotional pain.

But being on the pill and under stress for so long created some unwanted lasting effects: Nearly all of my sex hormones were at the bottom end of normal, while my cortisol was too high. My thyroid hormones were all low normal; my DHEA was below the reference range, with the DHEA-to-cortisol ratio even lower; my vitamin D level was dismally low at thirty-eight; plus my free testosterone was not detectable. That would explain much about my low energy, decreased libido, and frequent colds. To top it off, even though my estrogen was low, I was estrogen dominant. Perimenopause brought severe PMS that was reminiscent of puberty, with mood swings, easy irritability, and even nausea.

I started working with a holistic doctor who taught me a conservative approach to balancing hormones. He warned that taking hormones was a sledgehammer when what was needed was a delicate touch like herbs and adaptogens. At first, maca supplements did wonders for eliminating night sweats, but six weeks later, they were back with a vengeance. Three other supplements worked, with subtle albeit noticeable effects, and so I continue to use them in rotation: the adaptogenic herbs ashwagandha and Rhodiola rosea plus the brain-nourishing phosphatidylserine (PS). Together they help raise my daytime energy levels, promote a calmer mood, and improve my sleep. As for my thyroid, I was slightly hypothyroid but had no elevated antibodies, so it was not Hashimoto's. Nevertheless, I tried compounded thyroid medication for a time, but it turns out I was deficient in zinc and iodine, so adding both in supplement form, plus healing my gut, raised my T3 levels sufficiently without the need to continue thyroid meds.

While my stress levels were far reduced from their peak in the 2000s when I was caring for my aging parents while managing a sales team and dealing with unpredictable MS symptoms, I still suffered from what my husband calls "cortisol addiction." I was so used to being in a stressed state, I'd unconsciously create cortisol-stimulating situations like overfilling my schedule, drinking too much coffee, and being too quick to defend. It became imperative for me to find ways to pause and find peace every day. That led me to Muse, a neurofeedback headband that I often wear while I meditate. Chirping birds let me know I'm calm, while crashing waves indicate my mind is active.

Over time, my bird scores have consistently risen, the waves subsided, and even my husband can tell I'm more easygoing.

Even with a dialed-in, organic, sometimes ketogenic, Paleo-template diet, stress reduction, and supplements, as peri-menopause progressed I began to suffer from hot flashes, night sweats, and nighttime awakenings. I stopped drinking what little alcohol I drank and cut way back on caffeine. Still I remained sleep deprived and uncomfortably sweaty. I did more research and finally decided to work with a naturopath who was skilled in bioidentical hormones. We followed a "less is more" approach, and it took nearly a year to fill my depleted tank with just the right amounts of needed hormones. What worked for me was a combination of oral progesterone before bed, Biest—an estriol/estradiol cream—twice a day, and a testosterone cream compounded with a small amount of DHEA once in the morning. Today, all of my hormones—even cortisol—are finally in the normal range and my vitamin D levels are optimized in

---

Cholesterol Is Critical for Your Health

- Refined carbs, sugar, and vegetable oils found in processed foods are the primary dietary culprits causing heart disease, *not* saturated fat or cholesterol.
- Cholesterol is critical to optimize brain health and hormone levels, and even to *lower* heart disease risk.
- Studies confirm that higher cholesterol levels are associated with better health and longer life.
- Studies show that countries with the lowest cholesterol levels have the highest mortality rates!
- A better predictor of your heart disease risk is your HDL/total cholesterol ratio. Just divide your HDL level by your total cholesterol. This percentage should ideally be above twenty-four percent. Below ten percent, it's a significant indicator of risk for heart disease.
- Another good predictor is your triglyceride/HDL ratio: this percentage should ideally be below two.

the 75–90 ng/ml range. My blood sugar is now consistently in the low 90s ng/ml, which is better than it was but still not perfect (optimal fasting blood sugar is 70–85), and my insulin— finally tested—is safely under 2 uIU/mL (optimal fasting insulin is under 3 uIU/mL). I take biotin, also known as B7, after meals to help keep my blood sugar and insulin levels balanced. (Studies show that biotin may help with remyelination, which is especially helpful for people with MS.) I continue to monitor hormone levels twice a year and adjust as needed.

I hope my story motivates you to do what you can *today* to eliminate sugar and address stress so that you might balance your hormones as naturally, as early, and as easily as possible. If I was able to balance my hormones after dealing with all six major imbalances, then I know you can, too. The key is that you adopt the mindset that hormonal balance is possible, and diabetes and chronic disease are not inevitable.

Hormone Balance Toolkit

As tempting as it might be to jump straight to hormone supplementation, it's essential first to determine *why* your hormones are imbalanced. Unfortunately, it's not as simple as getting tested and then replacing what's low. Your body is too complicated, and there are way too many moving parts and mysterious metabolic pathways to mess with Mother Nature and win.

Take me as an example. If I had just taken progesterone rather than proactively managing my stress, the extra hormone may not have done any good, since cortisol blocks progesterone receptors. I could have easily written off progesterone altogether and missed out on its much-needed calming and cancer-protective benefits. Once I addressed stress, which is the root cause of cortisol imbalances, my levels found their normal daily rhythm so that when I added progesterone into my life I could experience its positive impact.

For men with low testosterone, supplementation without addressing root causes could come back to bite you. If it turns out that you're insulin resistant, the extra testosterone may be converted to belly fat–promoting and breast-enlarging estrogen instead. The optimal approach would be to address the cause of the low testosterone, in this case, insulin resistance. Once insulin resistance is addressed, testosterone naturally rises.

Hormone balance is a F.I.G.H.T.S.-first, upstream approach. Once you tackle the three biggest imbalances—high cortisol, high insulin, and high estrogen—by addressing stress, sugar, and toxins, all your hormones will naturally move toward balance.

The first step is to consider which of the imbalances you may be experiencing. Then I recommend getting tested, so you have a baseline on all your hormones, and reviewing the beneficial food and lifestyle strategies from the other F.I.G.H.T.S. chapters as they relate to hormones. Once you have the data about your hormone status and have implemented other key F.I.G.H.T.S. strategies, you may choose to try hormone-balancing herbs and supplements. For those who need extra help, I've included information on bioidentical hormones for you to discuss with a doctor who specializes in natural hormone therapy.

Step 1: Review hormone imbalance self-assessments.
Step 2: Get the data.
Step 3: Follow F.I.G.H.T.S. for hormone balance.
Step 4: Try herbs and adaptogens.
Extra Step: Consider bioidentical hormones.

Step 1: Review Hormone Imbalance Self-Assessments

Go back through the Six Major Hormonal Imbalances in America section (page 225) and consider the common symptoms associated with each. You'll notice some overlap—like fatigue, which is common to many and difficult to attribute to any one imbalance. Are there any categories that jump out at you? Did any include three or more symptoms that resonated with you? If so, chances are you're dealing with a hormonal imbalance. But the only way to know for sure is to get tested. To do so, you'll need to work with an experienced practitioner who is particularly skilled at recognizing patterns associated with hormone imbalance and its symptoms.

Which imbalance(s) do you believe you're dealing with?

1. High insulin
2. High cortisol
3. Estrogen dominance
4. Low thyroid

5. Low vitamin D*
6. Low DHEA

Note: Symptoms of vitamin D deficiency typically don't appear until levels are alarmingly low. Even if you don't have any symptoms, make sure to ask your doctor to run a vitamin D test a few times a year.

Now that you have a hypothesis, it's a good time to get the data.

Step 2: Get the Data

While it's often possible to order your own lab tests online, because this is such a complicated arena, I encourage you to work with a practitioner experienced in hormones. Some naturopaths, integrative physicians, and Functional Medicine practitioners also specialize in hormones, but many do not. If you're not sure, you need to ask.

To find a practitioner who specializes in hormone balancing, consider these websites, which you can search by zip code or state. Several provide an advanced search feature or pull-down menu for specialty, including: "Women or Men's Health and Aging," "Endocrinology, Diabetes, and Metabolism," "Female Disorders," or "Male Disorders." Other code names for hormones include "anti-aging" or just "BHRT" for bioidentical hormone replacement therapy.

FIND A HORMONE PRACTITIONER:
www.naturopathic.org/AF_MemberDirectory
www.a4m.com/find-a-doctor.html
network.foreverhealth.com/bioidentical-hormone-doctors/search
myzrt.zrtlab.com/tools/FindProvider

If you decide to go it alone, consider ordering your own labs through a company like TrueHealthLabs.com, which also offers one-on-one remote consultations with Functional Medicine doctors.

ONLINE DIRECT-TO-CONSUMER HORMONE TESTING:
www.truehealthlabs.com/Female-Hormones
www.mymedlab.com
www.walkinlab.com

www.canaryclub.org
www.directlabs.com
www.ultawellness.com
www.lifeextension.com
www.healthcheckusa.com
requestatest.com

INSULIN

Three blood tests provide a snapshot of your insulin and blood sugar status. Note these are fasting tests, which are available at most standard labs like LabCorp and Quest:

TESTS:	OPTIMAL RANGES:
Fasting serum insulin	3 uIU/mL or below
Fasting serum glucose	70–85 mg/dl or lower
Hemoglobin A1c (HA1c)	< 5.2

ON YOUR OWN: WAIST-TO-HEIGHT RATIO (WHTR)

The waist-to-height ratio is an excellent do-it-yourself predictor of insulin resistance in most people. Wrap a measuring tape around your waist evenly and align the bottom edge of the measuring tape with the top of your hip bones. Take the measurement at the end of a normal exhalation. Have a friend or family member help measure your height in inches. Then divide your height in inches by your waist in inches. You want your waist circumference to be less than half your height.

Waist-to-height ratio (WHtR) Less than 0.5

The caveat to this is that you can be thin and insulin resistant, as I was. Experts call this profile *TOFI* for "thin outside, fat inside," meaning harmful visceral fat is layered around vital organs in the abdomen. If you have signs of TOFI including family history of heart disease or diabetes (type 1 or 2), have a little potbelly, and/or deal with lots of stress, then you'll definitely want to get the above fasting blood tests done.

CORTISOL AND DHEA

Salivary cortisol and DHEA testing is a reliable, easy, at-home way to evaluate how your cortisol levels change throughout the day. Saliva testing measures the free, bioavailable hormones in the body, unlike blood tests, which represent total hormone level—both free and bound (not bioavailable). Ideally, your cortisol is highest in the morning when you wake, tapers during the day, and is lowest when you go to sleep.

Test: Salivary cortisol and DHEA sulfate (DHEA-S or DS)
Labs that offer saliva testing:
- ZRT: Adrenal Stress saliva—DS and Cx4
- Genova Diagnostics: Adrenocortex Stress Profile

Optimal ranges: saliva
- Cortisol: 3.7–9.5 ng/mL (morning); 1.2–3.0 ng/mL (noon); 0.6–1.9 ng/mL (evening); 0.4–1.0 ng/mL (night)
- DHEA-sulfate (DHEA-S): 2–23 ng/ml—age dependent:
  under thirty years old: 6.4–18.6 ng/ml
  thirty-one to forty-five years old: 3.9–11.4 ng/ml
  forty-six to sixty years old: 2.7–8 ng/ml
  sixty-one years old or older: 2–6 ng/ml

SEX HORMONES: ESTROGENS, PROGESTERONE, TESTOSTERONE

Dried urine testing is a relatively new and more comprehensive way to measure hormones than saliva or blood testing, since it also measures how estrogen is being excreted. Estrogen metabolism occurs via several pathways, including 2-hydroxyestrone, which is benign and protective for health, and 4-hydroxyestrone and 16-hydroxyestrone, which are potentially harmful to health. Too little of the protective type 2 and too much of the dangerous types, 4 and 16, can put people at risk for cancers and autoimmune conditions.

Test: Dried urine
Labs that offer dried urine testing:
- Precision Analytical's DUTCH (dried urine test for comprehensive hormones)
- ZRT's Urine Metabolites Profile
- Meridian Valley Lab's CompletePLUS hormone profile

Optimal ranges: dried urine
Please refer to the reference ranges provided on lab reports and discuss with your practitioner. Ranges will vary by gender; and estrogens (for women) will have four reference ranges: luteal, follicular, or midcycle and post-menopausal.

THYROID

There are eight key blood tests that can assess your thyroid function, and you may need to insist on getting a comprehensive thyroid panel instead of the typical TSH-only test, or order the full panel on your own. Most labs, like Quest and LabCorp, offer comprehensive panels. In addition to the full thyroid panel, consider getting tested for nutrient status, including zinc, selenium, and iodine, which are trace minerals essential for optimal thyroid function.

TESTS:	OPTIMAL RANGES:
TSH	.4–1.5 mIU/L
Free T3	2.3–4.2 pg/mL
Free T4	0.8–1.8 ng/dL
Reverse T3 (rT3)	<15 ng/dl (also expressed as <150)
Free T3/rT3 ratio	>2
TPO antibodies	< 2 IU/m
TG antibodies	< 2 IU/m
Ferritin	70–90 mg/dl

On your own at home:
basal body temperature on waking   97.8–98.6 degrees F

Keep a good, old-fashioned mercury thermometer right by your bed; shake it down and then place it under your armpit the moment you wake up and keep it there for ten minutes. Note and write down your temperature. If your temperature is lower than 98.6 (37°C) five mornings in a row, you may have low thyroid function and low metabolism. Check out the Infections Clearing Toolkit for ideas to help raise your metabolism while working with your health practitioner on addressing hypothyroid.

VITAMIN D

Many doctors still do not routinely check vitamin D status, so you need to request it or order it on your own.

TEST: 25(OH)D TEST   OPTIMAL RANGES:
For general health: 50–70 ng/ml
For reversing or preventing disease (autoimmune conditions, cancer, heart disease): 70–100 ng/ml

If you're waiting for test results, or just want to jump into action, there's lots you can you do to help bring your hormones into balance. Read on for a review of beneficial lifestyle changes that can improve your health and even prepare you for possible hormone supplementation.

Step 3: Follow F.I.G.H.T.S. for Hormone Balance

Follow these F.I.G.H.T.S. strategies to help balance your hormones naturally. If you've been making small changes already, this will be a quick review. I'm a huge fan of leverage, so these tips will assist you in balancing as many hormones as possible at the same time:

- ✔ **Remove SAD foods:** Sugar in all forms, processed grains, and starchy carbohydrates promote insulin resistance. Researchers have found that for every 150 calories of added sugar *per day*—about one can of soda—the risk for diabetes goes up about 1 percent.[15] Conventionally grown, pesticide-laden produce and commercially raised meats, poultry, and dairy products promote estrogen dominance.
- ✔ **Reduce alcohol and coffee:** Alcohol promotes estrogen dominance and significantly raises breast cancer risk. A 2015 study revealed the risk of breast cancer goes up 60 percent with each daily five-ounce glass of alcohol.[16] Studies have shown that caffeine spikes cortisol, raises insulin, and may even elevate estrogen. A clinical trial of five hundred women showed that women who consumed 500 mg of caffeine daily—the equivalent of four or five cups of coffee—had nearly 70 percent more estrogen than women who consumed less than 100 mg of caffeine a day.[17] Reduce by going half-caf, and then consider only organic, water-processed decaf. Or replace coffee with green or white teas, which are lower in caffeine, or herbal teas, which are caffeine-free.
- ✔ **Eat organic vegetables:** Leafy greens (e.g., dandelion root, kale, Swiss chard, spinach, arugula), cruciferous vegetables (e.g., broccoli, cauliflower, cabbage, Brussels sprouts), and sulfur-rich vegetables (onions and garlic) promote healthy liver function and help clear harmful estrogen metabolites.[18]
- ✔ **Enjoy healthy fats:** Despite the sugar industry's best attempts to convince us otherwise, healthy fats are essential for health and are the

foundational building blocks of hormones, cell membranes, and brain health. Replace processed vegetable oils like canola, corn, peanut, safflower, soybean, and sunflower with healthy saturated fats like coconut oil, ghee, and lard from pasture-raised animals; and increase consumption of omega-3 fats like wild salmon, 100 percent grass-fed animals, flax seed, and walnuts. Other nourishing fats include: extra virgin olive oil, hemp, flax seed, and pine nut oils (beneficial omega-6 fats), nuts, seeds, and avocados.

✓ **Increase your fiber intake:** Fiber feeds your beneficial gut bacteria, crowding out harmful bacteria, which can help optimize thyroid function and improve insulin sensitivity. Fiber also reduces estrogen dominance by binding toxins, like used-up estrogen, and helping to safely excrete them from the body. Aim for forty to fifty grams of fiber per day, remembering to ramp up slowly.

✓ **Heal your gut:** Probiotics (supplements and fermented foods) and prebiotics (fiber found in vegetables, flax, and chia seeds and supplemental powders like psyllium husk, acacia, and inulin) help balance your microbiome, which in turn helps with overall hormone balance, including optimizing thyroid function, lowering cortisol, increasing serotonin production, and even raising vitamin D levels.[19] If you take zinc, consider taking a low dose (5 or 10 mg) with each meal.

✓ **Avoid toxicants:** Our environment is loaded with estrogenic waste (xenoestrogens), like the herbicide Atrazine, which is turning male frogs into female frogs via aromatization—the same process that creates "man boobs" in men.[20] Do all you can to keep your home and body toxin-free. Use EWG's Skin Deep or the Think Dirty app to scan your cosmetics and determine which to keep and which to toss. Dispose of all chemical-based cosmetics, body care products, house cleaners, and pesticides at a local chemical waste drop-off facility; replace plastic storage containers with glass; swap plastic water bottles for stainless steel or glass; and filter your water for drinking and showering.

✓ **Get restorative sleep:** Make it a priority to get eight or more hours of high-quality sleep each night to balance your hormones, keep extra weight off, and reduce your risk of type 2 diabetes. Accumulating evidence indicates that chronic sleep deprivation—defined as less than seven or eight hours a night—causes hormonal imbalance, including elevated insulin levels, increased nighttime cortisol, and increased levels of the hormones that increase your hunger (ghrelin), and appetite (leptin).[21]

✔ **Move more:** Whatever form you choose, exercise can help balance your hormones—with one big caveat: if your adrenals are depleted with high or low cortisol, pass on the high intensity and endurance varieties in favor of gentle movement like easy walks, swims, or bike rides. Consider yoga, tai chi, or qi gong, which help to lower cortisol levels, reduce anxiety, and promote the brain-calming neurotransmitter GABA. If your adrenals are up for it, burst training, also called high intensity interval training (HIIT), improves insulin sensitivity and increases human growth hormone (HGH).

✔ **Get outside:** Whenever you can, get out in nature for a walk, a hike, or just to sit. Morning sunlight, especially, has been shown to help regulate your hormones, support brain function and mood, help you sleep better at night, and calm the stress response. When possible, go barefoot—on pesticide-free grass—to benefit from grounding (also called Earthing), which has been shown in studies to lower cortisol and lower stress by decreasing the sympathetic stress response and increasing the healing parasympathetic stress response.[22, 23]

✔ **Pause daily:** Make time to pause and move into the "rest and digest" healing state—in whichever way you choose—for just twenty minutes a day to help lower cortisol and improve sex hormone production. Revisit the Emotional Balance Toolkit for ideas to incorporate twenty minutes of stress-relieving strategies, like conscious breathing, meditating, dancing, yoga, forest bathing, listening to soothing music, or soaking in a hot Epsom salt bath with a few drops of lavender oil, to help lower cortisol.

ADVANCED CONSIDERATIONS:

✔ **Consider a cyclical ketogenic diet:** Periodically following a ketogenic diet that emphasizes vegetables and healthy fats, some meat, poultry, and fish, and restricts carbohydrates can be especially helpful in balancing hormones for peri- and menopausal women. When carbohydrate consumption is restricted, insulin resistance has been shown to improve or resolve entirely; estrogen levels decrease with reduction in body fat; risk for cardiovascular and neurodegenerative diseases decreases; daily energy levels stabilize; hunger is reduced; and mood swings even out. Before going keto, be sure to read the Consider Ketosis sidebar on page 70 and check out resources in Appendix F.

✔ **Practice intermittent fasting (IF):** Studies confirm that intermittent fasting, which can be defined as going without food periodically, has numerous health benefits like improving insulin sensitivity, boosting metabolism and energy levels, and reducing the risk of diabetes, cardiovascular disease, cancer, autoimmune conditions, and Alzheimer's.[24] Consider allowing fifteen hours between dinner and breakfast a few times per week. Or try skipping dinner a few times a week, and just eat breakfast and lunch.

Step 4: Try Herbs and Adaptogens

Sometimes beneficial lifestyle modifications aren't enough to balance hormones. If you find you need extra support, like I did, these are supplements that are scientifically proven to help.

To lower cortisol:

✔ **Adaptogens** are herbs that help your body adapt to stress and balance your hormones. Ashwagandha (*Withania somnifera*), also known as Indian ginseng, may be *the* superhero hormonal adaptogen, since it can help lower cortisol, optimize thyroid function, and increase both testosterone and DHEA. In a randomized, double-blind, placebo-controlled study, ashwagandha was shown to raise DHEA levels and reduce the stress hormone cortisol by up to 26 percent.[25, 26]

Caution: Ashwagandha is a nightshade, so avoid if sensitive to the *Solanaceae* (nightshade) family or if pregnant.

Dose: You might start with 500 mg organic ashwagandha twice a day and ramp up as needed to 3,000 mg twice a day of dried ashwagandha root, or 1 mL (~30 drops) of tincture in a few ounces of water, up to four times per day.

✔ **Rhodiola (Rhodiola rosea)** is a good option if nightshades are problematic or if you want an alternative that also offers belly fat–burning capabilities. Rhodiola has been studied extensively and has been shown to successfully improve stress-related fatigue, decrease cortisol, reduce anxiety, boost energy metabolism, burn belly fat, increase mental performance, and enhance immune function. It is often used in the treatment of chronic fatigue syndrome and fibromyalgia.[27, 28]

Caution: Avoid if you have bipolar spectrum or manic disorders; and discuss with your doctor if you are pregnant, breastfeeding, or taking antidepressant medication.

Dose: Take a 500 mg capsule twice daily between meals or 1 mL (~30 drops) of tincture in a few ounces of water, up to four times per day.

Notes: Choose organic or wildcrafted Rhodiola standardized to 3 percent rosavins and 1 percent salidroside for greatest efficacy. Consider taking by early afternoon to avoid interfering with sleep.

✔ **Phosphatidylserine (PS)** is a fat-soluble extract of cell membranes found in all cells but is most highly concentrated in brain cells. Supplementing with PS helps protect against dementia, cognitive decline, and depression. PS has been shown to normalize cortisol levels in chronically stressed individuals at a dose of 400 mg per day for six weeks.[29] You can find PS supplements derived from soy or sunflower lecithin. Avoid the soy version if sensitive to soy, and either way, choose a non-GMO variety.

Caution: Avoid taking PS together with other blood-thinning supplements or medications, such as gingko, kava, warfarin, and aspirin.

Dose: 200 mg twice per day, ideally with omega-3 fatty acids and food.

To lower insulin:

✔ **Berberine,** a yellow-colored extract found in several plants, including goldenseal and Oregon grape root, improves insulin resistance and blood sugar disorders and has been shown to be just as effective as the drug metformin for type 2 diabetics.[30]

Dose: 500 mg non-GMO or organic berberine two to three times per day with food.

Caution: Wait at least three hours between doses, as taking too much at once can increase the likelihood of gastrointestinal side effects.

✔ **Chromium picolinate** has been shown to stabilize blood sugar, reduce insulin resistance, and help reduce the risk of cardiovascular disease and type 2 diabetes.[31]

Dose: 200–500 mcg chromium picolinate two times per day with meals.

Caution: Chromium might make behavioral or psychiatric conditions worse; and chromium supplements may cause allergic reactions in people with chromate or leather contact allergy.

✔ **Biotin (B7)** has been shown to improve insulin sensitivity and blood sugar metabolism, lower triglycerides, and reduce LDL cholesterol. Studies also show that the combination of chromium and biotin significantly enhances blood sugar uptake and fat metabolism in people with diabetes. [32, 33]

Dose: 2–10 mg (2,000–10,000 mcg) of biotin two times per day with food.

Note: No adverse side effects have been reported for taking biotin dosages of up to 10 mg per day.

To lower estrogen:

✔ **Diindolylmethane (DIM)**, the metabolic byproduct of cruciferous vegetables like Brussels sprouts, cauliflower, and cabbage, helps encourage proper metabolism of estrogens in the body and helps to clear excess estrogen and xenoestrogens from the system.

Dose: Standard DIM dose is 150–300 mg per day with food. Liposomal form (an advanced delivery form for better absorption) in 20–25 mg units can be taken orally as two to four pumps two times per day on an empty stomach and should be held in the mouth for thirty seconds before swallowing.

Caution: Some reports of nausea or headache have been reported above doses greater than 300 mg/day.

✔ **Calcium-d-glucarate (CDG)**, like DIM, helps the body lower estrogen by ensuring that toxic estrogen metabolites don't get reabsorbed. They may work even better together. Extensive studies in animals show that CDG may reduce the risk of lung, breast, colon, prostate, liver, and skin cancers.[34]

Dose: 500 mg three times per day with or without food.

Caution: CDG may decrease effectiveness of certain medications, including statins and acetaminophen; and alcohol may reduce CDG's effectiveness.

✔ **Vitamin C**, also known as ascorbic acid, is a superstar vitamin that has many benefits, including helping to repair and regenerate tissues, protect against cancer, improve insulin sensitivity, support the adrenal glands, and raise progesterone levels, which counters estrogen dominance. Women who took 750 mg of vitamin C increased their progesterone levels by as much as 77 percent.[35]

Dose: 750–5,000 mg vitamin C daily in buffered or ascorbic acid form taken in divided doses with or without food. You can find capsules and/or powder to mix into water.

Note: Most vitamin C is made from corn. There are a few corn-free varieties (made from tapioca), like Ecological Formulas, Douglas Laboratories, and NutraMedix. The bottle must indicate "corn-free," otherwise, assume it's made from corn.

Caution: High doses of vitamin C can cause loose stools, so consider taking to bowel tolerance and then backing off 1,000 mg.

To support thyroid function:

✔ **Selenium**, an essential trace mineral with powerful anticancer effects, is found in high concentrations in the thyroid gland. It is also a catalyst for the production of the active thyroid hormone T3. In one randomized controlled study of 192 people with Hashimoto's or subclinical hypothyroid, treatment with 83 mcg selenomethionine per day restored normal thyroid function in 30 percent of participants compared to only 3 percent of controls.[36, 37]

Dose: 200 mcg per day selenomethionine form. Check your multivitamin to see if you're already getting selenium before adding more.

Note: Look for yeast-free brands of selenomethionine, like Pure Encapsulations or Solgar. Signs of selenium toxicity include nausea, diarrhea, skin rashes, or a metallic taste in the mouth.

✔ **Iodine** is a controversial element in the hypothyroid discussion. Worldwide, the most common cause of hypothyroidism is an inadequate dietary intake of iodine. However, studies show that both low and high levels of iodine increase the risk for Hashimoto's thyroiditis. My recommendation is to get tested for iodine status (e.g., Hakala Research or Doctor's Data, as opposed to the skin-absorption patch test) before supplementing with iodine. If you are deficient, take iodine along with selenium.

Dose: The key is to start low and go slow with iodine. Kelp tablets contain a relatively low dose (~225 mcg) of iodine per tablet. For larger doses, try a half tablet (6.25 mg) of Optimox Iodoral 12.5 mg tablets, and increase to the full tablet if that works for you.

Caution: Some people with hypothyroid or Hashimoto's may feel worse on iodine. The only way you will know for sure is to get tested and then try a small amount. Stop taking it if your symptoms worsen.

✔ **Zinc** is an all-star mineral that has multiple vital functions in the body, including supporting immune system function and tissue repair, preventing excess estrogen, improving insulin sensitivity, and converting T4 into active T3 thyroid hormone. Even if you have enough T3, if you are deficient in zinc, your thyroid won't function optimally.

Dose: 30 mg of zinc plus 1 mg copper per day with food unless your DIY zinc test results indicate otherwise (refer to page 102 in the Gut chapter). Low dose zinc: 5–10 mg with each meal may be more effective than one single 30 mg dose for healing and sealing the gut.

Notes: Taking zinc without copper may create a copper deficiency, so be sure to take 1 mg of copper for every 30 mg zinc. Stress and toxin exposure increase the need for zinc.

Caution: Like iodine, too much zinc may suppress thyroid function. Excess zinc may also interfere with copper absorption, so make sure you take adequate copper with zinc.

To raise your vitamin D:

Once you know your vitamin D level, choose a target goal. For general health: 50–70 ng/ml. For reversing or preventing disease like autoimmune conditions, cancer and heart disease: 70–100 ng/ml. Vitamin K2 works synergistically with D3, to make sure calcium gets absorbed in your bones and not in your arteries, so make sure to take K2 along with your D3.

✔ **Daily sun:** If weather permits and you are able to get your D from sun, that's ideal. Try to get ten to thirty minutes of midday sun daily without sunscreen—at least on your arms and legs. *Note:* Increase sun exposure gradually and back off if you get pink.

✔ **Vitamin D3:** Most of us are unable to get adequate sun exposure and need to supplement with D3. Dose varies by need, but many people need 5,000 or 10,000 IU per day. Studies show that people who are overweight or have dark skin may need greater levels to achieve optimal status.[38]

   Dose: 5,000-10,000 IU per day, depending on your needs (see Food chapter supplement section for calculation). Take D3 in the morning with food. It may take six months to a year to reach your goal. Remember to retest a few times a year to keep monitoring your levels.

   Note: Take 90 mcg of K2 per day along with D3, ideally in the MK7 form. K2 is found in grass-fed animals and fermented foods, so if you're getting your D from the sun, consider taking K2 or eating K2-rich foods.

If you have been diligent about your food, lifestyle, and supplements for several months and you're *still* experiencing symptoms of hormonal imbalance, it may be time to work with a practitioner well-versed in the fine art of bioidentical hormones.

Extra Step: Consider Bioidentical Hormones

If you're a woman over forty-five, odds are you've heard about HRT (hormone replacement therapy) and you don't want to touch it with a ten-foot pole. That's understandable, but we need to make a critical distinction between *synthetic* and *bioidentical* hormones.

SYNTHETIC VS. BIOIDENTICAL HORMONES: A QUICK DISTINCTION

In 1993, the Women's Health Initiative (WHI) began an eight-year study of more than 160,000 postmenopausal women, investigating the most common causes of disability, death, and decreased quality of life following menopause. The study used synthetic estrogen—called Premarin (derived from pregnant mares' urine)—both with and without a synthetic progestin called Provera, a fake progesterone replacement. The study was ended abruptly three years early due to the increased risk of breast cancer, heart disease, stroke, and pulmonary embolism (blood clots to the lungs). It turns out the highest risk was associated with the combination Premarin plus Provera drug, called Prempro.

Tens of thousands of women understandably halted their HRT.

On the other hand, *bioidentical* hormones—derived from a plant molecule found in wild yams and soybeans and converted in a lab into bioidentical progesterone and bioidentical estrogens—are identical to hormones produced by the human body. This makes all the difference in safety and effectiveness, but it is bad news to the pharmaceutical companies who cannot patent them.

There are many forms of bioidentical hormones: pills, patches, pellets, troches, injections, creams, and gels. It is beyond the scope of this book to discuss the merits of each, and I defer to natural hormone experts who work with multiple forms and have preferences and good reasons for when and how to use each.

I simply want to offer some key points for you to consider and discuss with your hormone doctor. I encourage you to do your homework, find a practitioner who is skilled in the fine art of hormones, and decide what's best for *you*.

BIOIDENTICAL HORMONES MAY IMPROVE AUTOIMMUNE CONDITIONS

Evidence is in that people with autoimmune conditions and Alzheimer's typically have low levels of hormones. Evidence is also emerging that restoring optimal levels of hormones in men and women can be anti-inflammatory and immune-protective, conferring benefits to people who already have autoimmune conditions and to those seeking to prevent chronic disease and cognitive decline. Here's a snapshot of the science highlighting the therapeutic benefits of taking bioidentical hormones:

- Treating with pregnancy levels of estrogen and estriol may have an immune-protective effect on microbiota and be neuroprotective for people with MS.[39]
- Rheumatoid arthritis tends to improve during pregnancy and during estrogen replacement therapy.[40]
- A randomized double-blind study of postmenopausal women with primary Sjögren's syndrome who had low levels of DHEA-S showed that DHEA levels were restored and dry mouth symptoms reduced by taking 50 mg oral DHEA per day for nine months.[41]
- In a patient satisfaction survey of 450 people being treated for hypothyroidism, 78 percent preferred treatment with Armour© Thyroid (desiccated thyroid that contains both T4 and T3 thyroid hormones) over T4-only (e.g., Synthroid) replacement strategies.[42]
- High vitamin D levels are associated with lower MS risk; and according to a recent review, the best serum 25-hydroxyvitamin D concentrations are between 75 and 100 nmol/L.[43]

BIOIDENTICAL HORMONES—KEY POINTS

Progesterone

- **Science:** One large study of 80,377 postmenopausal women with twelve years follow-up demonstrated that women who used bioidentical progesterone in combination with estrogen had a significant *reduction* in breast cancer risk.[44]
- **Note:** Bioidentical progesterone is often the only hormone experts provide in oral form since it bypasses the liver and, therefore, doesn't have the risk of being converted into unsafe metabolites.
- **Oral bioidentical progesterone helps with sleep and anxiety,** which are welcome benefits for many menopausal women.
- **On your own:** You can find over-the-counter progesterone creams online and in health food stores. Make sure the cream contains 450 mg of USP progesterone per ounce or 20 mg per quarter teaspoon and follow directions on the box. Note that menstruating women need to take a break from the cream each month.

- **Caution:** Do not confuse natural progesterone with synthetic *progestins* like Provera, where studies show increased risk for breast cancer and blood clots.

Estrogen

- **Science:** A five-year study of more than nine hundred post-menopausal women demonstrated the successful use of estriol in the treatment of menopausal symptoms. Seventy-one percent of the participants had complete elimination of hot flashes. Other benefits included reduction in depressive moods, forgetfulness, loss of concentration, irritability, migraines, and heart palpitations.[45]
- **Note:** Unlike progesterone, estrogen must be prescribed by a clinician.
- **Cautions:** Women who use estrogen must also use progesterone at least twelve days a month to protect against uterine cancer. Women who are pregnant or who have estrogen-sensitive cancers (e.g., breast, ovarian, endometrial); gallbladder, liver or heart disease; fibroids; or blood clots should avoid taking bioidentical estrogen and discuss with their doctor. Oral estrogens increase the risk for blood clots, so should be avoided if possible.

Testosterone

- **Science:** Testosterone has been shown to enhance libido in both men and women, improve heart health, reverse bone loss, alleviate depression, improve well-being and cognitive function, and reduce the risk for Alzheimer's.[46]
- **Dose:** Women typically start with 1–2 mg bioidentical testosterone replacement as a cream, up to 5 mg. Men have multiple options for bioidentical testosterone replacement (e.g., injections, topical gels, creams, implantations of long-lasting pellets or via buccal systems [between mouth and gums]) and should discuss dose and delivery methods with their doctor.
- **Caution:** Signs of too much testosterone in women include increased facial hair and acne. Signs of too much testosterone in men include acne, decreased sperm count, and breast enlarge-

ment—that's a sign that excess testosterone is being aromatized into estrogen.

Thyroid

- **Science:** Optimal thyroid function is vital for every system in the body. It's essential for optimal immune function, metabolism, brain health, and mood. Untreated hypothyroid increases the risk for heart disease and Alzheimer's disease in middle-aged women.[47, 48]
- **Note:** *All* thyroid hormone medications are bioidentical, but many people prefer the desiccated porcine (pig) thyroid gland form, like Armour Thyroid, Nature-Throid and Westhroid, which contains both T3 and T4 thyroid hormone.
- **Caution:** Too much thyroid hormone can cause hyperthyroid symptoms of feeling jittery, heart palpitations, anxiety, trouble falling asleep, diarrhea, etc.
- **Dose and risks:** Talk with your doctor about optimal doses, contraindications, and possible risks for you.

DHEA

- **Science:** Accumulating evidence shows that restoring optimal DHEA levels benefits immune function, reduces autoimmune symptoms, restores insulin sensitivity, improves cardiovascular health, bone health, metabolism, and psychological well-being, and supports healthy cognitive function.[49]
- **On your own:** DHEA is available over the counter, online, and in health food stores. DHEA is also available by prescription in creams, troches (dissolve between your cheek and gums), and liquid sublingual drops.
- **Dose:** Oral dose for women is usually 5 or 10 mg/day. Start low, go slow, and reduce dose if you develop facial hair or acne. For women with gut problems, you might consider topical cream or sublingual dosing. Do not take at night, as DHEA may interfere with sleep.
- **Caution:** Men should consult a hormone expert before taking DHEA, as it may be converted into unwanted estrogen. Women who have estrogen-dependent cancers should consult their physician before taking DHEA.

Hormones may be a complex and challenging arena, but they can also be a richly rewarding one, once dialed in. The key to hormonal balance is to live in harmony with nature and stop harming yourself with unnatural elements, which can be summed up in two words: stress and sugar.

Summary: Top Five Hormone Balancing Actions

1. **Address stress** to reduce cortisol and insulin levels. Pause for twenty minutes a day and prioritize sleep.
2. **Stop eating sugar** to improve your insulin sensitivity and immune function.
3. **Avoid toxicants** in your food, water, home, and body care products to reduce your load of xenoestrogens.
4. **Know your hormone levels** so you can track, manage, and optimize your levels over time.
5. **Consider bioidentical hormones**, especially calming progesterone, which can help balance estrogen dominance, support better sleep, and protect against autoimmune conditions and cancers.

CHAPTER 7

Keep Moving Forward

If you can't fly then run, if you can't run then walk, if you can't walk then crawl, but whatever you do, you have to keep moving forward.
—MARTIN LUTHER KING, JR.

We've come a long way in our understanding of why we develop autoimmune conditions and what we can do to reverse them. To appreciate the massive evolution we've undergone, let's contrast what we know today with our recent past:

Last century we believed our DNA was our destiny. What your parents or grandparents had would likely befall you, too. Viewed though this lens of genes as a static blueprint, your health outcomes were pretty much predestined. And if you were diagnosed with an autoimmune disease, it was common to assume that things would get progressively worse, and possibly even shorten your life. The only option presented by specialists was to manage your disease, often with immune-suppressing medications and/or steroids—each of which presents significant side effects, including, ironically enough, the possibility of developing an autoimmune condition. Furthermore, it's not uncommon to require more medications just to deal with symptoms brought on by autoimmune medications.

This bleak, fatalistic view would understandably have us blaming our ancestors and avoiding taking personal responsibility for our health outcomes. Why bother adjusting your lifestyle if your fate is already sealed?

Fast forward to the early 2000s, when research findings completely flipped our understanding of how health outcomes happen. In the beginning of the book, I shared my excitement about three of the biggest recent advances:

1. Epigenetics—the science of how environmental factors influence gene expression for better or worse—has been proven to supersede genetics, meaning we have way more control over our health outcomes than we ever imagined possible. Beyond ourselves, our choices today can even impact the genetic expression of our future *offspring*!

2. Studies show, and the CDC confirms, that our exposome—our total environment, not our genome—accounts for the vast majority of our health outcomes. What you eat, drink, think, believe, and do accounts for 90 percent, while your genes account for just 10 percent of the risk.

3. A breakthrough study led by Dr. Fasano of Harvard Medical School provides the equation for reversing autoimmune conditions: find and remove your root causes and heal your gut.

The implications of these findings are nothing less than revolutionary. Put simply, how you live determines your health outcomes. This is good news or bad news, depending on your perspective. If you're willing to examine your life and do what you can to live a more evolutionarily suited lifestyle, swapping SAD foods for a Paleo template and embracing nourishing habits like prioritizing sleep, moving more, stressing less, breathing more, having meaningful social connections, and getting out in nature, you will be on the healing or prevention path.

After reading the science and stories of people who have successfully changed their health outcomes by removing harmful elements and embracing beneficial lifestyle factors, I hope you share my enthusiasm and are encouraged and empowered to believe that you can do it, too.

I've categorized and tried to simplify the seemingly endless root causes into what I hope is a useful mnemonic, F.I.G.H.T.S., for Food, Infections, Gut health, Hormone balance, Toxins, and Stress. These six areas do not cover everything, but research shows they are the most important things to address. As a group, they provide a comprehensive strategy that is also easy to understand and pretty straightforward to implement. I believe you'll have most of what you need for healing and achieving optimal health.

I've included healing stories specifically suited to each F.I.G.H.T.S. chapter, but just because a story was placed in the Toxins chapter, for example, does not mean that the practitioner solely addressed toxins and healed. Each person tackled multiple areas, if not every area, of F.I.G.H.T.S. There's just no getting around it. Just as you can't exercise your way out of a bad diet, you can't supplement your way out of buried emotional trauma or heal your gut while you're crazy stressed.

Let's review my journey back to health as an example of addressing all of F.I.G.H.T.S.:

Food: I removed gluten in November 2010 and have not experienced a single MS symptom since (with MRI confirming the lessening or complete disappearance of lesions on my brain), despite six neurologists telling me "there's nothing you can do." My markers of inflammation have all improved since I eliminated grains, dairy, and sugar and started eating a green, Paleo-template, mildly ketogenic diet. I practice intermittent fasting daily, restricting eating to a six- or eight-hour window, and often eat two meals a day: brunch and dinner. I typically finish eating by six or six-thirty p.m. so my body can repair and restore while sleeping instead of being distracted with digestion.

Gut: After learning about my non-celiac gluten sensitivity (NCGS), I strictly followed the 5R Gut Restoration Program, doing a thirty-day elimination diet, taking probiotics once or twice a day, taking pancreatic enzymes with meals, eating fermented foods often, using ghee, MCT, and coconut oils frequently, sipping bone broth, slowly adding prebiotic fiber, and taking RESTORE along with zinc, omega-3s, and antioxidants like vitamins A, C, and E. Today I continue to follow much of the 5R protocol as part of my daily routine.

Infections: My infections-clearing journey involved reducing a heavy burden of *Candida* in my gut and addressing oral cavitations in all four wisdom teeth areas. I revved up my metabolism by restricting starchy carbs, adding more good fats, intermittent fasting most days, doing more HIIT workouts, and taking cold showers—at least for the last minute. By adopting nourishing lifestyle habits like prioritizing sleep, spending more time in nature, and using a rotation of herbal and other natural botanical remedies like berberine, mono-laurin, and wormwood, I was able to unburden my immune system and lower my infectious load.

Toxins: The first thing my husband and I did was to go all-organic with food purchases. We replaced plastic storage containers with glass, filtered our shower/bath water, and started drinking spring or filtered water we store in three-gallon glass carboys. We replaced all chemical-based home and body products with fragrance-free eco-friendly and biologically friendly cleaning products and organic soaps, and I swapped chemical-based cosmetics with nontoxic ones. To detox, I made sure to keep my detox pathways open with glutathione, omega-3s, and drainage formulas. Then I had my silver mercury fillings safely removed and replaced with composites. Because I had high levels of mercury, I continue to limit fish consumption; and several times per week, I use a far infrared sauna and take a binder cocktail of chlorella, cilantro, bentonite clay, and activated charcoal to continue lowering my load of heavy metals safely and gently.

Stress: While I have experimented with dozens of stress-reduction techniques since my MS diagnosis, five are standouts. The most powerful have been proactively surrendering my stressors (by creating a "stress surrender sheet" and deciding what to do about each perceived stressor), meditating daily using a neurofeedback device, practicing forgiveness and gratitude, hiking in nature, and laughing as often as possible with good friends, family, and my husband. Proactive stress reduction continues to be my top priority for preventing any recurrence of MS or any other illness.

Hormones: Getting off sugar and birth control pills and reducing my stress levels helped bring my hormones back into balance. But after so many years of living out of balance, I needed additional support and found the answer with a conservative regime of bioidentical hormones. By adding small quantities of physiologic levels of Biest, DHEA, testosterone, and progesterone, I've managed to find a hormonal homeostasis I can't remember ever experiencing before.

Of course, my takeaways from each category won't look exactly like yours, and that's okay. The goal isn't to mimic the healing stories that have been presented in these pages, but to use them as motivation to find the path that brings you back to balance and wellness. The key is to find and remove *your* sources of inflammation and imbalance. Dr. Vojdani has a useful mantra to keep in mind: *detect, remove, repair*!

Fortunately, as you likely gathered, there are some basic starting points that apply to almost everyone:

- ✔ Swap standard American diet (SAD) foods for a more evolution- arily suited diet of organic vegetables, 100 percent grass-fed (pastured) meats, wild small fish, and nourishing fats.
- ✔ Replenish nutrient deficiencies with quality supplements that complement a diet of nutrient-dense foods.
- ✔ Remove inflammatory elements like toxins—including the overuse of antibiotics and other medications, infections, and SAD foods that harm our guts and promote an inflamed, autoimmune state.
- ✔ Address childhood trauma and adopt relaxation practices that you do consistently to shift out of an always-on fight or flight state into a calming and healing rest and digest mode.
- ✔ Embrace foundational elements like having a bedtime that supports getting eight or more hours of sleep. Find ways to move throughout the day; pause to breathe or meditate, even for five minutes; do what you can to reduce or avoid potentially harmful effects of electromagnetic radiation (EMR) exposure; and proactively seek ways to deepen connections with others. How about making it more fun by finding a buddy to join you on the path to vitality?

While you've heard me repeat myself about working with an autoimmune expert, the top recommendations I can offer are things you can do on your own right away. Turns out the most profound ingredients for creating health are simple, straightforward, and pretty reasonably priced. And if you're still pushing back on the cost of organic food, consider the far higher cost of office visits, medications, and medical procedures that you'll hopefully avoid as you lower your toxic load.

Beat Autoimmune Top Six
Recommendations:

1. Remove grains, dairy, and sugar for good.
2. Buy organic and 100 percent grass-fed food—at least meat, poultry, and eggs, and avoid the "dirty dozen" fruits and vegetables, which is updated yearly by EWG: www.ewg.org/foodnews/list .php#.WrLyAq2ZP-Y.
3. Eat a variety of colorful and fiber-rich vegetables every day.
4. Set a bedtime for yourself, ideally by ten p.m., and do what you can to get restorative sleep. Follow sleep-hygiene guidelines, like total darkness, avoidance of blue light in the evening, and using red light at night.
5. Replace chemical-based cleaners and cosmetics with green eco- and body-friendly choices. This includes shifting to *unscented* laundry products and ditching the dryer sheets in favor of non-toxic varieties or reusable wool balls.
6. Reduce stress however you can. Think you don't have time? Just practice deep belly breathing a few times a day with one hand on your heart and one on your belly. Give yourself the gift of getting quiet for just five minutes, or even one! And spend a few minutes trying EFT (tapping) as a means to help you engage the relaxation response quickly and easily.

Harkening back to Dr. Hyman's lecture, we can simplify even further: remove the causes of imbalance and add what creates balance.

Next Steps

You've got all this information, and you may be wondering, now what? I'd say that depends on where you are and how you're feeling. Since everyone's at a different point, let's break things down a bit. Which category applies best to you?

For the ultramotivated self-starter: You're the kind of person who is so motivated that you've already begun to make changes. Perhaps you've cleaned out your pantry, disposed of your chemical-based cleaners and cosmetics, and jumped into the 30-Day Food Vacation. My message to you is great job! Keep going and keep up the positive forward momentum.

What's next: You might consider building a team to support you or joining a community of people like a local Meetup.com group that gathers regularly to discuss healing with food and other supportive self-care elements. Continue educating yourself, experimenting with nourishing lifestyle practices, and seeking support to assist you in your journey to vibrant health. If you get stuck at any point along the way, ask for help, ideally from someone who has already been there and back. The main thing is to keep moving forward toward optimal health and away from the elements that keep you in an inflamed, autoimmune state. You're doing it, so keep on keeping on the good F.I.G.H.T.S.! Soon you may have your own healing story to share with the BeatAutoimmune.com community.

For the completely overwhelmed: There's so much to take in, you're not even sure where to begin. While intellectually, it makes sense to start with food, you still can't fathom giving up sugar for a month. First of all, take a deep breath; you can do this. Maybe you resonate more with a baby steps approach and prefer a little more hand-holding. That's okay! My advice is to review the six Beat Autoimmune recommended actions above, then ask yourself what you're willing to try. The Chinese philosopher Lao Tzu offers sound advice: "Do the difficult things while they are easy and do the great things while they are small. A journey of a thousand miles must begin with a single step."

What's next: If giving up sugar in one fell swoop sounds too daunting, how about a smaller step of just cutting out sugary drinks like fruit juice, sodas, sweetened teas, or energy drinks? (That's not a pass for drinking diet drinks. "Diet" is code for artificial sweeteners, which are neurotoxic and, ironically, promote weight *gain*.) So that you don't feel deprived, find healthy swaps that sound good to you. How about making your own flavored water (filtered, of course) with lemon and/or a splash of unsweetened cranberry juice and stevia? Or, how about making spa water by adding organic peeled and sliced cucumbers to a glass pitcher you keep in the fridge? The key is finding healthy swaps you enjoy, at the pace that feels comfortable. As your taste buds adjust, soda might not taste so good anymore.

For every small stride, pay attention to how you feel and how you sleep. I bet as you start to feel a little better, you'll have more energy, and you'll naturally want to move more. How about getting a step-tracking device? What about finding a buddy to walk with? And don't forget to celebrate positive actions you're taking and consider writing about them in a gratitude journal. Remember Mary Ruddick, who, while suffering from twelve painful illnesses, kept a gratitude journal in which she wrote nightly? At one point, the most Mary could muster for exercise was thirty *seconds* on a stationary bike—but she got in the habit of feeling grateful for even the tiniest things and wrote them down. By noting her microprogress, she slowly built the momentum she needed to reach for and attain higher and higher levels of healing and vibrant health.

In other words, even the smallest gain is a step in the right direction.

If you'd prefer a partner in health, you might benefit from hiring a Functional Medicine health coach: someone who can assist you in envisioning a healthy future, who can motivate you, hold you ac-countable—without judgement—and help you create healthy lifestyle habits. (Find one at www.functionalmedicinecoaching.org/find-a-coach.) However you begin, the main thing is to have com-passion for yourself, keep learning, and do what you can when you're ready. Continue to ask yourself: what small step can I take toward a brighter future right now?

For the wellness pro: You're an experienced autoimmune person, and this was mostly a review for you. You've probably been at this healing thing a long time, and in doing so, worked your way through F.I.G.H.T.S. at least once, removing the inflammatory ele-ments and adding in the nourishing ones. You eat a green, Paleo, sometimes ketogenic diet, you've healed your gut, cleared an under-lying gut infection or two, exercise most days, take high-quality supplements, and have a daily stress reduction and gratitude prac-tice. You may even use bioidentical hormones, and yet you *still* feel less than optimal. Perhaps you're wondering, *what in the world am I missing*? First, know that you're not alone. I've personally struggled at this level for years, even following my MS reversal, as I've contin-ued to seek optimal health. I am simply not willing to settle for feeling pretty good.

What's next: My message to you is never stop seeking answers or settling for feeling okay when you know vibrant health is possible. For every effect, there is a cause, you just haven't found what that is for you *yet*. Check out the Advanced Considerations and Practitioners in Appendix D. With all your experience, knowledge, and determination, perhaps you would enjoy studying to becoming a health coach or finding some way to use your valuable knowledge to serve others. No matter what, never give up!

Your Turn

For those seeking to heal, I leave you with two questions:

1. Why do you think you got the autoimmune condition(s)?
2. And what will you do to address it or them *right now*?

For those on the prevention path who seek optimal health, I offer you these questions:

1. Which areas of your life require better balance?
2. And what will you do *today* to move toward optimal health and well-being?

30-Day Food Vacation Recipes

All recipes are autoimmune Paleo (AIP), i.e., free of grains (and gluten), dairy, sugar, chocolate, caffeine, eggs, soy, corn, nuts, seeds, and night-shades (tomatoes, peppers, eggplant, white potatoes, and goji berries). For a handy online version to print out, visit BeatAutoimmune.com/Recipes.

TEAS AND SMOOTHIES
- Dandelion Liver Detox Tea
- Coconut Chai Tea
- Golden Latte
- Very Berry Green Smoothie
- Keto Coconut Smoothie

SNACKS
- Brussels Sprouts Chips
- Curried Coconut Chips
- Guacamole
- Liver Pâté

BREAKFAST/LUNCH/DINNER
- Spiced Beef "Tacos"
- Thai Chicken Sausage Patties
- Turkey Meatballs with Artichoke Hearts
- Whole Roast Chicken
- Quick Chicken Curry

- Juicy Bison Burgers

FISH/SHELLFISH
- Broccoli Shrimp Stir-Fry
- Baked Cod with Thyme
- Salmon Stuffed Avocados

SOUPS AND STEWS
- Homemade Bone Broth
- Vibrant Green Soup
- Coconut Salmon Chowder
- Hearty Beef Stew

SALAD DRESSINGS AND SAUCES
- Everyday Salad Dressing
- Linda's No-Tomato Sauce

VEGGIES
- Spring Ferments
- Red Cabbage Coleslaw
- Cauliflower "Rice"
- Zucchini Pasta with Green Harissa Sauce
- Rainbow Roasted Root Veggies
- Massaged Kale Salad
- Simple Sautéed Greens

DESSERTS
- Keto Cinna-Bombs
- Keto Cardamom Custard
- Quick Creamed Coconut

EXTRA
- Homemade Coconut Milk

To reduce inflammation and lower your toxic load, make sure to use organic ingredients as much as you can. Many grocery stores, including Trader Joe's, Costco, and Walmart, are expanding their organic sections as consumers demand clean products. And, many stores offer their own organic brands, which can be less expensive. For those not close to stores with organic options or farmers' markets, I have included companies that deliver organic foods, pantry items, body and home care products in the Resources by Chapter section (Appendix F). And, if still not practical, consult with www.EWG.org for their Clean Fifteen and Dirty Dozen lists to ensure you're doing the best you can.

Teas and Smoothies

These teas and smoothies will support your liver, nourish your gut, calm inflammation, and help you kick your caffeine habit. If you choose to do intermittent fasting, that means *zero* calories during the fasting part, so go for white, green, black, or herbal teas like the Dandelion Liver Detox Tea, but wait for coconut milk, MCT oil, collagen, and smoothies until your eating window is open.

Dandelion Liver Detox Tea

Reprinted with permission from *Eating Clean: The 21-Day Plan to Detox, Fight inflammation and Reset Your Body,* by Amie Valpone, HHC, AADP

Makes 1 serving.

2 cups (filtered) water
2 roasted dandelion root tea bags
½ teaspoon ground cardamom
1 cinnamon stick
Freshly squeezed lemon juice, to taste, optional
Stevia* for serving, optional

1. Place the water, tea bags, cardamom, and cinnamon stick in a small saucepan. Cover and bring to a boil.
2. Reduce the heat and simmer for 15 minutes.
3. Pour into a large mug, add lemon juice and stevia, if desired, and serve.

*Note: The original recipe includes honey as an optional sweetener. I replaced with stevia for this elimination phase.

Coconut Chai Tea

By Jill Carnahan, MD

Makes 1 serving.

4 ounces filtered water
4 ounces coconut milk
1–2 teaspoons xylitol or whole leaf stevia
1 decaf chai tea bag

1. Bring water and coconut milk to a slow boil and pour into a mug.
2. Steep tea bag 3–5 minutes.
3. Add xylitol or stevia, stir, and savor.

Option: Add a dash of cinnamon like Dr. Jill does.

Golden Latte

By Palmer Kippola, FMCHC

Makes 1 serving.

1 cup full fat coconut milk
1 heaping tablespoon fresh turmeric root, grated, or 1.5 tsp. ground
    turmeric root
Optional: add 1 tablespoon grated fresh ginger root or 1 teaspoon
    ground ginger
1–2 teaspoons MCT or coconut oil
Stevia to taste (start with a few drops and increase as desired)
Pinch of ground cinnamon or nutmeg (optional)
1 scoop (1 tablespoon) grass-fed collagen powder (optional)

Variations: Masala rooibos chai (e.g., Blue Lotus brand) or decaffeinated
sencha or matcha green tea powder instead of turmeric

1. Gently heat coconut milk in a small saucepan. Do not boil.
2. Add turmeric (and optional ginger). Stir and simmer for about 5 minutes.

3. Add MCT or coconut oil, collagen powder, and stevia to taste. Whisk or use an immersion blender to create a foamy beverage.

Alternative method: To create an extra frothy well-blended latte, blend with high-speed blender instead of whisk or immersion blender.

Very Berry Green Smoothie
By Michelle Corey, CNWC, FMC

Makes 1 serving.

1 cup unsweetened coconut milk
1–2 scoops vanilla hypoallergenic protein powder, collagen, or
    medical food
1 cup mixed blackberries, blueberries, and raspberries
1 cup chopped dandelion greens or spinach
1 tablespoon coconut oil
Stevia to sweeten as necessary

Place all ingredients in a blender and blend until smooth.

Keto Coconut Smoothie
By Mary Ruddick, CNC

Makes 1 serving.

½ avocado
½–1 cup coconut milk (best if kept in fridge overnight)
1 tablespoon MCT oil
1–2 scoops collagen powder
Optional additions: 1 teaspoon vanilla and/or ¼ cup frozen berries
2–4 tablespoons water (optional, if needed for texture)
½–1 cup ice (optional)

Blend until creamy.

Snacks

Enjoy nutrient-dense alternatives to chips and salsa.

Brussels Sprouts Chips
By Jill Carnahan, MD

> 2 cups Brussels sprouts leaves (outer leaves) from 2 pounds of
>   Brussels sprouts
> 2 tablespoons melted ghee
> Kosher salt to taste
> Lemon zest (optional)

1. Preheat oven to 350°F.
2. Mix the leaves, ghee, and salt together in a large bowl.
3. Line two large baking trays with parchment. Divide the leaves evenly
   in a single layer on each tray.
4. Bake each tray for 8–10 minutes or until crispy and brown around the edges
   (careful not to burn). Microplane some lemon zest over the chips (optional).

Curried Coconut Chips
By Mary Ruddick, CNC

> 2–3 mature coconuts or 1 bag of unsweetened coconut flakes
> 2 limes
> 1 tablespoon curry powder
> Sea salt to taste

1. Crack open coconuts and scoop out the meat.
2. Shave the meat into strips using a vegetable peeler.
3. Place the strips or flakes into a bowl and toss with lime juice.
4. Sprinkle the strips with curry powder and add salt to taste.
5. Arrange strips onto dehydrator trays and dehydrate for 2–3 days. Or put
   them in your oven at the lowest heat setting until they are golden and
   crunchy, making sure not to burn.

These chips will keep for several weeks in a sealed container.

Guacamole
By Mary Ruddick, CNC

Makes 4 servings.

3 ripe avocados, halved, seeded, and peeled
2 limes, juiced
½ teaspoon sea salt
½ medium onion
¼ cup cilantro, chopped
3 garlic cloves, minced

1. In a large bowl, place the avocado and lime juice.
2. Toss to coat, then mash with all of the other ingredients.
3. Let sit at room temperature for an hour and then serve with sea salt to taste.

Serve with raw veggies (e.g., celery, cucumber, jicama), eat by the spoonful, add to Spiced Beef "Tacos," or serve atop Juicy Bison Burgers.

Note: Store covered in fridge with pit to keep from browning too fast. Eat within two days.

Liver Pâté
By Mary Ruddick, CNC

Makes 8 servings.

1 pound of grass-fed beef liver
1 cup of lemon juice
½ cup ghee
1 cup yellow onions, chopped
2 teaspoons minced garlic
2 bay leaves (optional)

1 tablespoon thyme
½ teaspoon sea salt

1. In a bowl, soak the livers in the lemon juice for 2 hours. Drain well.
2. In a large sauté pan or skillet, melt 4 tablespoons of the ghee over medium-high heat.
3. Add onions and cook, stirring, until soft, about 3 minutes.
4. Add garlic and cook until fragrant, about 30 seconds.
5. Add the livers, bay leaves, thyme, and salt and cook, stirring, until the livers are browned on the outside and still slightly pink on the inside, about 5 minutes.
6. Remove from the heat and let cool slightly.
7. Discard bay leaves.
8. In a food processor, puree the liver mixture. Add the remaining ghee slowly by tablespoon and pulse to blend.
9. Divide the pâté into two portions. Place one container in the freezer and the other in the fridge until firm.

Notes: The original recipe called for 2 tablespoons peppercorns, but I omitted pepper for the 30-Day Food Vacation.

Mary often advises her clients to eat a spoonful of pâté daily. She says if people don't care for liver, they can cut raw liver into small cubes, freeze, and swallow whole as a "liver pill" with food to get the benefits of vitamin A, B vitamins, and zinc.

Breakfast/Lunch/Dinner

No question about it, not having eggs, dairy, nuts, or seeds makes a typical American breakfast more challenging. Do what successful 30-Day Food Vacationers do: eat leftovers for breakfast! Or, do what I do and practice intermittent fasting (that means zero calories during your fasting window), making brunch or lunch your first meal. When buying poultry, remember that "organic" just means the chickens and turkeys are fed a "vegetarian diet" that includes organic or non-GMO corn, soy and other grains. To avoid eating the corn, soy and grains your chickens or turkeys ate, you have to search specifically for soy, corn and grain-free poultry.

Spiced Beef "Tacos"
By Palmer Kippola, FMCHC

Makes 2–4 servings.

1 pound ground 100 percent grass-fed beef (or substitute ground, pastured turkey, chicken, bison or lamb)
½ onion, diced
1–2 tablespoons cumin
1–2 teaspoons ground coriander
1 cup chopped greens (spinach, kale, dandelion greens, beet tops, or chard)
2 tablespoons chopped cilantro
1 sliced avocado (or guacamole)
Options: shaved red cabbage and/or chopped scallions (green onions)
Sea salt and lime wedges to taste
Large head of red or green leaf lettuce for taco shells
Ghee for cooking

1. In a large skillet over medium heat, add ghee and sauté onion in ghee for a few minutes to soften.
2. Add beef, cumin, and coriander and sauté for 5–10 minutes, until beef is cooked through but not dry.
3. Add greens near end of beef's cook time and cook until just tender.
4. Spoon the taco mixture into lettuce wrappers and top with avocado (or guacamole), cilantro, red cabbage, green onions, a squeeze of lime, and salt to taste.

Thai Chicken Sausage Patties
By Mary Ruddick, CNC

Makes 8 patties.

2 pounds ground pastured chicken thighs (or pastured turkey)
1 cup onion, minced
1 dropperful liquid stevia

2 teaspoons sea salt
¼ cup fresh basil
¼ cup fresh mint
¼ cup fresh cilantro
2 tablespoons fresh ginger, minced
Ghee for cooking

1. Mix all ingredients well in a medium size bowl with your hands and shape into 8 patties.
2. Preheat a large pan with enough ghee to cover the bottom.
3. Cook until one side is browned and it looks like it is cooked halfway up the sausage, turn over, and cook until the other side is browned as well. You may have to cook in several batches. Just make sure the middle is cooked. Place the cooled sausage between sheets of parchment paper and freeze. To reheat, take the number of patties desired out of the freezer and reheat with a skillet or toaster oven.

Option: Bake these in the oven on a greased cookie sheet at 375° F for 10 minutes, then flip and cook for another 10 minutes.

Turkey Meatballs with Artichoke Hearts
By Linda Clark, MA, CNC

Makes around 18 meatballs.

1 pound ground turkey
1 jar of artichoke hearts (non-GMO)
1 onion, finely chopped
4 tablespoon fresh basil
1 teaspoon coconut oil
Sea salt to taste

1. Heat oven to 350° F.
2. In a large skillet, add coconut oil to coat the bottom of the skillet.
3. On medium heat, lightly sauté the artichoke hearts and onion.
4. Remove from pan and let cool.

5. In a large bowl, mix the ground turkey, artichoke hearts, onion, basil, and sea salt.
6. Form meatballs (about 18).
7. Place on an oiled baking sheet or use parchment paper.
8. Bake for 15–20 minutes, or until thoroughly baked.

Try with Linda's No-Tomato Sauce and serve over spaghetti squash or zucchini noodles (zoodles); or try turkey meatball rollups with avocado in lettuce cups.

Whole Roast Chicken
By Palmer Kippola, FMCHC

Makes 4 servings or provides lots of leftovers for chicken curry or chicken tacos.

1 whole pastured fryer chicken (~4 pounds)
1 large onion, chopped into large chunks and separated
10–20 cloves unpeeled garlic (depends on how much you love
    roasted garlic)
Handful of fresh or dried herbs (e.g., thyme, rosemary, oregano)
Optional: add additional chunked vegetables (e.g., parsnips, carrots, or beets)
1 teaspoon sea salt
1 tablespoon grass-fed ghee
½ cup filtered water

1. Preheat oven to 400° F.
2. Place chicken into a 9-by-13-inch glass or ceramic roasting pan.
3. Spread the onion, garlic, herbs, and other veggies around the chicken on the bottom of the pan.
4. Generously sprinkle the whole chicken with coarse sea salt and dried herbs if using. Dot with ghee.
5. Add ½ cup of water to the bottom of the pan.
6. Place into the oven and bake for 10 minutes at 400° F to seal in the juices, then reduce heat to 325° F and cook for approximately 1–1½ more

hours. Note: If you're using a meat thermometer, you want it to read 165–180° F in the thickest part of the breast or thigh.
7. Let rest for 10 minutes before cutting into it to allow juices to integrate.
8. Save pan juices to add to your bone broth or pour over chicken and veggies.
9. Save the chicken carcass for making stock or bone broth.
10. Serve atop cauliflower rice and/or with sautéed greens.

Quick Chicken Curry

Reprinted with permission from *Beat Sugar Addiction Now! Cookbook* by Jacob Teitelbaum, MD

Makes 5 servings.

1 tablespoon extra-virgin olive oil, divided
3–4 garlic cloves, minced
1 large red or brown onion, chopped
1½ pounds boneless, skinless chicken breasts (or leftover roast chicken), cubed
1½ cups chicken stock or broth
1 can coconut milk
2–4 teaspoons curry powder
1–2 teaspoons ground ginger

1. Heat half the oil in a large saucepan over medium heat.
2. Sauté garlic and onion for 5–10 minutes.
3. Add remaining oil and sauté chicken until cooked through.
4. To the garlic-onion mixture, add chicken broth, coconut milk, and cooked chicken.
5. Add curry powder and ginger to taste.
6. Simmer until flavors meld and sauce is heated through, about 10 minutes.

Serve atop cauliflower rice and/or with sautéed greens.

Note: Carrots and peas were omitted from original recipe. Broccoli and cauliflower are always good additions to curries.

Juicy Bison Burgers*
by Palmer Kippola, FMCHC

Makes 4–6 servings.

2 pounds ground bison
2 tablespoons nutritional yeast flakes
1½ teaspoons salt
1 teaspoon dried onion flakes or powder
Large head of red or green leaf lettuce for burger "buns"
Ghee or avocado oil for cooking
Optional toppings: 1 cup sautéed onions, 1 cup sautéed mush-
    rooms, sliced avocado

1. If you are topping with onions and/or mushrooms, sauté them first, separately, in ghee. Keep warm in oven while cooking burgers.
2. Using your hands, mix the bison, yeast flakes, onion flakes, and salt in
   a bowl to combine. Divide into 6 patties.
3. Preheat the grill to medium high heat; or use a grill pan on the stove
   and cook with ghee or avocado oil.
4. Grill the burgers for 3 to 5 minutes per side, depending on your preferred degree of doneness.
5. Place the burgers on lettuce "buns." Top with mushrooms, onions, avocado, and sea salt to taste.

Serve with Massaged Kale Salad, Brussels Sprouts Chips, or Red Cabbage
Coleslaw.
    *Hat tip to True Food Kitchen in Santa Monica, California, for the orig-
inal, awesome bison burger.

Fish/Shellfish

Make sure your fish and seafood are wild-caught, not farmed. You
definitely don't want to be eating the GMO corn or soy your farmed
salmon ate!

Broccoli Shrimp Stir-Fry
By Mary Ruddick, CNC

Makes 4 servings.

4 cups broccoli
2 cups wild shrimp (raw, deveined, and peeled)
8 cloves of garlic
1 onion cut into thin, long slices
3 tablespoons ghee or coconut oil
¼ cup lemon juice
½ cup scallions

1. Place the ghee, garlic, and onion into a pan over medium heat. Stir continuously.
2. Once the onions are translucent, add in the shrimp and cook until slightly pink. Avoid overcooking the shrimp.
3. Remove from heat and place in a serving bowl with the lemon juice. Sprinkle with sea salt and scallions.

Baked Cod with Thyme
By Mark Hyman, MD

Makes 4 servings.

1½ pounds cod fillets
1 tablespoon extra virgin olive oil
1 teaspoon fresh thyme
½ teaspoon sea salt
¼ teaspoon onion powder

1. Preheat oven to 375° F.
2. Cut the cod into 5-ounce pieces or have your fish provider do this for you.
3. Combine the olive oil, thyme, salt, and onion powder in a bowl. Mix.

4. Rub or spray a cookie sheet with olive oil to prevent sticking (or cover the pan with parchment paper). Place cod fillets on the sheet pan. Evenly spread the herb and oil mixture over the cod.

5. Bake for approximately 12–15 minutes or until fish flakes easily with a fork; internal temperature of the cod should be 155° F.

Salmon Stuffed Avocados
By Mary Ruddick, CNC

Makes 2 servings.

2 avocados, sliced in half with pit removed
6 ounces wild salmon, cooked and flaked
1 cup cilantro, chopped
¼ cup lemon juice
2 tablespoons extra virgin olive oil
½ teaspoon cumin
Sea salt to taste

1. Add the salmon, cilantro, lemon juice, olive oil, and cumin to a bowl and mix well.

2. Place salmon mixture into the avocado halves and serve with salt to taste.

Soups and Stews

These soups and stews are easy to digest, nourishing, and comforting any time of year.

Homemade Bone Broth

Sourced with permission from *Minding My Mitochondria: How I Overcame Secondary Progressive Multiple Sclerosis (MS) And Got Out Of My Wheelchair*, 2nd Edition, by Terry Wahls, MD.

Bones, saved from previous cooking

Scraps of vegetables, such as celery, parsley, and any vegetable that looks past its prime

Large stockpot or soup pot half full of water

2–4 tablespoons vinegar

1 tablespoon dried powdered kelp or dulse, or part of a whole leaf

1 packet plain gelatin

1. Put all ingredients except seaweed and gelatin into the pot and simmer for 2 or more hours (ideally 24 hours).
2. Add water if needed.
3. Strain out the vegetables and bones and discard them.
4. Dissolve a packet of plain gelatin in the broth.
5. Freeze it in pint or quart batches for future use.

I leave one or two cups in the refrigerator to gently sauté vegetables in homemade broth. Because the broth has just a small amount of fat, sautéing with broth provides the benefits of sauté without the calories of using frying oil. Put three tablespoons in a pan whenever you wish to sauté or stir-fry fresh vegetables. That'll give you that stir-fry taste without losing the antioxidant capabilities in the food you're cooking!

Vibrant Green Soup
By Palmer Kippola, FMCHC

Makes 2–3 servings.

2 cups broccoli florets

1 bunch kale or chard

½ bunch cilantro

Optional: ~12 leaves dandelion greens or any other green leafy veggie

½ to 1 avocado

2½ cups beef or chicken bone broth or stock

¼–½ cup olive oil

1 teaspoon sea salt plus additional to taste

1. Heat bone broth or stock in saucepan.
2. In a separate saucepan, steam all veggies (first four ingredients) for about 6 minutes.
3. Immediately transfer broccoli and greens to high-speed blender to avoid overcooking.
4. Add avocado and broth, pulsing to mix.
5. Blend until smooth, adding more broth as needed.
6. Pulse in olive oil and salt to taste.

Coconut Salmon Chowder
By Michelle Corey, CNC

Makes 2–3 servings.

1 pound lightly poached salmon filet, skin and bones removed
1 medium onion, finely chopped, or 1½ cups leeks, sliced
2 cups carrots, diced into small pieces
1 tablespoon fresh dill, chopped
2 tablespoons olive or coconut oil
1 bay leaf
2 cups chopped cauliflower florets
3 cups chicken stock or chicken broth
1 can unsweetened, full-fat coconut milk
Sea salt to taste
Fresh dill to garnish

1. In a large stockpot, add olive oil, onions/leeks, and carrots; sauté 5 minutes or until tender.
2. Add the chicken broth, coconut milk, cauliflower, bay leaf, and dill; bring to a simmer. Add poached salmon filets and simmer until filets break apart easily. Stir well to break apart the salmon and cook until tender.
3. To poach salmon: Sprinkle salmon fillets with a dash of sea salt. Place salmon fillets skin-side down in a sauté pan. Cover with 1 cup chicken or fish stock and bring to a simmer on medium heat. Cook 5–10 minutes, depending on the thickness of the fillet.

Hearty Beef Stew
By Palmer Kippola, FMCHC

Makes 6–8 servings.

Can be cooked on the stove in a heavy pot like a Dutch oven or cast-iron pot, or in a slow cooker or instant pot.

> 3 pounds 100 percent grass-fed beef chuck roast, bottom round roast, or pot roast cubed into 1-inch chunks—the smaller the better (most butchers will do it for you with advance notice)
> 1 pound mushrooms cut into 1-inch chunks
> 2 cups peeled and cubed (1- to 2-inch chunks) turnips, radishes, carrots, celery, and/or celery root
> 1 large onion, chopped
> 3–5 cloves garlic, crushed
> 2 tablespoons ghee or avocado oil
> 1 teaspoon coconut aminos (Caution: coconut aminos are very salty, so go easy)
> 1 tablespoon red wine vinegar or Linda's No-Tomato Sauce (as swaps for traditional tomato paste)
> 5 cups beef bone broth or stock
> 1 large bay leaf
> 1 teaspoon dried thyme or 2 fresh thyme sprigs
> Olive oil for drizzling
> Sea salt to taste

1. Place beef in bowl and toss with 1 teaspoon sea salt. Allow beef to come to room temperature.
2. Chop mushrooms and set aside.
3. Chop the onion and other vegetables and set aside.
4. Heat Dutch oven or heavy-bottomed pot on the stove over medium heat, then add ghee or avocado oil. Sauté mushrooms for about 5 minutes, then remove from pot and set aside with other vegetables.
5. Brown the beef in the pot in batches, adding more oil or ghee as needed. Once browned, set aside. Should take about 15 minutes total.
6. Sauté onions and add pressed garlic in pot until golden and fragrant.
7. Place all of the beef back into the pot and stir in the coconut aminos, vinegar, bay leaf, and thyme. Simmer together for 5 minutes.

8. Add broth slowly and scrape browned bits from the bottom of the pot.
9. Cover, reduce heat, and simmer gently for 2 hours or until beef is fork tender.
10. Add all vegetables and simmer uncovered for another hour, allowing flavors to concentrate and broth to thicken.
11. Add salt and drizzle olive oil to taste.

Note: To thicken, simmer longer with lid off or add more vegetables. Serve over steamed cauliflower or broccoli.

Salad Dressing and Sauces

Get in the habit of making simple, delicious, and healthy dressings and sauces. When you go out, just ask for olive oil and lemon on the side. I carry a small Celtic salt travel-sized grinder in my purse.

Everyday Salad Dressing
By Palmer Kippola, FMCHC

> 1 clove raw garlic, crushed
> 4 tablespoons extra virgin olive oil (more or less, to taste)
> Juice of one lemon wedge
> Sea salt to taste
> Whisk together in small bowl.

Alternative: Omit lemon and add 1 teaspoon apple cider vinegar (ACV). Some people like to add 1–2 drops stevia with the ACV.

Linda's No-Tomato Sauce
By Linda Clark, MA, CNC

Use this as a substitute for tomato sauce.

> 6 carrots, scraped and diced
> 1 beet, peeled and diced
> 1 large onion, diced

3 celery stalks, diced
4 cloves of garlic, chopped
1 bay leaf, whole
1½ cups chicken broth or water
1 teaspoon Italian seasoning blend (usually a mix of oregano, basil, marjoram, thyme, rosemary, and sage)
2 tablespoons apple cider vinegar
3 teaspoons olive oil
Sea salt to taste

1. Put all ingredients except Italian seasoning blend, apple cider vinegar, and olive oil into a covered pot and bring to a boil.
2. Reduce heat and simmer until the vegetables are cooked. Take out the bay leaf.
3. Put ingredients into a blender and blend until smooth.
4. Stir in the Italian seasoning and apple cider vinegar. Blend. Taste. You may need to add more vinegar.
5. Put into a bowl and add salt to taste.

Use in place of tomato sauce. Serve with Turkey Meatballs with Artichoke Hearts or over baked spaghetti squash, steamed zucchini spears, or cauliflower rice.

Veggies

As a percentage of your plate, non-starchy vegetables should cover at least 50 percent. Rotate colorful vegetables, eat more fermented veggies, and have fun finding new greens, sprouts, and other vegetables at your farmers' market, or planting your own, if practical.

Spring Ferments
By Toréa Rodriguez, FDN-P

Spring Asparagus
1 bunch fresh asparagus
1 head green garlic, sliced

A few sprigs fresh dill
2 cups cold, filtered water
2 teaspoons fine sea salt
Mason jar with lid*

Herby Carrots and Turnips
1 carrot (purple is fun!)
4–5 small turnips, sliced
1 head green garlic, sliced
A few sprigs fresh dill
½ teaspoon coriander seed
¼ teaspoon fennel seed
2 cups cold, filtered water
2 teaspoons fine sea salt
Large mason jar with lid

1. For the asparagus, snap off at the ends with your hands, where asparagus naturally becomes tender rather than tough and stringy.
2. Cut to fit into the mason jar.
3. For the green garlic, use a mandoline or just slice thinly.
4. Place the ingredients into the jars. You can stack them on the ends or layer them however you like, as long as all the ingredient make it to beneath the shoulder of the jar.
5. Make a 2 percent brine by adding 2 teaspoons fine sea salt, like pink Himalayan, to every 2 cups cold, filtered water.
6. Pour enough brine to cover the veg by about an inch (2–3 cm).
7. Keep on your kitchen counter for approximately 3–7 days. You'll see the bubbles forming on the carrot/turnips 24 hours later, but the asparagus may take longer. Keep checking them visually each day and do a taste test every few days. Once they change from tasting salty to tangy, yet still have a bit of crispness, that is when you'll know they are done. Then swap out the tops for normal canning jar lids and store them in the fridge.

*Consider using Kraut Source lids, which are great at keeping the good bacteria in and keeping out everything you don't want with their water lock. They also help keep the veggies submerged under the brine (www.kraut source.com).

Red Cabbage Coleslaw
By Terry Wahls, MD

1 head red cabbage, tough bottom ribs removed, shredded
   (about 6 cups)
2 bulbs fennel, cored and julienned
3 carrots, grated
1 large jicama, julienned
1 red onion, very thinly sliced
1 cup apple cider vinegar
Kosher salt
1–2 tablespoons extra virgin olive oil per two cups
   serving
2–3 teaspoons horseradish or wasabi powder

1. Combine the cabbage, fennel, carrots, jicama, and onion in a large bowl.
2. Douse with the vinegar, season with salt, and let sit at least 1 hour. This will soften the cabbage and make it seem almost cooked, but it will still have a great texture.
3. Drain the cabbage of excess liquid but still keep it fairly juicy.
4. Stir in the olive oil and horseradish.
5. Taste for seasoning and add salt.
6. The result should be a creamy and tart slaw.

Serve with Juicy Bison Burgers or as a side with any main dish.

Cauliflower "Rice"
By Palmer Kippola, FMCHC

1 head cauliflower

1. Remove the leaves and the hard core of the cauliflower and save the florets.
2. Put florets in small batches into blender and pulse carefully until the florets resemble rice.

Cooking methods:

1   Steam: Place in a steamer over boiling water and cook for 5–7 minutes. Fluff with fork and add ghee and salt to taste.
2. Pan roast: Sauté the cauliflower rice with ghee for 6–10 minutes or until it softens and turns golden. Options: Sauté with diced onion, garlic, and mushrooms and top with chopped cilantro for a "fried rice" version.

Zucchini "Pasta" with Green Harissa Sauce
By Susan Blum, MD, MPH

For the green harissa sauce:
1 packed cup flat leaf parsley leaves
½ cup cilantro leaves
¼ cup mint leaves
2 medium cloves garlic
Juice from half a lemon
1 teaspoon ground cumin
⅓ cup extra virgin olive oil
½ teaspoon sea salt

For the zucchini "pasta":
2 tablespoons extra virgin olive oil
3 scallions, trimmed and thinly sliced
3 cups shaved or spiralized zucchini (If you don't own a spiralizer, you can use a vegetable peeler and peel long, thin strips of zucchini.)
2 cups baby spinach, stems trimmed
Sea salt to taste

To make the sauce:

1. Place all ingredients except the olive oil into a blender and blend until smooth.
2. While the blender is running, slowly add the oil until incorporated.
3. Stir in salt to taste and set aside.

To make the pasta:

1. Heat the olive oil in a large skillet over medium heat until shimmering, about 3 minutes.
2. Add the scallions and sauté for about 3 minutes.
3. Stir in the zucchini and spinach and cook for another 5 minutes.
4. Add salt to taste.
5. Add the Green Harissa Sauce and stir well to mix the sauce throughout the vegetables.

Rainbow Roasted Root Veggies
By Palmer Kippola, FMCHC

These are higher-carb veggies, so go easy on portion size and complement with a larger portion of sautéed greens or salad.

   1 pound Brussels sprouts, halved, or 1 head cauliflower, cut into
       bite-sized florets
   1 medium onion cut into 1-inch chunks
   Optional additional veggies: chopped parsnips, turnips, fennel,
       beets, carrots, mushrooms
   10–15 cloves garlic, peeled and sliced
   1–2 tablespoons avocado or coconut oil (melted)
   ½ teaspoon sea salt
   2–3 sprigs of fresh rosemary or thyme or 1 teaspoon dried
       rosemary or thyme and/or any other spice you'd like to add:
       oregano, sage, marjoram, etc.
   Optional: I like to use liberal amounts of dried turmeric powder.
       Caution: It will turn your baking sheet, counter top, and hands
       temporarily orange.

1. Preheat oven to 350° F.
2. Line a baking sheet with parchment paper and place the veggies on the sheet. Add the avocado or coconut oil onto the veggies along with the herbs and salt and mix to combine.
3. Bake in the oven for 20 minutes, then flip veggies.

4. Bake another 15–25 minutes (oven temps vary) until veggies have softened and become golden brown.

Serve with protein (meat, fish, poultry) and a salad or sautéed greens.

Massaged Kale Salad
By Palmer Kippola, FMCHC

Makes 2–4 servings.

¼ cup extra virgin olive oil
Juice of 1 lemon
2 garlic cloves, crushed
Optional: 1 tablespoon nutritional yeast flakes to add a nutty-
    cheesy flavor
½ teaspoon salt
1 big bunch dino kale, ribs removed and leaves torn into
    bite-sized pieces

1. In a bowl, whisk together oil, lemon juice, garlic, salt, and yeast flakes.
2. Pour over kale and knead or massage to break down tough fibers until kale is tender. Let kale sit at room temperature for 15–30 minutes.
3. Store in airtight container and refrigerate for up to 2 days.

Note: After the 30-Day Food Vacation, if you can tolerate peppers and like a little heat, add ½ teaspoon crushed red pepper flakes.

Simple Sautéed Greens
By Palmer Kippola, FMCHC

1 tablespoon coconut or avocado oil or 3 tablespoons broth
4 ounces mixed greens (kale, collard, mustard, or greens of your
    choice), about 3–4 cups chopped and well packed
1 clove garlic, minced

1. Heat oil or broth in a large skillet over medium-low heat.
2. Add garlic and stir until fragrant.
3. Add greens, mixing to coat with oil. Cook until greens are barely wilted and tender.
4. Add salt and olive oil to taste.

Desserts

Keto Cinna-Bombs
By Palmer Kippola, FMCHC

Makes 12–18 cinna-bombs, depending on size of silicone molds.

You'll probably want to double this recipe and store in freezer for snacks or dessert!

½ cup coconut butter (manna)
1 cup coconut oil
1 tablespoon cinnamon
1 teaspoon vanilla
1 tablespoon MCT oil (optional)
1 squirt stevia extract (to taste)
⅛ teaspoon sea salt
Silicone candy molds

1. Melt the above ingredients in a saucepan on low heat and stir well with a whisk. Taste to see if you need more stevia or salt.
2. Pour into silicone candy molds and place in the freezer.
3. Keep frozen or refrigerated, as these will melt if kept at room temperature.

Variation: Swap ginger for cinnamon to make Ginger-Bombs.

Keto Cardamom Custard
By Palmer Kippola, FMCHC

Makes 3–4 servings, depending on pudding cup size.

1 can (just under 2 cups) full fat coconut milk
1 heaping tablespoon cardamom
1 squirt stevia
2 tablespoons water
1 tablespoon grass-fed gelatin

1. Add coconut milk, cardamom, and stevia to a pan over low-medium heat and stir with a whisk until integrated.
2. Mix the gelatin and water in small bowl.
3. Add the gelatin to the pan and whisk until dissolved.
4. When the coconut milk mixture is smooth and warm, transfer into 3–4 small ramekins or pudding cups.
5. Place in the fridge for 30–45 minutes or freeze for faster setting.

Variations: Swap ginger, cinnamon, or vanilla for cardamom

Quick Creamed Coconut
By Palmer Kippola, FMCHC

1 can coconut milk, refrigerated overnight
1 teaspoon vanilla extract
Several drops to 1 squirt stevia to taste

1. Place the can of coconut milk into a mixer bowl, add stevia and vanilla.
2. Beat the mixture with a hand mixer on high until the cream is light and fluffy.

Note: For thicker cream, only use hard cream that has risen to top of can. For lighter cream, use whole can. Serve atop berries or enjoy by the spoonful.

Extra

Homemade Coconut Milk
By Palmer Kippola, FMCHC

Makes 4–6 servings

2 cups unsweetened, shredded coconut
4 cups hot (not boiling), purified water
1 teaspoon vanilla extract (optional)
6 drops stevia (optional)

1. Place shredded coconut in a bowl of very hot (not boiling), pure water. Let soak for 1–2 hours and save the water.
2. In a Vitamix or blender, combine coconut, saved water, vanilla, and stevia. Blend on the highest speed for about a minute.
3. Strain liquid through a nut milk bag or very fine cheesecloth, squeezing out all the liquid into a glass mason jar.
4. Discard solids or save for adding to smoothies.
5. Use immediately or store in the fridge up to 3 days.
6. Since there are no preservatives or fillers, the fat in the coconut milk may rise to the top if stored in the fridge. Just shake or stir before using.

Food Symptom Tracker

Reintroduce foods and beverages one at a time over two days (48 hours).
See page 44 for details. The main thing is to go slow, reintroducing one food
at a time. Pay attention. How do you feel?

DATE	TIME	FOOD	SYMPTOM(S)

DATE	TIME	FOOD	SYMPTOM(S)

What's Your ACE Score?

The ten questions below were designed by ACEs study coprincipal investigators, Robert Anda, MD, MS of the CDC, and Vincent Felitti, MD, of Kaiser-Permanente.[1]

PRIOR TO YOUR EIGHTEENTH BIRTHDAY:

1. Did a parent or other adult in the household often or very often swear at you, insult you, put you down, or humiliate you, or act in a way that made you afraid that you might be physically hurt?
   No _____   If Yes, enter 1 _____

2. Did a parent or other adult in the household often or very often push, grab, slap, or throw something at you, or ever hit you so hard that you had marks or were injured?
   No _____   If Yes, enter 1 _____

3. Did an adult or person at least five years older than you ever touch or fondle you or have you touch their body in a sexual way or attempt or actually have oral, anal, or vaginal intercourse with you?
   No _____   If Yes, enter 1 _____

4. Did you often or very often feel that no one in your family loved you or thought you were important or special, or your family

didn't look out for each other, feel close to each other, or support each other?

No _____   If Yes, enter 1 _____

5. Did you often or very often feel that you didn't have enough to eat, had to wear dirty clothes, and had no one to protect you, or your parents were too drunk or high to take care of you or take you to the doctor if you needed it?

No _____   If Yes, enter 1 _____

6. Were your parents ever separated or divorced?

No _____   If Yes, enter 1 _____

7. Was your mother or stepmother:

Often or very often pushed, grabbed, slapped, or had something thrown at her?

Sometimes, often, or very often kicked, bitten, hit with a fist, or hit with something hard?

Ever repeatedly hit over at least a few minutes or threatened with a gun or knife?

No _____   If Yes, enter 1 _____

8. Did you live with anyone who was a problem drinker or alcoholic, or who used street drugs?

No _____   If Yes, enter 1 _____

9. Was a household member depressed or mentally ill, or did a household member attempt suicide?

No _____   If Yes, enter 1 _____

10. Did a household member go to prison?

No _____   If Yes, enter 1 _____

Now add up your "Yes" answers: _____ This is your ACE Score.

Your score does not define who you are. It just presents a risk for possible negative coping behaviors and health outcomes. *No matter your score, resilience and healing are possible!* The first step is to have an awareness of how ACEs may be impacting you today. My hope is that you choose to put yourself first, to embrace the possibility of healing, and to move forward into a better future that *you* get to create. Revisit the Emotional Well-Being Toolkit (page 198) for healing strategies.

Advanced Considerations
and Practitioners

Any one of these mind-body-spirit elements can block healing, and in combination may sabotage your best efforts. I have personally explored and addressed each with varying but mostly positive results and higher levels of my own healing. Review this list, see what resonates with you, and explore solutions:

- **Dehydration:** Seventy-five percent of Americans may be chronically dehydrated, a state which can contribute to a wide array of medical complications, including fatigue, headaches, joint pain, weight gain, high blood pressure, and kidney disease.[1] Urine should be light and straw-colored. If your urine is dark, you need to drink more pure water. A good rule of thumb is to drink half your body weight in ounces of water every day. Herbal teas, vegetable juices, and broth count. This is one of the simplest yet most powerful things you can do to help your body perform optimally.

- **Exposure to mold:** If your home, office, or other building you frequent has ever had water damage, there's a chance you've been exposed to mycotoxins—toxic mold waste. Find information, resources, and doctors who specialize in environmental illness at the website of mold expert Ritchie Shoemaker, MD, www.surviving mold.com, and at the International Society for Environmentally Acquired Illness, iseai.org.

- **Mast cell activation syndrome (MCAS):** Mast cells are immune cells that release histamine, which is involved in allergic reactions. While we can't live without them, many people, especially those dealing with CIRS (chronic inflammatory response syndrome), suffer from overactive mast cells and the inflammation they produce. Environmental biotoxins like mold, heavy metals, Lyme, and bartonella are common triggers of MCAS, creating a host of symptoms, including brain fog, memory issues, headaches, skin rashes, abdominal pain, diarrhea, and anxiety. If this resonates, read the piece by Jill Carnahan, MD, "Mast Cell Activation Syndrome (MCAS): When Histamine Goes Haywire…": www.jillcarnahan .com/2016/10/31/mast-cell-activation-syndrome-mcas-when-histamine-goes-haywire and check out the interview with Dr. Jill by Sandeep Gupta, MD: www.moldillnessmadesimple.com/mast-cells-and-mold-illness-with-dr-jill-carnahan.

- **Hidden Lyme and coinfections:** The Lyme spirochete and coinfections are super stealthy and may not show up on standard lab tests, resulting in frequent false negatives. People who suffer from persistent Lyme may experience numerous confounding symptoms like the ones described here: www.lymedisease.org/lyme-disease-symptom-checklist/.

  Find a Lyme-literate doctor near you who is familiar with more advanced tests by contacting LymeDisease.org, www.lyme disease.org/members/lyme-disease-doctors or the International Lyme and Associated Diseases Society (ILADS), ilads.org/ilads_ media/physician-referral. Because persistent Lyme is a politically charged issue, you have to sign up to receive recommendations.

- **Kryptopyrroluria (KPU) aka pyroluria:** KPU is a condition, possibly inherited or brought on by trauma or chronic infections, that results in a dramatic loss of zinc, vitamin B6, biotin, and other important nutrients via the kidneys. Dr. Klinghardt notes that four out of five patients he treats for persistent Lyme, as well as many of his patients with MS, heavy metal toxicity, autism, and Parkinson's, test *highly* positive for KPU. If you are dealing with any of these conditions, or have symptoms of depression, nail spots (leukodynia), parasites, or poor dream recall, read Scott Forsgren,

FDN-P, and Dietrich Klinghardt, MD, Ph.D.'s piece in the *Townsend Letter,* www.betterhealthguy.com/kpu-2017, and consider getting tested for KPU at either DHA Laboratory, www.dhalab.com/shop/kryptopyrrole-quantitative/, or Health Diagnostics and Research Institute (HDRI), www.hdri-usa.com/tests/kryptopyrrole.html.

- **Parasites:** Parasite problems are much more common than you may imagine—most people coexist with parasites to some degree. But, in excess, they can cause disturbing symptoms and be the ultimate root cause of many unexplained illnesses. Watch the webinar on parasites by health educator Ann Louise Gittleman, Ph.D., author of the book *Guess What Came to Dinner: Parasites and Your Health*: annlouise.com/2016/04/13/parasites-101; check out the comprehensive information from Susan Luschas, Ph.D., who, with her family, has been there and back: www.debugyourhealth.com/parasites-in-humans; listen to podcast interviews with Ann Louise, Susan Luschas, and Jay Davidson, DC, on www.BetterHealthGuy.com; and consider getting tested by www.ParawellnessResearch.com, a lab available direct to consumers as well as through health practitioners. Some practitioners have found that parasites may only be discovered with various forms of energetic testing, so keep an open mind and keep searching.

- **Electromagnetic frequencies (EMF)/electromagnetic radiation (EMR):** Excessive free radicals triggered by low-frequency microwave exposure from cellphones and Wi-Fi networks have been linked to chronic diseases such as cardiac arrhythmias, anxiety, depression, autism, Alzheimer's, and infertility.[2] A growing body of research from Europe shows that EMFs both amplify the virulent effects of pathogenic microbes, including Lyme and mold toxins, and reduce the growth of beneficial bacteria, leaving you more vulnerable to immune challenges. Some practitioners, like Dr. Klinghardt, will not work with patients until they address chronic EMF exposure. To learn more about potential harm and simple steps you can take to protect yourself, read investigative health journalist Nicolas Pineault's book *The Non-Tinfoil Guide to EMFs: How to Fix Our Stupid Use of*

Technology. To explore the science of EMF/EMR, check out numerous studies at www.powerwatch.org.uk/science/studies.asp.

- **Oral cavitations (osteonecrosis) and infections:** If you've had your wisdom teeth removed, root canals, dental implants, other oral surgery, or gingivitis, there is a chance that the site has become infected, even if you don't feel any symptoms. If you have had *any* invasive dental work done and are not healing from a chronic illness, do yourself a favor and see a dental surgeon who can take a 3-D cone beam scan and determine whether you are a candidate for cavitation surgery. Susan Luschas, Ph.D., once again offers comprehensive information about cavitation surgery with a checklist you can print out: www.debugyourhealth.com/cavitation-surgery.

- **Subconscious beliefs:** PSYCH-K, a combination of *psyche* and *kinesiology* (muscle testing), is an effective way to change disempowering beliefs. Bruce Lipton, Ph.D., author of *The Biology of Belief* endorses and coteaches PSYCH-K. Consider working with a PSYCH-K instructor or facilitator in person or remotely to help you identify and shift subconscious beliefs: psych-k.com/instructors. You may also benefit from Dr. Mario Martinez's book *The MindBody Code: How to Change the Beliefs that Limit Your Health, Longevity, and Success,* which shines a light on healing the archetypal wounds of shame, abandonment, and betrayal that may be sabotaging your health.

- **Unresolved or subconscious emotional trauma:** Lee Cowden, MD, and Dietrich Klinghardt, MD, Ph.D., assert that the primary root cause of chronic physical conditions may be deeply held emotions that get trapped in the body during traumatic events like adverse childhood experiences (ACEs). This may be the toughest yet most rewarding part of any healing journey. Consider extra-strength therapies highlighted in the Emotional Well-Being Toolkit of neurofeedback, EMDR, and DNRS. Additional therapies that address subconscious traumas include Recall Healing (RH), recall healing.com; Family Constellation therapy, www.family-constellation.net/trainings/family-constellation; and Applied

Psycho-Neurobiology (APN); www.sophiahi.com/what-is-apn-dr-jennifer-grushon.

- **Unforgiveness:** Holding onto grudges, bitterness, resentment, anger, hostility, animosity, and hatred is powerfully corrosive and can take a huge toll on one's physical, emotional, mental, and spiritual health. On the other hand, research demonstrates a significant relationship between forgiveness and positive health outcomes. Explore the science of forgiveness at the Greater Good Science Center, greatergood.berkeley.edu/article/item/the_new_science_of_forgiveness, and the book *Forgive for Good: A Proven Prescription for Health and Happiness* by Frederic Luskin, Ph.D., founder of the Stanford Forgiveness Project.

- **Scars:** Most of us have scars, byproducts of wound healing from cuts, scrapes, surgeries, or even our own birth (belly button) or episiotomy (vaginal scar from childbirth). According to Dietrich Klinghardt, MD, scars can create abnormal electrical signals that can alter the function of the autonomic nervous system (ANS) and interfere with healing. A practitioner trained in Autonomic Response Testing (ART) or Nutrition Response Testing (NRT) can use muscle testing to see if scars are impeding your healing. Scar treatments often include acupuncture, cold laser therapy, pelotherapy (mud or clay therapy), and/or topical wheat germ or sesame oil.

- **Subluxations of the spine:** Your nervous system controls every function in your body, so it stands to reason that if your spine is out of alignment, you may have functional problems ranging from aches and pains to loss of organ function. Visit with a doctor of osteopathy (DO) or Network Spinal Analysis (NSA) chiropractic practitioner for an assessment and techniques that aim to re-establish alignment *gently*: doctorsthatdo.org or www.chiropractorspinalanalysisnetwork.com.

- **Temporal mandibular disorder (TMD):** The structure and position of the jaw may be contributing to your health issues. Read Sophia Health Institute's piece, "Jaw Health as it Relates to Overall Health":

www.sophiahi.com/jaw-health-relates-overall-health; if it resonates, find a dentist trained in dental occlusion, jaw function, and
orthopedic dysfunction (TMJ/TMD) at members.iccmo.org.

- **Genetic mutations (SNPs):** Remember, genes aren't your destiny,
  but they do indicate a *tendency*. While MTHFR, CYP, COMT,
  GSTM1 are all mysterious and complicated-sounding acronyms,
  it is pretty common for people with autoimmune conditions to
  have mutations in these genes that are critically important for
  detoxification, methylation, mitochondrial function, and more.
  Learn about important genetic mutations from Ben Lynch's book
  Dirty Genes and check out Suzy Cohen, RPh's primer on mutations: suzycohen.com/articles/snpsmethylation.

Advanced Practitioners

These doctors specialize in complex multifactorial illnesses and often have
bigger toolkits than their Functional Medicine/naturopathic/integrative
counterparts. They are considered "destination doctors," as people often fly
to see them, usually after seeing numerous other doctors.

Several factors distinguish them from most docs:

- They consider and treat the full gamut of mind-body-spirit root
  causes: mold, metals, Lyme, parasites, other environmental toxins,
  oral health, and subconscious emotional trauma.
- They offer energetic testing to prioritize treatments.
- They believe total recovery from autoimmune conditions is possible.
- They can prescribe medication but have a nutrition- and lifestyle-
  first approach to treatment and prevention of illness.
- They offer a variety of holistic treatments which may include:
  - Allergy desensitization
  - Biocommunication devices (e.g., ZYTO scan and EVOX percep-
    tion reframing technology)
  - Colon hydrotherapy
  - Far infrared (FIR) sauna
  - Frequency specific microcurrent (FSM)
  - Heavy metal detoxification

○ Homeopathy
○ Hyperbaric oxygen therapy (HBOT)
○ IV nutrition therapy
○ Kinesiology (muscle testing)
○ Laser Energetic Detoxification (LED)
○ Neural therapy
○ Ozone
○ Pulsed electromagnetic field therapy (PEMF)

Dietrich Klinghardt, MD, Ph.D., Christine Schaffner, ND, and the team at Sophia Health Institute, north of Seattle in Woodinville, Washington
www.sophiahi.com/services
Find a Dr. Klinghardt-certified practitioner:
www.klinghardtacademy.com/images/stories/event/certified_instructors_may_2013.pdf
www.klinghardtacademy.com/images/stories/event/klinghardt_certified_practitioners.pdf?v=2018

W. Lee Cowden, MD, MD(H), cardiologist and founder of the Academy of Comprehensive Integrative Medicine (ACIM)
Unfortunately, Dr. Cowden is no longer seeing patients one on one but offers a resource to find an ACIM-trained practitioner:
www.acimconnect.com/Resources/FindHealthProfessional.aspx

The team at Holistic Healing Arts: Amy Derksen, ND, Katherine (Katie) Dahlgren, ND, Michele Grindstaff, ND, and Christopher Wakely, ND
Holistic Healing Arts, Edmonds, Washington
www.holistichealingarts.org

Marie Matheson, ND
Hampton Wellness Centre, Ottawa, Ontario, Canada
hamptonwellnesscentre.com/dr-marie-matheson

Beth McDougall, MD
Clear Center of Health, Mill Valley, California
clearcenterofhealth.com

David Minkoff, MD

LifeWorks Wellness Center, Clearwater, Florida

www.lifeworkswellnesscenter.com

Dave Ou, MD

Bridges to Health, LLC, Atlanta, Georgia

www.drdaveou.com

Sonia Rapaport, MD

Keith Berndtson, MD

Haven Medical, Chapel Hill, North Carolina

havenmedical.com

Simon Yu, MD

Prevention and Healing, Inc., St. Louis, Missouri

www.preventionandhealing.com

Sanoviv Medical Institute

Integrative medical team, Baja California, Mexico

www.sanoviv.com

Find a Practitioner and Become a Practitioner Yourself!

Functional/integrative/naturopathic doctors have more in common than not. Unlike conventional (allopathic) doctors, who focus on diagnosing symptoms, usually by body part, and prescribing medications for symptom relief, functional/integrative/naturopathic doctors focus on getting to the root causes of health challenges and attempt to bring the body back to balance as naturally and completely as possible. Many functional/integrative/naturopathic doctors were also trained in conventional medicine first and then went beyond to study a more holistic approach. Many have bigger toolkits than most conventionally trained doctors, since they may start with nutrition but also prescribe medication if needed.

Please consult these websites to find a holistic practitioner who suits your needs and geography:

Find a Functional Medicine physician: Functional Medicine is a systems-oriented approach to finding and resolving the root causes underlying surface symptoms and chronic disease, thereby returning a body back to a state of optimal *function.* The Institute for Functional Medicine describes Functional Medicine as "an individualized, patient-centered, science-based approach that empowers patients and practitioners to work together to address the underlying causes of disease and promote optimal wellness."

  Institute for Functional Medicine (IFM): www.ifm.org/find-a-practitioner

Find a naturopathic physician: As their name suggests, naturopathic physicians have a nature-first approach. According to Naturopathic.org, "Naturopathic medicine recognizes an inherent self-healing process in people that is ordered and intelligent. Naturopathic physicians act to identify and remove obstacles to healing and recovery, and to facilitate and augment this inherent self-healing process. Naturopathic physicians treat each patient by taking into account individual physical, mental, emotional, genetic, environmental, social, and other factors."

American Association of Naturopathic Physicians (AANP): www.naturopathic.org/AF_MemberDirectory.asp?version=2

Find an integrative physician: Integrative physicians are educated in both conventional and holistic medicine and are therefore able to use natural approaches or pharmaceuticals when necessary. The University of Arizona Center for Integrative Medicine (ACAIM) defines integrative medicine (IM) as "healing-oriented medicine that takes account of the whole person, including all aspects of lifestyle. It emphasizes the therapeutic relationship between practitioner and patient, is informed by evidence, and makes use of all appropriate therapies."

American College for Advancement in Medicine (ACAM): acam.site-ym.com/search/custom.asp?id=1758

Find an environmental medicine physician: From the International Society for Environmentally Acquired Illness (ISEAI), "Environmentally acquired illness (EAI) refers to serious chronic health problems caused by exposure to mold and other biotoxins, Lyme and other persistent infections, toxic chemicals such as pesticides, heavy metals, air pollution, dust, and other irritants found in the environment. Unhealthy indoor air and persistent infections are the two primary causes of EAIs." Conditions often seen by environmental medical experts include: CIRS (also called mold illness), persistent Lyme and coinfections, MCAS, and multiple chemical sensitivities (MCS).

International Society for Environmentally Acquired Illness: iseai.org

American Academy of Environmental Medicine (AAEM): www.aaemonline.org/find.php

Ritchie Shoemaker, MD—trained practitioners (mold): www
.survivingmold.com/shoemaker-protocol/Certified-Physicians-
Shoemaker-Protocol

Become a Practitioner Yourself!

There are an increasing number of opportunities for people without advanced medical degrees to become health coaches or integrative practitioners. These are some well-regarded, comprehensive, holistic programs, most of which are online:

- Become a certified Academy of Comprehensive Integrative Medicine (ACIM) Fellow at Dr. Cowden's ACIM Connect integrative health and wellness community: www.acimconnect.com/Certifications.
- Become a Functional Medicine certified health coach (FMCHC) with the Functional Medicine Coaching Academy (FMCA): www.functionalmedicinecoaching.org.
- Become a certified integrative health coach with Duke Integrative Medicine: www.dukeintegrativemedicine.org/integrative-health-coach-training/about-the-certification-course.
- Become a certified gluten practitioner with Tom O'Bryan, DC: certifiedglutenpractitioner.com.
- Become a certified human potential coach at the Bulletproof Training Institute: www.humanpotentialinstitute.com.
- Become an autonomic response testing (ART) practitioner at the Klinghardt Academy: www.klinghardtacademy.com/Seminars-Workshops.
- Become a CHEK holistic lifestyle coach: chekinstitute.com/chek-holistic-lifestyle-coach-program.
- Become a Functional Diagnostic Nutrition practitioner (FDN-P) with the Functional Diagnostic Nutrition Course and Community: functionaldiagnosticnutrition.com.
- Become a nutrition therapy consultant (NTC) or nutrition therapy practitioner (NTP) with the Nutritional Therapy Association: nutritionaltherapy.com/nutritional-therapy-programs.

Resources and Recommended Reading by Chapter

Please visit Beat Autoimmune.com for more resources.

Introduction: Overview

The Autoimmune Epidemic by Donna Jackson Nakazawa
The Biology of Belief 10th Anniversary Edition: Unleashing the Power of Consciousness, Matter & Miracles, by Bruce Lipton, Ph.D.
Grain Brain: The Surprising Truth about Wheat, Carbs, and Sugar—Your Brain's Silent Killers by David Perlmutter, MD
Gluten Freedom: The Nation's Leading Expert Offers the Essential Guide to a Healthy, Gluten-Free Lifestyle by Alessio Fasano, Ph.D.

Chapter 1: Start with Food

There are an increasing number of mail order companies that supply organic and wild meats, fish, home and personal care products straight to you or to a community drop-off location:

US Wellness Meats: Find 100 percent grass-fed (never grain finished) beef, lamb, bison, and venison; pasture-raised (soy-free) chicken and duck; fish; and even an autoimmune Paleo-friendly foods section. Note that US Wellness Meats has a minimum seventy-five dollar order. Consider stocking up your freezer or sharing with friends and family: grasslandbeef.com.

Vital Choice: A socially conscious supplier of sustainably harvested wild seafood from the Pacific Northwest, Vital Choice provides a 100 percent guarantee on all foods within thirty days of purchase. Note that frozen products must total sixty-five dollars to prevent thawing during shipping: www.vitalchoice.com.

Vitacost: A non-subscription-based provider of below-retail-priced supplements (including the discounted Vitacost brand), organic and non-GMO foods, pantry items, and household products. Even offers products for pets and kids: www.vitacost.com.

Thrive Market: A yearly membership model, like Costco, for lower-cost organic food and home products. A ding against Thrive is that they don't share prices until you provide your email address. On the plus side, Thrive donates a membership to a family in need from every membership that is purchased: thrivemarket.com/landing/tmhome.

Azure: Another lower-cost option for organic food delivery, Azure drops off organic and non-GMO once a month at a designated drop-off location. Compare prices, groceries, and convenience with Thrive to see which one is better for your needs: www.azurestandard.com/healthy-living/about-us/get-organic-products-delivered.

Pharmaca: A holistic pharmacy that has both brick and mortar stores and online shopping for discounted organic and non-GMO supplements, health and beauty products, and cosmetics. Offers free shipping on orders over thirty-five dollars: www.pharmaca.com.

Food Documentaries and Videos

Sugar: The Bitter Truth: Robert H. Lustig, MD, professor of pediatrics at UCSF, explores the damage caused by sugary foods. He argues that too much fructose and not enough fiber appear to be driving high insulin, which is fueling the obesity epidemic: www.youtube.com/watch?v=dBnniua6-oM.

Food, Inc.: An informative, educational and downright disturbing examination of America's food and agricultural industries: amzn.to/2LEdqiN.

King Corn: An entertaining and eye-opening film by college buddies who follow the food chain from the farm to nearly every product Americans consume today: www.kingcorn.net.

Paleo Diet and Cookbooks

Wheat Belly: Lose the Wheat, Lose the Weight, and Find Your Path Back to Health and *Wheat Belly Slim Guide: The Fast and Easy Reference for Living and Succeeding on the Wheat Belly Lifestyle* by William Davis, MD

Primal Fat Burner: Live Longer, Slow Aging, Super-Power Your Brain, and Save Your Life with a High-Fat, Low-Carb Paleo Diet by Nora Gedgaudas, CNS, NTP, BCHN

Paleo Principles: The Science Behind the Paleo Template, Step-by-Step Guides, Meal Plans, and 200+ Healthy & Delicious Recipes for Real Life by Sarah Ballantyne, Ph.D.

Practical Paleo, 2nd Edition (Updated and Expanded): A Customized Approach to Health and a Whole-Foods Lifestyle by Diane Sanfilippo

The Autoimmune Paleo Cookbook by Mickey Trescott, NTP

Wired to Eat: Turn Off Cravings, Rewire Your Appetite for Weight Loss, and Determine the Foods That Work for You and *The Paleo Solution: The Original Human Diet* by Robb Wolf

No Grain, No Pain: A 30-Day Diet for Eliminating the Root Cause of Chronic Pain by Dr. Peter Osborne, DC

Epi-paleo Rx: The Prescription for Disease Reversal and Optimal Health by Jack Kruse, MD

Ketogenic Diet Information and Cookbooks

The Keto Reset Diet: Reboot Your Metabolism in 21 Days and Burn Fat Forever, The Primal Kitchen Cookbook: Eat Like Your Life Depends On It! and *The New Primal Blueprint: Reprogram Your Genes for Effortless Weight Loss, Vibrant Health and Boundless Energy* by Mark Sisson

Keto Clarity: Your Definitive Guide to the Benefits of a Low-Carb, High-Fat Diet by Jimmy Moore with Eric Westman, MD

The Keto Diet: The Complete Guide to a High-Fat Diet, by Leanne Vogel

KetoDietApp.com

CharlieFoundation.org

Nutrition

In Defense of Food, An Eater's Manifesto by Michael Pollan

The Big Fat Surprise: Why Butter, Meat and Cheese Belong in a Healthy Diet by Nina Teicholz

Eat Fat, Get Thin: Why the Fat We Eat Is the Key to Sustained Weight Loss and Vibrant Health by Mark Hyman, MD

Good Calories, Bad Calories: Fats, Carbs, and the Controversial Science of Diet and Health and *The Case Against Sugar* by Gary Taubes

Deep Nutrition: Why Your Genes Need Traditional Food, by Catherine Shanahan, MD

Nourishing Traditions: The Cookbook that Challenges Politically Correct Nutrition and the Diet Dictocrats by Sally Fallon and Mary Enig, Ph.D.

Nutrition and Physical Degeneration by Weston A. Price, DDS

Fasting

The Complete Guide to Fasting: Heal Your Body Through Intermittent, Alternate-Day, and Extended Fasting by Jason Fung, MD with Jimmy Moore

The Longevity Diet: Discover the New Science Behind Stem Cell Activation and Regeneration to Slow Aging, Fight Disease, and Optimize Weight by Valter Longo, Ph.D.

Mitochondrial Health

Radical Metabolism: A Powerful New Plan to Blast Fat and Reignite Your Energy in Just 21 Days by Ann Louise Gittleman, Ph.D., CNS

Mitochondria and the Future of Medicine: The Key to Understanding Disease, Chronic Illness, Aging, and Life Itself by Lee Know, ND

Fat for Fuel: A Revolutionary Diet to Combat Cancer, Boost Brain Power, and Increase Your Energy by Joseph Mercola, DO

The Bulletproof Diet: Lose up to a Pound a Day, Reclaim Energy and Focus, Upgrade Your Life and *Head Strong: The Bulletproof Plan to Activate Untapped Brain Energy to Work Smarter and Think Faster—In Just Two Weeks* by Dave Asprey, founder and CEO of Bulletproof

Chapter 2: Heal Your Gut

The Good Gut: Taking Control of Your Weight, Your Mood, and Your Long-term Health by Justin and Erica Sonnenburg, Ph.D.s

The Microbiome Solution: A Radical New Way to Heal Your Body from the Inside Out by Robynne Chutkan, MD

The Microbiome Diet: The Scientifically Proven Way to Restore Your Gut Health and Achieve Permanent Weight Loss by Raphael Kellman, MD

Brain Maker: The Power of Gut Microbes to Heal and Protect Your Brain for Life by David Perlmutter, MD

Eat Dirt: Why Leaky Gut May Be the Root Cause of Your Health Problems and 5 Surprising Steps to Cure It by Josh Axe, DNM, DC, CNS

Gut and Psychology Syndrome: Natural Treatment for Autism, Dyspraxia, A.D.D., Dyslexia, A.D.H.D., Depression, Schizophrenia by Natasha Campbell-McBride, MD

Chapter 3: Clear Infections

Lyme disease

New Paradigms in Lyme Disease Treatment: 10 Top Doctors Reveal Healing Strategies That Work by Connie Strasheim

How Can I Get Better?: An Action Plan for Treating Resistant Lyme & Chronic Disease and *Why Can't I Get Better? Solving the Mystery of Lyme and Chronic Disease* by Richard Horowitz, MD

The Lyme Solution: A 5-Part Plan to Fight the Inflammatory Auto-Immune Response and Beat Lyme Disease by Darin Ingels, MD

How To Fix Lyme Disease: 3 Secrets to Improve Any Lyme Disease Treatment by Jay Davidson, DC, PScD

Unlocking Lyme: Myths, Truths, and Practical Solutions for Chronic Lyme Disease by William Rawls, MD

Parasites

Accidental Cure: Extraordinary Medicine for Extraordinary Patients by Simon Yu, MD

Guess What Came to Dinner?: Parasites and Your Health by Ann Louise Gittleman, Ph.D., CNS

Infections Interviews

Nikolas Hedberg, DC, DABCI, DACBN: drhedberg.com/autoimmune-disease-infection-connection

Dietrich Klinghardt, MD: www.sophiahi.com/demystifying-lyme

Lee Cowden, MD: www.betterhealthguy.com/episode29

Scott Forsgren, FDN-P multiple podcast interviews: www.BetterHealthGuy.com

Chapter 4: Minimize Toxins

Toxicants in Home, Food, and Body Care Products

Organizations that monitor home, food, and body care products for safety can help you figure out what to avoid and what to buy:

Environmental Working Group (EWG) is a nonprofit, nonpartisan organization dedicated to protecting human health and the environment. EWG conducts

research, does advocacy work in Washington D.C., and provides reports online free of charge. EWG focuses on food, water, consumer products, energy,
farming, toxins, and children's health. Check out their Clean 15 and Dirty
Dozen yearly reports to evaluate which produce to definitely buy organic.
And, if you are motivated, consider supporting their important work with
a donation: www.ewg.org.

EWG's Consumer Guide to Seafood is the output of EWG's investigation into existing data amassed by the government and third-party scientific sources on
mercury contamination and omega-3 levels in seafood: www.ewg.org/
research/ewgs-good-seafood-guide#.Wt4q3a2ZPqo.

EWG's Skin Deep Cosmetics Database is an online resource that provides a rating
scale from one to ten (fewest to most toxicants) on more than 74,000 products. See how well your skin care, sunscreen, and cosmetics rate on the
safety scale at www.ewg.org/skindeep/#.WtEUe62ZPqo.

Think Dirty was started by a woman whose family was impacted by breast cancer
and who wanted to understand possible connections between cosmetics and
cancer. The Think Dirty mobile app empowers users to make informed decisions at the point of purchase by scanning bar codes of nearly 1 million
products and more than four thousand brands: www.thinkdirtyapp.com.

Toxicant and Disease Database

Collaborative on Health and the Environment (CHE), a nonprofit that seeks to share
evidence-based science and resources and help improve individual and collective health, offers a Toxicant and Disease Database where you can search
by toxicant or disease to learn which chemicals have what degree of evidence for causing specific diseases: www.healthandenvironment.org/
our-work/toxicant-and-disease-database.

Books

*Toxic: Heal Your Body from Mold Toxicity, Lyme Disease, Multiple Chemical Sensi-
tivities, and Chronic Environmental Illness* by Neil Nathan, MD

*The Toxin Solution: How Hidden Poisons in the Air, Water, Food, and Products We
Use Are Destroying Our Health—And What We Can Do To Fix It* by Joseph
Pizzorno, ND

*Clinical Environmental Medicine: Identification and Natural Treatment of Diseases
Caused by Common Pollutants* (textbook) by Walter Crinnion, ND, and
Joseph Pizzorno, ND

TOX-SICK: From Toxic to Not Sick by Suzanne Somers

Detoxify or Die by Sherry A. Rogers, MD

The Non-Tinfoil Guide to EMFs: How to Fix Our Stupid Use of Technology by Nicolas Pineault

Vaccines and Autoimmunity by Yehuda Shoenfeld, MD FRCP (Hon.), Nancy Agmon-Levin, MD & Lucija Tomljenovic, Ph.D.

Silent Spring by Rachel Carson, MA

Films

Unacceptable Levels: An important and informative film about the chemicals in our bodies, how they got there, and what we can do about it: www.amazon.com/Unacceptable-Levels-Ralph-Nader/dp/B00JDB4I4G.

Moldy: An important overview of the topic of toxic mold illness, with interviews with a variety of doctors as well as patients by Dave Asprey, founder of Bulletproof, who was personally affected by mold. Sign up to watch for free: moldymovie.com/index?affiliate=3983.

Trade Secrets: A Moyers Report: Journalist Bill Moyers investigates the chemical industry and finds secrets the chemical industry doesn't want us to see, including the negative consequences of the chemical revolution on our bodies: www.pbs.org/tradesecrets/problem/bodyburden.html.

Chapter 5: Address Stress

Books

Why Zebras Don't Get Ulcers by Robert Sapolsky, Ph.D.

The Last Best Cure: My Quest to Awaken the Healing Parts of My Brain and Get Back My Body, My Joy, and My Life and *Childhood Disrupted: How Your Biography Becomes Your Biology, and How You Can Heal* by Donna Jackson Nakazawa

The Body Keeps the Score: Brain, Mind, and Body in the Healing of Trauma by Bessel van der Kolk, MD

When the Body Says No: Exploring the Stress-Disease Connection by Gabor Maté MD

Full Catastrophe Living: Using the Wisdom of Your Body and Mind to Face Stress, Pain, and Illness by Jon Kabat-Zinn, Ph.D.

Resilient: How to Grow an Unshakable Core of Calm, Strength, and Happiness by Rick Hanson, Ph.D. and Forrest Hanson

Stressaholic: 5 Steps to Transform Your Relationship with Stress by Heidi Hanna, Ph.D.

The Upside of Stress: Why Stress Is Good for You, and How to Get Good at It by Kelly McGonigal, Ph.D.

Mindfulness: An Eight-Week Plan for Finding Peace in a Frantic World by Mark Williams, D.Phil., and Danny Penman, Ph.D.

You Are the Placebo: Making Your Mind Matter by Joe Dispenza, DC

Loving What Is: Four Questions That Can Change Your Life by Byron Katie

The Power of Now: A Guide to Spiritual Enlightenment by Eckhart Tolle (I prefer the audio version.)

Meditation Resources

Guided meditations may be the easiest way for you to ease into meditation. These are a few of my favorites for relaxing, healing, and getting better sleep:

Benson-Henry Institute for Mind Body Medicine offers an effective and free six-minute Relaxation Response guided meditation with Peg Baim, MS, NP: www.youtube.com/watch?v=gAIYm6wpzw4&index=1&list=PLxQozQsqi Ikh8FXeQJm-ZBdbCatIpYeuu&t=0s.

Kelly Howell offers powerful guided meditations like Mind Body Healing, Healing Meditation, Guided Relaxation, and more for purchase at: www.brains ync.com.

Davidji offers soothing guided meditations for free and for purchase at: davidji .com/meditation/free-guided-meditations.

Mobile Meditation Apps

These apps are available for your iOS or Android device. Each offers some free meditations and optional monthly subscriptions.

Calm: Apple's 2017 App of the Year, Calm comes with a "7 Days of Calm" intro program to get you started, as well as seven- and twenty-one–day meditation programs. The meditations range from three to twenty-five minutes long, there are nature sound options, and many are guided by a soothing female voice.

Headspace: Headspace is another a great option for beginners and for people who want to make meditation a habit. Get started with the ten-day free meditation pack on the basics. From there, you can explore meditation packs about health, happiness, work, performance, and more. Guided meditations are led by the soothing British voice of Andy Puddicombe, a cofounder of Headspace.

Meditation Tracking Technology

Muse: Muse is a headband with sensors that track your brain activity in real time. When your mind is calm, you hear peaceful weather sounds like gentle waves lapping on the shore and chirping birds; when your mind is active, you hear more intense weather sounds like crashing waves or heavy rain. Immediate neurofeedback gives you the opportunity to choose a more peaceful state. www.choosemuse.com

Mindfulness Meditation

Studies show that this form of meditation, which could be described as non-judgmental present moment awareness, reduces stress, anxiety, pain, and depression; improves memory, attention, and empathy; and even increases the brain's gray matter density.[1] Top mindfulness meditation teachers Tara Brach, Ph.D., and Jack Kornfield, Ph.D., offer daily fifteen-minute mindfulness training and practice: www.soundstrue.com/store/mindfulness-daily/free-access.

Mindfulness-based stress reduction (MBSR) training: An eight-week program originally founded by Jon Kabat-Zinn, Ph.D., in 1979 is now offered by many hospitals and medical centers worldwide. MBSR helps to reduce physical symptoms and psychological distress while helping people live with greater awareness and peace.
Find an in-person MBSR training: www.umassmed.edu/cfm/mindfulness-based-programs/mbsr-courses/find-an-mbsr-program.
Online and donation-based MBSR training: palousemindfulness.com.

Chapter 6: Balance Your Hormones

Books

The Hormone Fix: Burn Fat Naturally, Boost Energy, Sleep Better, and Stop Hot Flashes, the Keto-Green Way by Anna Cabeca, DO, OBGYN, FACOG
The Diabetes Code: Prevent and Reverse Type 2 Diabetes Naturally and *The Obesity Code: Unlocking the Secrets of Weight Loss* by Jason Fung, MD
The Hormone Cure: Reclaim Balance, Sleep and Sex Drive; Lose Weight; Feel Focused, Vital, and Energized Naturally with the Gottfried Protocol and *Younger: A Breakthrough Program to Reset Your Genes, Reverse Aging, and Turn Back the Clock 10 Years* by Sara Gottfried, MD

The Wisdom of Menopause (Revised Edition): Creating Physical and Emotional Health During the Change and *Goddesses Never Age: The Secret Prescription for Radiance, Vitality, and Well-Being* by Christiane Northrup, MD

Why Do I Still Have Thyroid Symptoms? when My Lab Tests Are Normal: a Revolutionary Breakthrough in Understanding Hashimoto's Disease and Hypothyroidism by Datis Kharrazian, DHSc, DC, MS, FAACP, DACBN, DABCN, DIBAK, CNS

HormoneSynergy by Kathryn Retzler, ND

Dr. John Lee's Hormone Balance Made Simple: The Essential How-To Guide to Symptoms, Dosage, Timing, and More by John Lee, MD and Virginia Hopkins

Hormone Videos

Barbara O'Neill, naturopath and health educator: www.youtube.com/watch?v=MGmpq43YxMA&list=PLxQozQsqiIkhibPQAosQALDb3oBmWchg4&index=3&t=os

Shari Caplan, MD, on Mike Mutzel, MSc's High Intensity Health podcast: www.youtube.com/watch?v=VkWwNoqDgJY&list=PLxQozQsqiIkhibPQAosQALDb3oBmWchg4&index=18&t=2s

Kathryn Retzler, ND, on Mike Mutzel, MSc's High Intensity Health podcast: www.youtube.com/watch?v=NhfvrXM7tBw&t=1343s

ABOUT THE PRACTITIONERS
PROFILED IN THE BOOK

Susan Blum, MD, MPH, is a preventive medicine and chronic disease specialist. Dr. Blum is the founder and director of Blum Center for Health in Rye Brook, New York. She is also assistant clinical professor in the Department of Preventive Medicine at the Icahn School of Medicine at Mount Sinai, a member of the medical advisory board for both *The Dr. Oz Show* and the Institute for Integrative Nutrition (IIN), and is senior teaching faculty with the Center for Mind-Body Medicine (CMBM) in Washington, D.C. Her books include: *Healing Arthritis: Your 3-Step Guide to Conquering Arthritis Naturally* and *The Immune System Recovery Plan: A Doctor's 4-Step Program to Treat Autoimmune Disease.*
www.blumcenterforhealth.com

Jill Carnahan, MD, ABFM, ABIHM, IFMCP, is a Functional Medicine expert and founder of Flatiron Functional Medicine in Louisville, Colorado. Dr. Jill specializes in complex disorders including mold illness, CIRS (chronic inflammatory response syndrome), and mast cell activation syndrome (MCAS). Dr. Jill is board-certified in both family medicine and integrative holistic medicine. Visit her website for video and podcast interviews, blog posts, and recipes.
www.jillcarnahan.com

Linda Clark, MA, CNC, is a holistic health expert, educator, and founder of Universal Wellness Associates in Sacramento, California. Linda is an adjunct professor at John F. Kennedy University, where she teaches numerous courses for the holistic health master's program. She created the Detox 360 program for functional nutrition company Apex Energetics and is a speaker for them. She is also author of the *Gluten-Free Life* booklet, which makes it easy for people to create a gluten-free lifestyle.

www.uwanutrition.com

Michelle Corey, CNWC, FMC, is a functional mind-body practitioner, nutritionist, and medical advocate. Michelle offers Total Recovery programs for patients worldwide who suffer from complex autoimmune and inflammatory conditions, and is based in Taos, New Mexico. Michelle is an advisor to the Academy of Functional Medicine and Genomics and the Functional Medical University, and she is a member of the Institute for Functional Medicine and the National Association of Healthcare Advocacy Consultants. She is the author of *The Thyroid Cure: The Functional Mind-Body Approach to Reversing Your Autoimmune Condition and Reclaiming Your Health!*

www.michellecorey.com

Mark Hyman, MD, is a practicing family physician, ten-time number-one *New York Times* bestselling author, and internationally recognized leader, speaker, educator, and health advocate. Dr. Hyman is the director the Cleveland Clinic Center for Functional Medicine, founder and medical director of The UltraWellness Center in Lenox, Massachusetts, and chairman of the board of the Institute for Functional Medicine. His latest books include: *Food: What the Heck Should I Eat?*; *Eat Fat, Get Thin: Why the Fat We Eat Is the Key to Sustained Weight Loss and Vibrant Health*; and *The Eat Fat, Get Thin Cookbook: More Than 175 Delicious Recipes for Sustained Weight Loss and Vibrant Health.*

www.drhyman.com

www.ultrawellnesscenter.com

Jacob Teitelbaum, MD, is a board-certified internist and nationally known expert in the fields of chronic fatigue syndrome, fibromyalgia, sleep, and pain. Dr. T. consults with patients both by phone and in person in Kona, Hawaii. He is the lead author of four studies on effective treatment for fibromyalgia and chronic fatigue syndrome and a study on effective treatment of autism using NAET (Nambudripad's Allergy Elimination Techniques). Dr. T's S.H.I.N.E. Protocol has helped tens of thousands of CFS/FMS sufferers reclaim their vitality. Dr. T. is also director of the Practitioners Alliance Network (PAN) and author of numerous books, including *The Fatigue and Fibromyalgia Solution: The Essential Guide to Overcoming Chronic Fatigue and Fibromyalgia, Made Easy!; From Fatigued to Fantastic;* and *The Complete Guide to Beating Sugar Addiction: The Cutting-Edge Program That Cures Your Type of Sugar Addiction and Puts You on the Road to Feeling Great—and Losing Weight!*

www.secure.endfatigue.com

Toréa Rodriguez is a certified Functional Diagnostic Nutrition practitioner and vitality transformation coach. She lives in Santa Cruz, California, and works with clients all over the world who are ready to achieve breakthroughs in any area of their lives. Toréa offers a Transform Your Vitality program tailored to each client that incorporates nutrition, stress reduction, mindfulness, and movement. She also appears on numerous podcast interviews, which you can find on her website.

www.torearodriguez.com

Mary Ruddick, CNC, is a healing diet expert, owner of Enable Your Healing and director of nutritional healing at Alive Holistic Counseling, in Eugene, Oregon. Mary sees clients both locally in Eugene and worldwide via Skype. Mary teaches her clients to follow a variety of healing diets, including the ketogenic diet, GAPS (Gut and Psychology Syndrome) diet, and many other tailored healing diets and nourishing lifestyle practices.

www.enableyourhealing.com
www.aliveholisticcounseling.com/clinical-nutritionists

Amie Valpone, HHC, AADP, is a Functional Medicine nutrition and wellness expert, chef, nutritionist, columnist, spokesperson, motivational speaker, and author of the best-selling *Eating Clean: The 21-Day Plan to Detox, Fight Inflammation, and Reset Your Body.* Amie lives in New York City and works with and cooks healthy, organic whole food meals for a variety of clients all over the world, including celebrities and athletes. She founded TheHealthyApple.com, and her work has been featured on Martha Stewart, ABC News, Fox News Health, WebMD, the *Huffington Post*, the Food Network, *Glamour* magazine, *Clean Eating Magazine*, *SELF* magazine, *Prevention* magazine, and PBS.

www.thehealthyapple.com

Terry Wahls, MD, is a clinical professor of medicine at the University of Iowa Carver College of Medicine in Iowa City, Iowa, where she teaches internal medicine residents in their primary care clinics. Dr. Wahls also does clinical research and has published more than sixty peer-reviewed scientific abstracts, posters, and papers. Her inspirational TED talk, entitled, "Minding Your Mitochondria," in which she recounts her healing journey from progressive MS back to health, has gotten three million views. Dr. Wahls is the author of the best-selling, *The Wahls Protocol: A Radical New Way to Treat All Chronic Autoimmune Conditions Using Paleo Principles* and the cookbook *The Wahls Protocol Cooking for Life: The Revolutionary Modern Paleo Plan to Treat All Chronic Autoimmune Conditions*.

www.terrywahls.com

ENDNOTES

Introduction: Overview

1. Rappaport, Stephen M., "Implications of the Exposome for Exposure Science," *Journal of Exposure Science and Environmental Epidemiology*, volume 21, pages 5–9 (2011) doi:10.1038/jes.2010.50, www.nature.com/articles/jes201050

2. Anand, P., et al., "Cancer is a Preventable Disease that Requires Major Lifestyle Changes," *Pharm Res.* 2008 Sep; 25(9): 2097–2116. doi: 10.1007/s11095-008-9661-9

3. "Exposome and Exposomics," National Institute for Occupational Safety and Health (NIOSH), Centers for Disease Control and Prevention (CDC), www.cdc.gov/niosh/topics/exposome/

4. Fasano, A., "Mechanisms of Disease: the Role of Intestinal Barrier Function in the Pathogenesis of Gastrointestinal Autoimmune Diseases," *Nat Clin Pract Gastroenterol Hepatol.* 2005 Sep;2(9):416-22. www.ncbi.nlm.nih.gov/pubmed/16265432

Chapter 1: Start with Food

1. National Center for Chronic Disease Prevention and Health Promotion, Centers for Disease Control and Prevention (CDC), www.cdc.gov/chronicdisease/overview/index.htm#ref1

2. Farrell, R.J. and Kelly, C.P., "Celiac Sprue," *N Engl J Med.* 2002 Jan 17; 346(3):180-8; www.nejm.org/doi/full/10.1056/NEJMra010852

3. 213 Abstracts with Roundup (herbicide) research, *GreenMedInfo.com*, www.greenmedinfo.com/article/specific-agricultural-pesticides-solvents-and-chemical-fertilizers-may-increase

4. Kleinewietfeld, et al., "Sodium Chloride Drives Autoimmune Disease by the Induction of Pathogenic TH17 Cells," *Nature* (2013); doi:10.1038/nature11868, www.ncbi.nlm.nih.gov/pmc/articles/PMC3746493/

5. Vojdani, A., Tarash, I., "Cross-Reaction Between Gliadin and Different Food and Tissue Antigens," *Scientific Research*, www.scirp.org/Journal/PaperInformation.aspx?paperID=26626#.VVykUc5ZabA

6. Procaccini, C., et al., "Obesity and Susceptibility to Autoimmune Diseases," *Expert Rev Clin Immunol.* 2011;7(3):287–294., www.ncbi.nlm.nih.gov/pubmed/21595595

7. De Punder, K., Pruimboom, L., "The Dietary Intake of Wheat and Other Cereal Grains and Their Role in Inflammation," *Nutrients.* 2013;5(3):771-787. doi:10.3390/nu5030771, www.ncbi.nlm.nih.gov/pmc/articles/PMC3705319/

8. Sarah Ballantyne, Ph.D., "The Whys Behind the Autoimmune Protocol: Eggs," www.thepaleomom.com/whys-behind-autoimmune-protocol-eggs/

9. Eigenmann, P.A., et al., "Managing Nut Allergy: a Remaining Clinical Challenge," *J Allergy Clin Immunol Pract.* 2017 Mar - Apr;5(2):296-300. doi: 10.1016/j.jaip.2016.08.014. www.ncbi.nlm.nih.gov/pubmed/27793601

10. Freed, David L.J., "Do Dietary Lectins Cause Disease? The Evidence is Suggestive—and Raises Interesting Possibilities for Treatment," *BMJ.* 1999 Apr 17; 318(7190): 1023–1024. www.ncbi.nlm.nih.gov/pmc/articles/PMC1115436/

11. Studer-Rohr, I., et al., "The Occurrence of Ochratoxin A in Coffee," *Food Chem Toxicol.* 1995 May;33(5):341-55., www.ncbi.nlm.nih.gov/pubmed/7759018

12. Vojdani, A., Tarash, I. "Cross-Reaction Between Gliadin and Different Food and Tissue Antigens," *Scientific Research*, www.scirp.org/Journal/PaperInformation.aspx?paperID=26626#.VVykUc5ZabA

13. Pérez-Cano, Francisco J., et al., "The Effects of Cocoa on the Immune System," *Front Pharmacol.* 2013; doi: 10.3389/fphar.2013.00071, www.ncbi.nlm.nih.gov/pmc/articles/PMC3671179/

14. Mellberg, C., et al, "Long-Term Effects of a Palaeolithic-Type Diet in Obese Postmenopausal Women: a 2-Year Randomized Trial," *European Journal of Clinical Nutrition*, 2014; doi:10.1038/ejcn.2013.290 www.ncbi.nlm.nih.gov/pubmed/24473459

15. Jonsson, T., et al., "A Paleolithic Diet Confers Higher Insulin Sensitivity, Lower C-Reactive Protein and Lower Blood Pressure Than a Cereal-Based Diet in Domestic Pigs," *Nutr Metab* (Lond). 2006; 3: 39., doi: 10.1186/1743-7075-3-39, www.ncbi.nlm.nih.gov/pmc/articles/PMC1635051/

16. Lindeberg, S., Jönsson, T., Granfeldt, Y. et al., "A Palaeolithic Diet Improves Glucose Tolerance More Than a Mediterranean-Like Diet in Individuals with Ischaemic Heart Disease," *Diabetologia*, 2007; 50: 1795. doi:10.1007/s00125-007-0716-y, link.springer.com/article/10.1007%2Fs00125-007-0716-y

17. Frassetto, L.A., et al., "Metabolic and Physiologic Improvements from Consuming a Paleolithic, Hunter-Gatherer Type Diet," *Eur J Clin Nutr.* 2009 Aug;63(8):947-55. doi: 10.1038/ejcn.2009.4. www.ncbi.nlm.nih.gov/pubmed/19209185

18. Carrera-Bastos, P., et., al., "The Western Diet and Lifestyle and Diseases of Civilization," *Dovepress*, 9 March 2011, Volume 2011:2 Pages 15–35, doi.org/10.2147/RRCC.S16919, www.dovepress.com/the-western-diet-and-lifestyle-and-diseases-of-civilization-peer-reviewed-article-RRCC

19. Baranski, M., et al., "Higher Antioxidant and Lower Cadmium Concentrations and Lower Incidence of Pesticide Residues in Organically Grown Crops: a Systematic Literature Review and Meta-Analyses," *British Journal of Nutrition*, Volume 112, Issue 5 14 September 2014, pp. 794-811; www.cambridge.org/core/journals/british-journal-of-nutrition/article/higher-antioxidant-and-lower-cadmium-concentrations-and-lower-incidence-of-pesticide-residues-in-organically-grown-crops-a-systematic-literature-review-and-metaanalyses/33F09637EAE6C4ED119E0C4BFFE2D5B1

20. *The American Nutrient Gap: What the Data Says We're Missing*, medcitynews.com/2015/12/the-american-nutrient-gap-what-the-data-says-were-missing/?rf=1

21. Schwalfenberg, G., and Genuis, S., "The Importance of Magnesium in Clinical Healthcare," *Scientifica*, Volume 2017 (2017), doi.org/10.1155/2017/4179326, www.hindawi.com/journals/scientifica/2017/4179326/

22. Tam, M., et al., "Possible Roles of Magnesium on the Immune System," *European Journal of Clinical Nutrition* volume 57, pages 1193–1197 (2003) doi:10.1038/sj.ejcn.1601689, www.nature.com/articles/1601689

Chapter 2: Heal Your Gut

1. Quigley, Eamonn M.M., "Gut Bacteria in Health and Disease," *Gastroenterol Hepatol* (NY). 2013 Sep; 9(9): 560–569, www.ncbi.nlm.nih.gov/pmc/articles/PMC3983973/

2. Vaarala, O., et al., "The 'Perfect Storm' for Type 1 Diabetes: the Complex Interplay Between Intestinal Microbiota, Gut Permeability, and Mucosal Immunity," *Diabetes*. 2008 Oct; 57(10): 2555–2562. doi: 10.2337/db08-0331, www.ncbi.nlm.nih.gov/pmc/articles/PMC2551660/

3. "Study Suggests Altering Gut Bacteria Might Mitigate Lupus," American Society for Microbiology (ASM), www.eurekalert.org/pub_releases/2014-10/asfm-ssa102014.php

4. Miyake, S., et al., "Dysbiosis in the Gut Microbiota of Patients with Multiple Sclerosis, with a Striking Depletion of Species Belonging to Clostridia XIVa and IV Clusters," *PLOS One*, September 14, 2015, doi.org/10.1371/journal.pone.0137429

5. Xhan, Z., et al., "Gram-Negative Bacterial Molecules Associate with Alzheimer Disease Pathology," *Neurology*, November 2016: 10.%u200B1212/%u200BWNL.%u200B0000000000003391

6. Gevers, D., et al., "The Treatment-Naive Microbiome in New Onset Crohn's Disease," *Cell Host & Microbe*, March 2014 DOI: 10.1016/j.chom.2014.02.005 www.cell.com/cell-host-microbe/abstract/S1931-3128(14)00063-8;

7. Viaud, S., et al., "Gut Microbiome and Anticancer Immune Response: Really Hot Sh*t!" *Cell Death Differ.* 2015 Feb;22(2):199-214. doi: 10.1038/cdd.2014.56. www.ncbi.nlm.nih.gov/pubmed/24832470

8. Bailey, M.T., et al., "Exposure to a Social Stressor Alters the Structure of the Intestinal Microbiota: Implications for Stressor-Induced Immunomodulation," *Brain, Behavior, and Immunity*, 2011; 25 (3): 397 DOI: 10.1016/j.bbi.2010.10.023

9. Wang, S., et al., "Effects of Psychological Stress on Small Intestinal Motility and Bacteria and Mucosa in Mice," *World J Gastroenterol.* 2005 Apr 7; 11(13): 2016–2021. doi: 10.3748/wjg.v11.i13.2016, www.sciencedirect.com/science/article/pii/S0889159110005295

10. Vanuytsel, T., et al., "Psychological Stress and Corticotropin-Releasing Hormone Increase Intestinal Permeability in Humans by a Mast Cell-Dependent Mechanism," *Gut.* 2014 Aug;63(8):1293-9. doi: 10.1136/gutjnl-2013-305690. www.ncbi.nlm.nih.gov/pubmed/24153250

11. Maroon, J.C., et al., "Natural Anti-Inflammatory Agents for Pain Relief," *Surg Neurol Int.* 2010; 1: 80. doi: 10.4103/2152-7806.73804

12. Chedid, V., et. al, "Herbal Therapy Is Equivalent to Rifaximin for the Treatment of Small Intestinal Bacterial Overgrowth," *Glob Adv Health Med.* 2014 May; 3(3): 16–24. doi: 10.7453/gahmj.2014.019, www.touroinstitute.com/natural%20bactericidal.pdf

13. Seto, C., et al., "Prolonged Use of a Proton Pump Inhibitor Reduces Microbial Diversity: Implications for *Clostridium Difficile* Susceptibility," *Microbiome*, 20142:42, DOI: 10.1186/2049-2618-2-42, microbiomejournal.biomedcentral.com/articles/10.1186/2049-2618-2-42

14. Campbell, Andrew W., "Autoimmunity and the Gut," *Autoimmune Dis.* 2014; 2014: 152428. doi: 10.1155/2014/152428, www.ncbi.nlm.nih.gov/pmc/articles/PMC4036413/

15. "Fermented Foods Contain 100 TIMES More Probiotics Than a Supplement," Natasha Campbell-McBride, MD, on GAPS Diet, *Mercola.com,* articles.mercola.com/sites/articles/archive/2012/05/12/dr-campbell-mcbride-on-gaps.aspx

16. Chapman, C.M., et al., "In Vitro Evaluation of Single- and Multi-Strain Probiotics: Inter-Species Inhibition Between Probiotic Strains, and Inhibition of Pathogens," *Anaerobe.* 2012 Aug;18(4):405-13. doi: 10.1016/j.anaerobe.2012.05.004. www.ncbi.nlm.nih.gov/pubmed/22677262

17. Kelesidis, Theodoros, "Efficacy and Safety of the Probiotic *Saccharomyces Boulardii* for the Prevention and Therapy of Gastrointestinal Disorders," *Therap Adv Gastroenterol,* 2012 Mar; 5(2): 111–125. doi: 10.1177/1756283X11428502, www.ncbi.nlm.nih.gov/pmc/articles/PMC3296087

18. Alander, Minna, et al., "Persistence of Colonization of Human Colonic Mucosa by a Probiotic Strain, *Lactobacillus rhamnosus* GG, after Oral Consumption," *Appl Environ Microbiol*, 1999 Jan; 65(1): 351–354, www.ncbi.nlm.nih.gov/pmc/articles/PMC91031/

19. Yong, Ed, "At Last, a Big, Successful Trial of Probiotics," *The Atlantic*, Aug 16, 2017, www.theatlantic.com/science/archive/2017/08/at-last-a-big-successful-trial-of-probiotics/537093/

20. Bader, J., Albin, A., and Stahl, U., "Spore-Forming Bacteria and Their Utilisation as Probiotics," *Beneficial Microbes*, (2012) 3(1), 67–75. doi:10.3920/BM2011.0039, www.wageningenacademic.com/doi/abs/10.3920/BM2011.0039

21. Gildea et al., "Protection Against Gluten-Mediated Tight Junction Injury with a Novel Lignite Extract Supplement," *J Nutr Food Sci*, (2016), 6:5, DOI: 10.4172/2155-9600.1000547, www.omicsonline.org/open-access/protection-against-glutenmediated-tight-junction-injury-with-a-novellignite-extract-supplement-2155-9600-1000547.php?aid=78597

22. Bodammer, P., et al., "Bovine Colostrum Increases Pore-Forming Claudin-2 Protein Expression but Paradoxically Not Ion Permeability Possibly by a Change of the Intestinal Cytokine Milieu," *PLoS One*, May 23, 2013, doi.org/10.1371/journal.pone.0064210

23. Skrovanek, S., et al., "Zinc and Gastrointestinal Disease," *World J Gastrointest Pathophysiol*, 2014 Nov 15; 5(4): 496–513. doi: 10.4291/wjgp.v5.i4.496, www.ncbi.nlm.nih.gov/pmc/articles/PMC4231515/

24. Larson, Shawn D., et al., "Molecular Mechanisms Contributing to Glutamine-Mediated Intestinal Cell Survival," *Am J Physiol Gastrointest Liver Physiol*, 2007 Dec; 293(6): G1262–G1271. doi: 10.1152/ajpgi.00254.2007, www.ncbi.nlm.nih.gov/pmc/articles/PMC2432018/

25. Suzuki, Takuya, and Hara, Hiroshi, "Role of Flavonoids in Intestinal Tight Junction Regulation," *The Journal of Nutritional Biochemistry*, Volume 22, Issue 5, May 2011, Pages 401-408, www.sciencedirect.com/science/article/pii/S0955286310001877

26. Rohlke, Faith, and Stollman, Neil, "Fecal Microbiota Transplantation in Relapsing *Clostridium Difficile* Infection," *Therap Adv Gastroenterol*, 2012 Nov; 5(6): 403–420., doi: 10.1177/1756283X12453637, www.ncbi.nlm.nih.gov/pmc/articles/PMC3491681/

27. Sachs, Rachel E., and Edelstein, Carolyn A., "Ensuring the Safe and Effective FDA Regulation of Fecal Microbiota Transplantation," *J Law Biosci*, 2015 Jul; 2(2): 396–415. 10.1093/jlb/lsv032, www.ncbi.nlm.nih.gov/pmc/articles/PMC5034381/#fn13

28. Mattner, J., et al., "Faecal Microbiota Transplantation—a Clinical View," *Int J Med Microbiol*. 2016 Aug;306(5):310-5. doi: 10.1016/j.ijmm.2016.02.003, www.ncbi.nlm.nih.gov/pubmed/26924753

Chapter 3: Clear Infections

1. Buchwald, D., et al., "A Chronic Illness Characterized by Fatigue, Neurologic and Immunologic Disorders, and Active Human Herpesvirus Type 6 Infection," *Ann Intern Med.* 1992 Jan 15;116(2):103-13, www.ncbi.nlm.nih.gov/pubmed/1309285

2. Scher, J., et al., "Expansion of Intestinal *Prevotella Copri* Correlates with Enhanced Susceptibility to Arthritis," *eLife.* 2013; 2: e01202. doi: 10.7554/eLife.01202, www.ncbi.nlm.nih.gov/pmc/articles/PMC3816614/

3. Kang, Insoo, et al., "Defective Control of Latent Epstein-Barr Virus Infection in Systemic Lupus Erythematosus," *J Immunol,* January 15, 2004, 172 (2) 1287-1294; doi, doi.org/10.4049/jimmunol.172.2.1287

4. Petru, G., et al., "Antibodies to Yersinia Enterocolitica in Immunogenic Thyroid Diseases," *Acta Med Austriaca,* 1987;14(1):11–14, www.ncbi.nlm.nih.gov/pubmed/3618088

5. Ascherio, Alberto, "Environmental Factors in Multiple Sclerosis," *Expert Review of Neurotherapeutics,* Vol. 13, Iss. sup2,2013, Harvard School of Public Health, www.tandfonline.com/doi/figure/10.1586/14737175.2013.865866?scroll=top&needAccess=true

6. "Herpes Simplex Virus, Key Facts," World Health Organization (WHO), www.who.int/news-room/detail/28-10-2015-globally-an-estimated-two-thirds-of-the-population-under-50-are-infected-with-herpes-simplex-virus-type-1

7. *The Journal of Investigative Medicine,* 2014;62:280-281, Presented at the Western Regional Meeting of the American Federation for Medical Research, Carmel, CA, January 25, 2014, www.prweb.com/releases/2014/01/prweb11506441.htm

8. Johnson, L., et al., "Severity of Chronic Lyme Disease Compared to Other Chronic Conditions: a Quality of Life Survey," *PeerJ.* 2014; 2: e322., doi: 10.7717/peerj.322, www.ncbi.nlm.nih.gov/pmc/articles/PMC3976119/

9. "Blue Light Has a Dark Side," *Harvard Health Letter,* updated: August 13, 2018, www.health.harvard.edu/staying-healthy/blue-light-has-a-dark-side

10. Aly, Salah Mesalhy, Ph.D., "Role of Intermittent Fasting on Improving Health and Reducing Diseases," *Int J Health Sci (Qassim),* 2014 Jul; 8(3): V–VI., www.ncbi.nlm.nih.gov/pmc/articles/PMC4257368/#b4-ijhs-8-3-v

11. Aird, T.P., et al., "Effects of Fasted Vs Fed-State Exercise on Performance and Post-Exercise Metabolism: a Systematic Review and Meta-Analysis," *Scand J Med Sci Sports.* 2018 Jan 6. doi: 10.1111/sms.13054. www.ncbi.nlm.nih.gov/pubmed/29315892

12. Sanchez, A., et al., "Role of Sugars in Human Neutrophilic Phagocytosis," *American Journal of Clinical Nutrition,* Nov 1973; 261:1180-1184; ajcn.nutrition.org/content/26/11/1180.abstract

13. Karuppiah, Ponmurugan, and Rajaram, Shyamkamur, "Antibacterial Effect of *Allium Sativum* Cloves and *Zingiber Officinale* Rhizomes Against Multiple-

Drug Resistant Clinical Pathogens," *Asian Pac J Trop Biomed,* 2012 Aug; 2(8): 597–601. doi: 10.1016/S2221-1691(12)60104-X, www.ncbi.nlm.nih.gov/pmc/articles/PMC3609356/

14. Kumamoto, Carol, et al., "Manipulation of Host Diet To Reduce Gastrointestinal Colonization by the Opportunistic Pathogen Candida Albicans," *mSphere,* November 2015, doi: 10.1128/mSphere.00020-15, msphere.asm.org/content/1/1/e00020-15

15. Jagetia, G.C. and Aggarwal, B.B., " 'Spicing Up' of the Immune System by Curcumin," *J Clin Immunol.* 2007 Jan;27(1):19-35, www.ncbi.nlm.nih.gov/pubmed/17211725

16. Parvez., S., et al., "Probiotics and Their Fermented Food Products Are Beneficial for Health," *Journal of Applied Microbiology,* onlinelibrary.wiley.com/doi/10.1111/j.1365-2672.2006.02963.x/full

17. Wilmot, E.G., et al., "Sedentary Time in Adults and the Association with Diabetes, Cardiovascular Disease and Death: Systematic Review and Meta-Analysis," *Diabetologia,* November 2012, Volume 55, Issue 11, pp 2895–2905; www.ncbi.nlm.nih.gov/pubmed/22890825

18. Nieman, David, "Moderate Exercise Improves Immunity and Decreases Illness Rates," *American Journal of Lifestyle Medicine,* July 1, 2011, doi.org/10.1177/1559827610392876

19. Lieberman, S., et al., "A Review of Monolaurin and Lauric Acid, Natural Virucidal and Bactericidal Agents," *Alternative and Complementary Therapies,* Dec. 2006, www.touroinstitute.com/natural%20bactericidal.pdf

20. Ponce-Macotela, M., et al., "Oregano (Lippia spp.) Kills Giardia Intestinalis Trophozoites in Vitro: Antigiardiasic Activity and Ultrastructural Damage," *Parasitol Res.* 2006 May; 98(6):557-60, www.ncbi.nlm.nih.gov/pubmed/16425064

21. Pozzatti, P., et al., "In Vitro Activity of Essential Oils Extracted from Plants Used as Spices Against Fluconazole-Resistant and Fluconazole-Susceptible Candida Spp.," *Can J Microbiol.* 2008 Nov;54(11):950-6. doi: 10.1139/w08-097., www.ncbi.nlm.nih.gov/pubmed/18997851

22. Sudjana, A.N., et al., "Antimicrobial Activity of Commercial Olea Europaea (Olive) Leaf Extract," *Int J Antimicrob Agents.* 2009 May;33(5):461-3. doi: 10.1016/j.ijantimicag.2008.10.026, www.ncbi.nlm.nih.gov/pubmed/19135874

23. Chedid, V., et al., "Herbal Therapy Is Equivalent to Rifaximin for the Treatment of Small Intestinal Bacterial Overgrowth," *Glob Adv Health Med.* 2014 May;3(3):16-24. doi: 10.7453/gahmj.2014.019., www.ncbi.nlm.nih.gov/pubmed/24891990

24. Wu, Y., et al., "In Vivo and In Vitro Antiviral Effects of Berberine on Influenza Virus," *Chin J Integr Med.* 2011 Jun;17(6):444-52. doi: 10.1007/s11655-011-0640-3, www.ncbi.nlm.nih.gov/pubmed/21660679

25. Morones-Ramirez, J.R., et al., "Silver Enhances Antibiotic Activity Against Gram-Negative Bacteria," *Science Translational Medicine,* 19 Jun 2013: Vol. 5, Issue 190, pp. 190ra81 doi: 10.1126/scitranslmed.3006276

26. Kamala, Tirumalai, immunologist, Ph.D., mycobacteriology, "Meet The Parasites That Might Cure Crohn's Disease, MS, and More," *Forbes,* April 11, 2016, www.forbes.com/sites/quora/2016/04/11/meet-the-parasites-that-might-cure-crohns-disease-ms-and-more/#643257c859c3

27. Fife, William P., Freeman, D.M., "Treatment of Lyme Disease With Hyperbaric Oxygen Therapy," Undersea and Hyperbaric Medical Society Annual Meeting Abstract (1998), www.hbotnova.com/resources/lyme_disease/Fife_Effectsof HyperbaricOxygenTherapyOnLymeDisease.pdf

Chapter 4: Minimize Toxins

1. McGinn, Anne Platt, POPs Culture, Worldwatch Institute, www.world watch.org/system/files/EP132C.pdf

2. Onstot, J., et al., Characterization of HRGC/MS Unidentified Peaks from the Analysis of Human Adipose Tissue. Volume 1: Technical Approach. Washington, DC: U.S. Environmental Protection Agency Office of Toxic Substances (560/6-87-002a), 1987, pubmedcentralcanada.ca/pmcc/articles/PMC1497458/pdf/12477912.pdf

3. Environmental Working Group analysis of tests of 10 umbilical cord blood samples conducted by AXYS Analytical Services (Sydney, BC) and Flett Research Ltd. (Winnipeg, MB), www.ewg.org/research/body-burden-pollution-newborns#.WhCRRBNSz3Q

4. "New government survey pegs autism prevalence at 1 in 45," Autism Speaks, Nov. 13, 2015, www.autismspeaks.org/science/science-news/new-government-survey-pegs-autism-prevalence-1-45

5. "Half of All Children Will Be Autistic by 2025, Warns Senior Research Scientist at MIT," 386, Dec. 23, 2014, www.anh-usa.org/half-of-all-children-will-be-autistic-by-2025-warns-senior-research-scientist-at-mit/

6. Main, Douglas, "Glyphosate Now the Most-Used Agricultural Chemical Ever," *Newsweek,* Feb. 2, 2016, www.newsweek.com/glyphosate-now-most-used-agricultural-chemical-ever-422419

7. Mercola, Joseph, DO, EMF, "Controversy Exposed," Mercola.com, articles .mercola.com/sites/articles/archive/2016/01/20/emf-controversy-exposed.aspx

8. Zhan, X., et al., "Gram-Negative Bacterial Molecules Associate with Alzheimer Disease Pathology," *Neurology,* Nov. 29, 2016, n.neurology.org/content/87/22/2324.full?sid=c000aa94-129a-4598-b83f-efb674336bed

9. EWG's Skin Deep Cosmetics Database, www.ewg.org/skindeep/2004/06/15/exposures-add-up-survey-results/#.WZSLOtPyuzk

10. Villanueva, Cristina M., et al., "Assessing Exposure and Health Consequences of Chemicals in Drinking Water: Current State of Knowledge and Research Needs," *Environ Health Perspect.*, 2014 Mar.; 122(3): 213–221., www.ncbi.nlm.nih.gov/pmc/articles/PMC3948022/

11. Hayes, T., et al., "Hermaphroditic, Demasculinized Frogs After Exposure to the Herbicide Atrazine at Low Ecologically Relevant Doses," *PNAS*, April 16, 2002, 99 (8) 5476-5480; doi.org/10.1073/pnas.082121499, www.pnas.org/content/99/8/5476.full

12. "The Toxin Solution, with Dr. Joseph Pizzorno," on Dr. Joe Tatta's podcast, March 23, 2017: DrJoeTatta.com.

13. Thompson, S.T., "Preventable Causes of Male Infertility," *World J Urol.*, 1993;11(2):111–9, www.ncbi.nlm.nih.gov/pubmed/8343795

14. Carre, J., et al., "Does Air Pollution Play a Role in Infertility? A Systematic Review," *Environ Health*, 2017; 16: 82. doi: 10.1186/s12940-017-0291-8

15. Parks, Christine G., et al., "Insecticide Use and Risk of Rheumatoid Arthritis and Systemic Lupus Erythematosus in the Women's Health Initiative Observational Study," *Arthritis Care Res* (Hoboken), 2011 Feb; 63(2): 184–194. doi: 10.1002/acr.20335, www.ncbi.nlm.nih.gov/pmc/articles/PMC3593584/

16. Kharrazian, Datis, "The Potential Roles of Bisphenol A (BPA) Pathogenesis in Autoimmunity," *Autoimmune Diseases,* Volume 2014 (2014), Article ID 743616, dx.doi.org/10.1155/2014/743616

17. Chen, D., et al., "Bisphenol Analogues Other Than BPA: Environmental Occurrence, Human Exposure, and Toxicity—A Review," *Environ. Sci. Technol.*, 50 (11), pp 5438–5453, doi: 10.1021/acs.est.5b05387, May 4, 2016, pubs.acs.org/doi/abs/10.1021/acs.est.5b05387?journalCode=esthag

18. "Multiple Sclerosis and Mercury Exposure: Summary and References," International Academy of Oral Medicine and Toxicology (IAOMT), iaomt.org/mercury-ms-summary-references/

19. "Multiple Sclerosis—Poisoning In Slow Motion," *What Doctors Don't Tell You*, (Volume 7, Issue 11), www.healthy.net/Health/Article/MULTIPLE_SCLEROSIS/3105/2 PCBs (20-21)

20. Bill Moyers, Trade Secrets: PCBs, *PBS.org,* www.pbs.org/tradesecrets/problem/popup_group_02.html

21. Choi, Y.J., et al., "Polychlorinated Biphenyls Disrupt Intestinal Integrity Via NADPH Oxidase-Induced Alterations of Tight Junction Protein Expression," Environmental Health Perspectives, 2010, dx.doi.org/10.1289./ehp.0901751. Medications (22-25)

22   Bjarnason, I., et al., "Effect of Non-Steroidal Anti-Inflammatory Drugs on The Human Small Intestine," *Drugs*. 1986, 32 Suppl 1:35-41, www.ncbi.nlm.nih.gov/pubmed/3780475

23. Garza, Anyssa, PharmD, "Drug-Induced Autoimmune Diseases," *Pharmacy Times,* www.pharmacytimes.com/publications/issue/2016/january2016/drug-induced-autoimmune-diseases

24. Mammen, A., "Statin-Associated Autoimmune Myopathy," *New England Journal of Medicine*, 2016;374:664-669. PMID: 26886523. 2016, www.ncbi.nlm.nih.gov/pubmed/26886523

25. Hart, F.D., "Drug-Induced Arthritis and Arthralgia," *Drugs*. 1984 Oct;28(4):347-54., www.ncbi.nlm.nih.gov/pubmed/6386428

26. Nassan, F., et al., "Personal Care Product Use in Men and Urinary Concentrations of Select Phthalate Metabolites and Parabens: Results from the Environment and Reproductive Health (EARTH) Study," *Environ Health Perspect*; doi:10.1289/EHP1374, ehp.niehs.nih.gov/EHP1374/Food Additives (27-28)

27. Lerner, A., et al., "Changes in Intestinal Tight Junction Permeability Associated with Industrial Food Additives Explain the Rising Incidence of Autoimmune Disease," *Autoimmunity Reviews*, Volume 14, Issue 6, June 2015, pages 479-489, www.sciencedirect.com/science/article/pii/S1568997215000245

28. Blaylock, Russell, MD, board-certified neurosurgeon and author of "Excitotoxins: The Taste that Kills," interview with Mike Adams: www.naturalnews.com/035555_Russell_Blaylock_interview_excitotoxins.html

29. EWG Tap Water Database, www.ewg.org/tapwater/contaminant.php?contam-code=1005#.WZDdOdPyuu4 Mold (30-31)

30. Hope, Janette, "A Review of the Mechanism of Injury and Treatment Approaches for Illness Resulting from Exposure to Water-Damaged Buildings, Mold, and Mycotoxins," *The Scientific World Journal,* Volume 2013, Article ID 767482, 20 pages, dx.doi.org/10.1155/2013/767482

31. Campbell, A., et al., "Mixed Mold Mycotoxicosis: Immunological Changes in Humans Following Exposure in Water-Damaged Buildings," *Arch Environ Health*. 2003 Jul;58(7):410-20., pdfs.semanticscholar.org/b439/5e4b0fa38841c5215e76682fff5556c6d6f4.pdf

32. Crinnion, Walter, ND, "Reduce 80% of Your Body's Toxins in 3 Weeks with These Tips," on iHealthTube.com.

33. Bradman, A., et al., "Effect of Organic Diet Intervention on Pesticide Exposures in Young Children Living in Low-Income Urban and Agricultural Communities," *Environ Health Perspect*, doi:10.1289/ehp.1408660, ehp.niehs.nih.gov/1408660

34. Göen, Thomas, "Greenpeace-Japan-Study of the Effect of Nutrition Change on the Pesticide Exposure of Consumers," Institute and Outpatient Clinic of Occupational, Social and Environmental Medicine, storage.googleapis.com/

p4-production-content/international/wp-content/uploads/2016/12/2c866e2e-201612_greenpeace_pesticide_study.pdf

35. Lau, C., et al., Perfluoroalkyl acids: a review of monitoring and toxicological findings. Toxicol Sci. 2007 Oct; 99(2):366-94. Epub 2007 May 22. PMID: 17519394, www.greenmedinfo.com/article/perfluoroalkyl-acids-review-monitoring-and-toxicological-findings

36. Sears, M.E., et al., "Arsenic, Cadmium, Lead, and Mercury in Sweat: a Systematic Review," *J Environ Public Health*, 2012; 184745. doi: 10.1155/2012/184745 PMCID: PMC3312275

37. Mercola, Joseph, DO, "How Cellphones Can Cause Brain Tumors and Trigger Chronic Disease," Mercola.com, articles.mercola.com/sites/articles/archive/2017/05/23/cellphones-cause-brain-tumors-trigger-chronic-disease.aspx

38. Klinghardt Academy, "Metal Detoxification Agents and Common Dosages," 2010 www.klinghardtacademy.com/images/stories/powerpoints/mercury%20detoxification%20agents.pdf EDTA (39-40)

39. Ferrero, Maria Elena, "Rationale for the Successful Management of EDTA Chelation Therapy in Human Burden by Toxic Metals," *Biomed Res Int*.: 8274504. 2016 Nov 8. doi: 10.1155/2016/8274504, www.ncbi.nlm.nih.gov/pmc/articles/PMC5118545/

40. Mosayebi, G., et al., "Therapeutic Effect of EDTA in Experimental Model of Multiple Sclerosis," *Immunopharmacol Immunotoxicol*. 2010 Jun;32(2):321-6. doi: 10.3109/08923970903338367., www.ncbi.nlm.nih.gov/pubmed/20233106

Chapter 5: Address Stress

1. Segerstrom, S.C., Miller, G.E. "Psychological Stress and the Human Immune System: a Meta-Analytic Study of 30 Years of Inquiry," *Psychol Bull*, 2004;130:601–30., www.ncbi.nlm.nih.gov/pmc/articles/PMC1361287/

2. Institute of Medicine (US) Committee on Health and Behavior: Research, Practice, and Policy, *Health and Behavior: the Interplay of Biological, Behavioral, and Societal Influences*, Washington (DC): National Academies Press (US); 2001. www.ncbi.nlm.nih.gov/books/NBK43743/

3. Hanna, Heidi, Ph.D., executive director, American Institute of Stress (AIS), "America's #1 Health Problem," *Stress.org*, www.stress.org/americas-1-health-problem/

4. 2015 Stress in America, *American Psychological Association (APA)*, www.apa.org/news/press/releases/stress/2015/snapshot.aspx

5. An NIH video, "A Nation Under Pressure: The Public Health Consequences of Stress in America," with Dr. Vivek Murthy, www.facebook.com/nih.gov/videos/10155434203121830

6. Cohen, Sheldon, et al., "Chronic Stress, Glucocorticoid Receptor Resistance, Inflammation, and Disease Risk," *PNAS*, April 2, 2012 doi: 10.1073/pnas .1118355109; www.pnas.org/content/109/16/5995.abstract

7. Stojanovich, L., et al., "Stress as a Trigger of Autoimmune Disease," *Autoimmun Rev.* 2008 Jan;7(3):209-13. doi: 10.1016/ j.autrev.2007.11.007, www.ncbi.nlm.nih .gov/pubmed/18190880

8. Roberts, A., et al., "Association of Trauma and Posttraumatic Stress Disorder With Incident Systemic Lupus Erythematosus in a Longitudinal Cohort of Women," *Arthritis & Rheumatology*, September 28, 2017, onlinelibrary .wiley.com/doi/full/10.1002/art.40222

9. Boscarino, J.A., "Posttraumatic Stress Disorder and Physical Illness: Results from Clinical and Epidemiologic Studies," *Ann N Y Acad Sci.* 2004 Dec;1032:141-53, www.ncbi.nlm.nih.gov/pubmed/15677401

10. Winsa, B., et al., "Stressful Life Events and Graves' Disease," *Lancet.* 1991 Dec 14;338(8781):1475-9., www.ncbi.nlm.nih.gov/pubmed/1683917

11. Hassett, Afton L., and Clauw, Daniel J., "The Role of Stress in Rheumatic Diseases," *Arthritis Res Ther.*, 2010; 12(3): 123. doi: 10.1186/ar3024, www.ncbi.nlm .nih.gov/pmc/articles/PMC2911881

12. Sgambato, D., et al., "The Role of Stress in Inflammatory Bowel Diseases," *Curr Pharm Des.*, 2017 Feb 28. doi: 10.2174/1381612823666170228123357, www.ncbi .nlm.nih.gov/pubmed/28245757

13. Mohr, D.C., "Moderating Effects of Coping on the Relationship Between Stress and the Development of New Brain Lesions in Multiple Sclerosis," *Psychosom Med.*, 2002; 64(5): 803–809. doi: 10.1097/01.PSY.0000024238.11538.EC, www.ncbi.nlm.nih.gov/pmc/articles/PMC1893006/

14. Dube, S.R., et al., "Cumulative Childhood Stress and Autoimmune Disease in Adults," *Psychosom Med*, 2009; 71:243–250. doi: 10.1097/PSY.0b013e3181907888.

15. Felitti, V., et al., "Relationship of Childhood Abuse and Household Dysfunction to Many of the Leading Causes of Death in Adults, the Adverse Childhood Experiences (ACE) Study," *American Journal of Preventive Medicine*, May 1998 Volume 14, Issue 4, Pages 245–258, www.ajpmonline.org/article/S0749-3797(98) 00017-8/fulltext

16. Sasso, F.C., et al., "Ultrastructural Changes in Enterocytes in Subjects with Hashimoto's Thyroiditis," *Gut*, Vol. 53, No. 12 (2004): 1878–1880, www.ncbi .nlm.nih.gov/pmc/articles/PMC1774342/

17. Stahl, J., et al., "Relaxation Response and Resiliency Training and Its Effect on Healthcare Resource Utilization," *PLoS One*, 2015, doi.org/10.1371/journal.pone .0140212

18. Gharib, S.A., et al., "Loss of Sleep, Even for a Single Night, Increases Inflammation in the Body; Elsevier; Transcriptional Signatures of Sleep Duration

Discordance in Monozygotic Twins," *Sleep*, January 2017, doi: 10.1093/sleep/zsw019, www.sciencedaily.com/releases/2008/09/080902075211.htm

19. Lin, I.M., et al., "Breathing at a Rate of 5.5 Breaths Per Minute with Equal Inhalation-to-Exhalation Ratio Increases Heart Rate Variability," *Int J Psychophysiol.* 2014 Mar;91(3):206-11. doi: 10.1016/j.ijpsycho.2013.12.006. www.ncbi.nlm.nih.gov/pubmed/24380741

20. Biswas, A., "Sedentary Time and its Association with Risk for Disease Incidence, Mortality, and Hospitalization in Adults: a Systematic Review and Meta-Analysis," *Ann Intern Med.* 2015 Jan 20;162(2):123-32. doi: 10.7326/M14-1651, www.ncbi.nlm.nih.gov/pubmed/25599350

21. Perandini, L.A., et al., "Exercise as a Therapeutic Tool to Counteract Inflammation and Clinical Symptoms in Autoimmune Rheumatic Diseases," *Autoimmunity Reviews*, Volume 12, Issue 2, December 2012, pages 218-224, doi.org/10.1016/j.autrev.2012.06.007

22. Friedman, Lauren F., and Loria, Kevin, "11 Scientific Reasons You Should Be Spending More Time Outside," *Business Insider*, Apr. 22, 2016, www.businessinsider.com/scientific-benefits-of-nature-outdoors-2016-4/#1-improved-short-term-memory-1

23. Livni, Ephrat, "The Japanese Practice of 'Forest Bathing' Is Scientifically Proven to Improve Your Health," *Quartz*, qz.com/804022/health-benefits-japanese-forest-bathing/

24. Williams, Florence, "Take Two Hours of Pine Forest and Call Me in the Morning," *Outside Online*, 2012, www.outsideonline.com/1870381/take-two-hours-pine-forest-and-call-me-morning

25. Millard, Elizabeth, "6 Reasons You Need More Sun, According To Science," *SELF.com*, www.self.com/story/sunlight-benefits

26. EFT Tapping Research, www.EFTUniverse.com, www.eftuniverse.com/research-studies/eft-research#anxiety

27. Bhasin, M., et al., "Relaxation Response Induces Temporal Transcriptome Changes in Energy Metabolism, Insulin Secretion and Inflammatory Pathways," *PLoS One*, 2013, doi.org/10.1371/journal.pone.0062817

28. Ortiz, Robin, and Sibing, Erica M., "The Role of Mindfulness in Reducing the Adverse Effects of Childhood Stress and Trauma," *Children*, 2017, 4(3), 16; doi:10.3390/children4030016

29. Xu, Mengran, et al., "Mindfulness and Mind Wandering: The Protective Effects of Brief Meditation in Anxious Individuals," *Consciousness and Cognition*, 2017; 51: 157 DOI: 10.1016/j.concog.2017.03.009

30. Baumeister, R.F., et al., "Bad is Stronger Than Good," *Review of General Psychology*, 2001, assets.csom.umn.edu/assets/71516.pdf

31. Holt-Lunstad, Julianne, et al., "Loneliness and Social Isolation as Risk Factors for Mortality, a Meta-Analytic Review," *Sage Journals*, Volume: 10 issue: 2, page(s): 227-237, March 1, 2015, doi.org/10.1177/1745691614568352

32. Seppala, Emma, Ph.D., Stanford University, The Center for Compassion and Altruism Research and Education, ccare.stanford.edu/uncategorized/connectedness-health-the-science-of-social-connection-infographic/

33. Hamilton, D., *Why Kindness Is Good for You* (Hay House, 2010); www.psychologytoday.com/blog/wired-success/201503/8-reasons-why-we-need-human-touch-more-ever

34. Mercola, Joseph, DO, "Fun Facts About Hugging," February 06, 2014, Mercola.com, articles.mercola.com/sites/articles/archive/2014/02/06/hugging.aspx

35. Grimm, David, "How Dogs Stole Our Hearts," *Science Magazine*, 2015, www.sciencemag.org/news/2015/04/how-dogs-stole-our-hearts

36. John Hopkins Medicine, "Forgiveness, Your Health Depends on It," *Healthy Aging*, www.hopkinsmedicine.org/health/healthy_aging/healthy_connections/forgiveness-your-health-depends-on-it

37. Breines, J., et al., "Self-Compassion as a Predictor of Interleukin-6 Response to Acute Psychosocial Stress," *Brain Behav Immun.*, 2014 Mar; 37: 109–114. doi: 10.1016/j.bbi.2013.11.006

38. van der Kolk, B.A., et al., "A Randomized Controlled Study of Neurofeedback for Chronic PTSD," *PLoS One.*, 2016 Dec 16;11(12):e0166752. doi: 10.1371/journal.pone.0166752, www.ncbi.nlm.nih.gov/pubmed/2799243

Chapter 6: Balance Your Hormones

1. Brogan, Kelly, MD, and Ji, Sayer, "Cracking the Cholesterol Myth: How Statins Harm the Body and Mind," kellybroganmd.com/cracking-cholesterol-myth-how-statins-harm-body-and-mind

2. Chitnis, T., et al., "Distinct Effects of Obesity and Puberty on Risk and Age at Onset of Pediatric MS," *Ann Clin Transl Neurol.*, 2016 Dec; 3(12): 897–907. doi: 10.1002/acn3.365, www.ncbi.nlm.nih.gov/pmc/articles/PMC5224818/

3. Park, Alice, "You Won't Believe How Much Processed Food Americans Eat," *Time Magazine*, March 9, 2016 time.com/4252515/calories-processed-food/

4. Sugar Science, UCSF, sugarscience.ucsf.edu/dispelling-myths-too-much.html#.WlFCua2ZN-U

5. Mercola, Joseph, D.O., "Puberty Before Age 10: a New 'Normal'?" Mercola.com, articles.mercola.com/sites/articles/archive/2012/04/16/early-precocious-puberty.aspx

6. Nielsen, N., et al., "Age at Menarche and Risk of Multiple Sclerosis: a Prospective Cohort Study Based on the Danish National Birth Cohort," *American*

Journal of Epidemiology, Volume 185, Issue 8, 15 April 2017, pages 712–719, doi.org/10.1093/aje/kww160

7. Bajaj, Jagminder K., et al., "Various Possible Toxicants Involved in Thyroid Dysfunction: a Review," *J Clin Diagn Res.*, 2016 Jan; 10(1): FE01–FE03. doi: 10.7860/JCDR/2016/15195.7092 www.ncbi.nlm.nih.gov/pmc/articles/PMC4740614/

8. Canaris, G.J., et al., "The Colorado Thyroid Disease Prevalence Study," *Arch Intern Med.*, 2000;160(4):526-534. doi:10.1001/archinte.160.4.526, jamanetwork .com/journals/jamainternalmedicine/fullarticle/415184

9. Kim, D., "Low Vitamin D Status is Associated with Hypothyroid Hashimoto's Thyroiditis," *Hormones* (Athens). 2016 Jul;15(3):385-393. doi: 10.14310/horm .2002.1681., www.ncbi.nlm.nih.gov/pubmed/27394703

10. Pfotenhauer, Kim M., and Shubrook, Jay H., "Vitamin D Deficiency, its Role in Health and Disease, and Current Supplementation Recommendations," *The Journal of the American Osteopathic Association*, 2017; 117 (5): 301 doi: 10.7556/jaoa.2017.055, jaoa.org/article.aspx?articleid=2625276

11. Munger, K., et al., "25-Hydroxyvitamin D Deficiency and Risk of MS Among Women in the Finnish Maternity Cohort," *Neurology*, September 13, 2017, doi: n.neurology.org/content/early/2017/09/13/WNL.0000000000004489

12. Forsblad-d'Elia, H., et al., "Low Serum Levels of Sex Steroids Are Associated with Disease Characteristics in Primary Sjogren's Syndrome; Supplementation with Dehydroepiandrosterone Restores the Concentrations," *The Journal of Clinical Endocrinology & Metabolism,* Vol. 94, No. 6 2044-2051(2009), www.ncbi.nlm.nih.gov/pubmed/19318446

13. Sawalha, Amr H., and Kovats, Susan, "Dehydroepiandrosterone in Systemic Lupus Erythematosus," *Curr Rheumatol,* Rep. 2008 Aug; 10(4): 286–291, www.ncbi.nlm.nih.gov/pmc/articles/PMC2701249/

14. Tellez, Nieves, et al., "Fatigue in Progressive Multiple Sclerosis Is Associated with Low Levels of Dehydroepiandrosterone," *Multiple Sclerosis,* 2006; 12: 487-494, citeseerx.ist.psu.edu/viewdoc/download?doi=10.1.1.842.31&rep=rep1&type=pdf

15. Basu, S., et al., "The Relationship of Sugar to Population-Level Diabetes Prevalence: an Econometric Analysis of Repeated Cross-Sectional Data," *PLoS One.*, 2013; 8(2): e57873. 2013 Feb 27. doi: 10.1371/journal.pone.0057873, www.ncbi .nlm.nih.gov/pmc/articles/PMC3584048/]

16. "Alcohol intake and breast cancer in the European prospective investigation into cancer and nutrition," Romieu, I., et al., *International Journal of Cancer*, Volume 137, Issue 8, pages 1921–1930, 15 October 2015, onlinelibrary.wiley.com/wol1/doi/10.1002/ijc.29469/abstract

17. Lucero, J., et al., "Early Follicular Phase Hormone Levels In Relation to Patterns of Alcohol, Tobacco, and Coffee Use," *Fertility and Sterility,* Vol 76, No. 4. Oct 2001, www.fertstert.org/article/S0015-0282(01)02005-2/pdf

18. Hofmekler, Ori, *The Anti-Estrogenic Diet: How Estrogenic Foods and Chemicals Are Making You Fat and Sick*

19. Sarkar, A., et al., "Psychobiotics and the Manipulation of Bacteria-Gut-Brain Signals," *Trends Neurosci.*, 2016 Nov; 39(11): 763–781. doi: 10.1016/j.tins.2016.09 .002, www.ncbi.nlm.nih.gov/pmc/articles/PMC5102282/

20. Murphy, M.B., et al., "Plasma Steroid Hormone Concentrations, Aromatase Activities and GSI in Ranid Frogs Collected from Agricultural and Non-Agricultural Sites in Michigan (USA)," *Aquat Toxicol.*, 2006 May 1;77(2):153-66. www.ncbi.nlm.nih.gov/pubmed/16427146

21. Won, Kim T., "The Impact of Sleep and Circadian Disturbance on Hormones and Metabolism," *Int J Endocrinol.* 2015; 2015: 591729. 2015 Mar 11. doi: 10.1155/2015/591729, www.ncbi.nlm.nih.gov/pmc/articles/PMC4377487/

22. Gabel, V., et al., "Effects of Artificial Dawn and Morning Blue Light on Daytime Cognitive Performance, Well-Being, Cortisol and Melatonin Levels," *Chronobiol Int.*, 2013 Oct;30(8):988-97. doi: 10.3109/07420528.2013.793196. www.ncbi .nlm.nih.gov/pubmed/23841684; and Mead, M. Nathaniel, "Benefits of Sunlight: a Bright Spot for Human Health," *Environ Health Perspect.*, 2008 Apr; 116(4): A160–A167. www.ncbi.nlm.nih.gov/pmc/articles/PMC2290997/

23. Chevalier, G., et al., "Earthing: Health Implications of Reconnecting the Human Body to the Earth's Surface Electrons," *J Environ Public Health.*, 2012; 2012: 291541. doi: 10.1155/2012/291541, www.ncbi.nlm.nih.gov/pmc/articles/ PMC3265077/#B13

24. Aly, Salah Mesalhy, Ph.D., "Role of Intermittent Fasting on Improving Health and Reducing Diseases," *Int J Health Sci* (Qassim). 2014 Jul; 8(3): V–VI., www.ncbi.nlm.nih.gov/pmc/articles/PMC4257368/#b4-ijhs-8-3-v

25. Ambiye, A., et al., "Clinical Evaluation of the Spermatogenic Activity of the Root Extract of Ashwaganda (*Withania somnifera*) in Oligospermic Males: A Pilot Study," *Evid Based Complement Alternat Med.*, 2013; 2013: 571420. doi: 10.1155/2013/571420, www.ncbi.nlm.nih.gov/pmc/articles/PMC3863556/

26. Chandrasekhar, K., et al., "A Prospective, Randomized Double-Blind, Placebo-Controlled Study of Safety and Efficacy of a High-Concentration Full-Spectrum Extract of *Ashwaganda* Root in Reducing Stress and Anxiety in Adults," *Indian J Psychol Med.*, 2012 Jul-Sep; 34(3): 255–262. doi: 10.4103/0253-7176.106022, www.ncbi.nlm.nih.gov/pmc/articles/PMC3573577/

27. Anghelescu, I.G., et al., "Stress Management and the Role of Rhodiola Rosea: a Review," *Int J Psychiatry Clin Pract.*, 2018 Jan 11:1-11. doi: 10.1080/13651501 .2017.1417442, www.ncbi.nlm.nih.gov/pubmed/29325481

28. Olsson, E.M., et al., "A Randomised, Double-Blind, Placebo-Controlled, Parallel-Group Study of the Standardised Extract Shr-5 of the Roots of Rhodiola Rosea in the Treatment of Subjects with Stress-Related Fatigue," *Planta Med.*,

2009 Feb;75(2):105-12. doi: 10.1055/s-0028-1088346. www.ncbi.nlm.nih.gov/pubmed/19016404

29. Hellhammer, J., et. at., "A Soy-Based Phosphatidylserine/Phosphatidic Acid Complex (PAS) Normalizes the Stress Reactivity of Hypothalamus-Pituitary-Adrenal-Axis in Chronically Stressed Male Subjects: A Randomized, Placebo-Controlled Study," *Lipids Health Dis,* 13:121, 2014, www.ncbi.nlm.nih.gov/pmc/articles/PMC4237891/

30. Chen, C., et al., "Berberine Inhibits PTP1B Activity and Mimics Insulin Action," *Biochem Biophys Res Commun,* Jul 2 2010;397(3):543-7, www.ncbi.nlm.nih.gov/pubmed/20515652

31. Hummel, M., et al., "Chromium in Metabolic and Cardiovascular Disease," *Horm Metab Res.,* 2007 Oct;39(10):743-51., www.ncbi.nlm.nih.gov/pubmed/17952838

32. Revilla-Monsalve, C., et al., "Biotin Supplementation Reduces Plasma Triacylglycerol and VLDL in Type 2 Diabetic Patients and in Nondiabetic Subjects with Hypertriglyceridemia," *Biomed Pharmacother.* 2006 May;60(4):182-5. www.ncbi.nlm.nih.gov/pubmed/16677798

33. Singer, Gregory M., and Geohas, Jeff, "The Effect of Chromium Picolinate and Biotin Supplementation on Glycemic Control in Poorly Controlled Patients with Type 2 Diabetes Mellitus: a Placebo-Controlled, Double-Blinded, Randomized Trial," *Diabetes Technol Ther.,* 2006 Dec;8(6):636-43. PMID: 17109595, www.ncbi.nlm.nih.gov/pubmed/17109595

34. Hanausak, M., et al., "Detoxifying Cancer-Causing Agents to Prevent Cancer," *Integrative Cancer Therapies,* Volume: 2 issue: 2, page(s): 139-144, Issue published: June 1, 2003, journals.sagepub.com/doi/pdf/10.1177/1534735403002002005

35. Henmi, H., et al., "Effects of Ascorbic Acid Supplementation on Serum Progesterone Levels in Patients with a Luteal Phase Defect," *Fertility and Sterility,* August 2003 Volume 80, Issue 2, Pages 459–461, www.fertstert.org/article/S0015-0282(03)00657-5/fulltext#References

36. Pirola, I., et al., "Selenium Supplementation Could Restore Euthyroidism in Ubclinical Hypothyroid Patients with Autoimmune Thyroiditis," *Endokrynol Pol.,* 2016;67(6):567-571. doi: 10.5603/EP.2016.0064., www.ncbi.nlm.nih.gov/pubmed/28042649

37. Rayman, M.P., "The Importance of Selenium to Human Health," *Lancet,* 2000 Jul 15;356(9225):233-41., www.ncbi.nlm.nih.gov/pubmed/10963212

38. Tovey, Amber, *Vitamin D Council,* May 22, 2017, www.vitamindcouncil.org/how-much-vitamin-d-is-needed-to-achieve-optimal-levels/

39. Benedek, G., et al., "Estrogen Protection Against EAE Modulates the Microbiota and Mucosal-Associated Regulatory Cells," *J Neuroimmunol,* 2017 Sep 15;310:51-59. doi: 10.1016/j.jneuroim.2017.06.007. www.ncbi.nlm.nih.gov/pubmed/28778445

40. Van Vollenhoven, R.F., and McGuire, J.L., "Estrogen, Progesterone, and Testosterone: Can They Be Used to Treat Autoimmune Diseases?" *Cleve Clin J Med.*, 1994 Jul-Aug;61(4):276-84, www.ncbi.nlm.nih.gov/pubmed/7923746

41. Forsblad-d'Elia, H., "Low Serum Levels of Sex Steroids are Associated with Disease Characteristics in Primary Sjögren's Syndrome; Supplementation with Dehydroepiandrosterone Restores the Concentrations," *J Clin Endocrinol Metab.*, 2009 Jun;94(6):2044-51. doi: 10.1210/jc.2009-0106, www.ncbi.nlm.nih.gov/pubmed/19318446

42. Pepper, Gary M., and Casanova-Romero, Paul Y., "Conversion to Armour Thyroid from Levothyroxine Improved Patient Satisfaction in the Treatment of Hypothyroidism," *Journal of Endocrinology, Diabetes and Obesity,* 11 September 2014, jeffreydachmd.com/wp-content/uploads/2013/06/Conversion-to-Armour-Thyroid_endocrinology-2-1055.pdf

43. Munger, K.L., et al., "Serum 25-Hydroxyvitamin D Levels and Risk of Multiple Sclerosis," *JAMA.* 2006 Dec 20;296(23):2832-8., www.ncbi.nlm.nih.gov/pubmed/17179460

44. Fournier, A., et al., "Unequal Risks for Breast Cancer Associated with Different Hormone Replacement Therapies: Results from the E3N Cohort Study," *Breast Cancer Res Treat.*, 2008 Jan; 107(1): 103–111. doi: 10.1007/s10549-007-9523-x, www.ncbi.nlm.nih.gov/pmc/articles/PMC2211383/

45. Lauritzen, C., "Results of a 5 Years Prospective Study of Estriol Succinate Treatment in Patients with Climacteric Complaints," *Horm Metab Res.*, 1987 Nov;19(11):579-84, www.ncbi.nlm.nih.gov/pubmed/3428874

46. Bolour, S., and Braunstein, G., "Testosterone Therapy in Women: a Review," *Int J Impot Res.*, 2005 Sep-Oct;17(5):399-408., www.ncbi.nlm.nih.gov/pubmed/15889125

47. Tan, Z., et al., "Thyroid Function and the Risk of Alzheimer's Disease: the Framingham Study," *Arch Intern Med.*, 2008 Jul 28; 168(14): 1514–1520. doi: 10.1001/archinte.168.14.1514, www.ncbi.nlm.nih.gov/pmc/articles/PMC2694610/

48. Luboshitzky, R., "Risk Factors for Cardiovascular Disease in Women with Subclinical Hypothyroidism," *Thyroid.*, 2002 May;12(5):421-5., www.ncbi.nlm.nih.gov/pubmed/12097204

49. Life Extension Foundation, "DHEA Restoration Therapy," www.lifeextension.com/Protocols/Metabolic-Health/Dhea-Restoration/Page-03

Appendix C: What's Your ACE Score?

1. Felitti, V.J., et al., "Relationship of Childhood Abuse and Household Dysfunction to Many of the Leading Causes of Death in Adults: the Adverse Childhood

Experiences (ACE) Study," *American Journal of Preventive Medicine*, 1998; 14:245–258., www.ncbi.nlm.nih.gov/pubmed/9635069?dopt=Abstract

Appendix D: Advanced Considerations and Practitioners

1. "75% of Americans May Suffer from Chronic Dehydration According to Doctors," www.medicaldaily.com/75-americans-may-suffer-chronic-dehydration-according-doctors-247393
2. Joseph Mercola, DO, articles.mercola.com/sites/articles/archive/ 2017/09/03/ electromagnetic-fields-harmful-effects.aspx

Appendix F: Resources and Recommended Reading by Chapter

1. *The Harvard Gazette*, April 17, 2018, news.harvard.edu/gazette/story/2018/04/ less-stress-clearer-thoughts-with-mindfulness-meditation

GRATITUDE

This book has been a labor of love, and I am so grateful to the many amazing people who shared in its evolution from idea to fruition.

First, I want to thank Marilyn Allen, my superb agent, who eagerly embraced the book concept and provided stewardship throughout. Heartfelt appreciation to Jacob Teitelbaum, MD, for the generous intro to Marilyn. To Denise Silvestro, talented editor at Kensington Publishing, who believed in me from the get-go and helped shape the book beautifully; to Ann Pryor and the entire team at Kensington books.

Huge thanks to Lauren Parvizi, magnificent freelance editor (and writer in her own right), who helped make everything in this book better, and for providing much-needed encouragement along the way. To Betsy Bigelow-Teller, my very first client, who became my first collaborator and content editor at BeatAutoimmune.com, and who I'm delighted has become a friend.

To Tom O'Bryan, DC, CCN, who generously introduced me to Mark Hyman MD's team. To Dhru Purohit, CEO, Dr. Hyman Enterprises, for openness and kindness, to Kaya Purohit, Head of Content, for eagerly embracing the book, and to Mark Hyman, MD, for your powerful foreword and support.

I am grateful for the courageous and pioneering functional and integrative doctors, practitioners, authors, and scientists who were generous with their time and healing stories: Susan Blum, MD, MPH; Jill Carnahan, MD; Linda Clark, MA, CNC; Michelle Corey, CNWC, FMC; Mark Hyman, MD; Toréa Rodriguez, FDN-P; Mary Ruddick, CNC; Jacob Teitelbaum, MD; Amie Valpone, HHC, AADP; Aristo Vojdani, Ph.D.; and Terry Wahls, MD. Your inspirational stories, passion for empowering people to thrive, and the powerful work you do every day offer hope and healing for everyone.

To Donna Jackson-Nakazawa, for important and beautifully written books and for advancing the understanding of the autoimmune epidemic—thank you.

I am so grateful for the functional/integrative/naturopathic giants who have paved the way for us all and from whom I've learned so much: Jeffrey Bland, Ph.D.; Ann Louise Gittleman, MS, CNS; Sara Gottfried, MD; Mark Hyman, MD; Christiane Northrup, MD; David Perlmutter, MD; Joseph Pizzorno, ND; Sherry Rogers, MD; Bob Rountree, MD; Tom Sult, MD. Thank heavens for the internet and the opportunity to learn from tippy-top health educators: Zach Bush, MD; Lee Cowden, MD; Dietrich Klinghardt, MD, Ph.D.; and Joseph Mercola, DO. And to stellar health educators John Bergman, DC, and Barbara O'Neill, naturopath and nutritionist.

To the women who warmly welcomed me at my first IFM training: Heather Moday, MD; Heidi Rasmussen, MD; and Karen Rout, MD—I sure sat in the right place—thank you! And thank yous to the Functional Medicine and naturopathic docs who kindly offered guidance and support early on: Nathalie Bera-Miller, MD, MPH, Rich Stagliano, MD, and Rebecca Green, ND, LAc, MSOM. To Russell Jaffe, MD, Ph.D., CCN, for generous conversations and kind introductions to kindred spirits. To Mary Ruddick, CNC, thank you for mentoring me on healing diets and helping to build my confidence to consult with my own clients. To the wonderful teachers at the Functional Medicine Coaching Academy (FMCA), led beautifully by Sandi Scheinbaum, Ph.D., and to our super kind cohort leader, Shelby Garay, FMCHC.

Huge thank yous to experts who were incredibly generous with their time to provide chapter feedback: Zach Bush, MD; Scott Forsgren, FDNP; Steve Fowkes, organic chemist and nanotechnologist; Heidi Hanna, Ph.D.; Courtney Jonson, LAc; Joseph Pizzorno, ND; and Aristo Vojdani, Ph.D. Deep bows to each of you.

A special thank you to Dr. Ari Vojdani, who saw this book before I did! I am so grateful for your support, humor, and humility.

I am enormously appreciative for Steve Fowkes, pioneering biohacker, for being a patient biochemistry mentor and outstanding scientific editor. I am also grateful for biohacker and Bulletproof founder Dave Asprey, and to Susan Downs, MD, for their leadership of the Silicon Valley Health Institute (SVHI), an excellent nonprofit resource and community of health-seekers.

A big thank you to Gerald Cohen, DHom, DC, FIHI, for his big heart and for staying after hours to mentor me on the truth of autoimmune conditions.

I'm so grateful for my original Functional Medicine nutritionist, Courtney Jonson, LAc, who I'm now honored to collaborate with in service of autoimmune clients and whom I'm happy to call a dear friend.

I'm privileged to work with amazing clients who are reversing their autoimmune conditions and sharing the wealth of good health with their families and friends and beyond. I'm so grateful for loyal readers of my blog at BeatAutoimmune.com, my Facebook page, Facebook/palmerkippola, our engaged private Facebook group community, Transcend Autoimmune, and to all who have shared their inspirational autoimmune healing journeys.

So much love and gratitude for dear friends who were totally there for me when the MS struck at nineteen and remain close today, John Denny, Carolyn Haldeman Hansen, Liza Kirkbride, and Elsa Lambert. Elsa, thank you for asking me the question that put me on the healing quest!

In 2014, I found my birth father on 23andMe by happy accident. It's a magical story and I remain awed and enormously grateful for the instant embrace, love, and support of my big, new family. To go from being an only child recently orphaned to having new, loving parents, two wonderful brothers, four awesome nieces and nephews, and a host of amazing aunts and uncles is beyond imagination. Special thanks to my "comma momma," JeriMom, for being an eager and very helpful early reader, and to my nephew, Taylor, for insightful and spot-on feedback.

I'm very lucky to have loving and wonderfully supportive in-laws. Special thanks to Mary Ann for ongoing encouragement from Michigan. We are so thankful for you and Wayne and can't wait to hang out at the lake, cook good food, laugh, and play endless Scrabble and cards.

For my husband, Tom, who graciously let me take over our kitchen table for much of the writing of this book, thank you for your patience and for being my number one cheerleader. Your understanding, strategic advice, love, and friendship fuel everything. I think it's time for a road trip with some great music!

None of this would have been possible without the love and support of my parents, Edgar and Beverly Beyer Rabey, pioneering travel writers who eagerly adopted me at three days old, whisked me off to a world of adventure, and sacrificed everything to give me the opportunities of a lifetime. You taught me the values of travel, education, equality, and humor. I am forever grateful for everything. I love you and miss your physical presence but know you are with me, always. And, dad, you were right: *We beat this thing!*

INDEX

Connect with Us

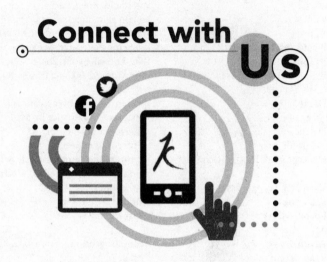

Visit us online at
KensingtonBooks.com
to read more from your favorite authors, see books
by series, view reading group guides, and more.

for sneak peeks, chances to win books and prize packs,
and to share your thoughts with other readers.

facebook.com/kensingtonpublishing
twitter.com/kensingtonbooks

Tell us what you think!

To share your thoughts, submit a review,
or sign up for our eNewsletters, please visit:
KensingtonBooks.com/TellUs.